Percutaneous Treatment of Cardiovascular Diseases in Women

Patrizia Presbitero • Julinda Mehilli
Anna Sonia Petronio
Editors

Percutaneous Treatment of Cardiovascular Diseases in Women

Springer

Editors
Patrizia Presbitero
Interventional Cardiology
Humanitas Research Hospital
Rozzano (Milan)
Italy

Julinda Mehilli
Interventional Cardiology
Klinik der Universität München
München
Bayern
Germany

Anna Sonia Petronio
Hemodynamic Laboratory
Azienda Ospedaliero Universitaria Pisana
Pisa
Italy

ISBN 978-3-319-81922-8 ISBN 978-3-319-39611-8 (eBook)
DOI 10.1007/978-3-319-39611-8

Softcover reprint of the hardcover 1st edition 2016

Printed on acid-free paper

This Springer imprint is published by Springer Nature
The registered company is Springer International Publishing AG Switzerland

Preface

For over a decade, the scientific community has been attempting to shed light on whether the disparities in clinical presentation and response to treatment for many cardiovascular diseases in men and women are due to variations in biological patterns or to social and cultural conventions leading to different attitudes toward diagnosis and treatment of cardiac diseases.

Since the first percutaneous interventions in the cardiovascular system, it was observed that women experience more procedural complications such as arterial dissections, bleeding, spasm etc. This raises the question of whether this is due to late presentation and mismanagement or to a different arterial disease pathophysiology.

It is now well known that compared to their male counterparts, women diagnosed with cardiovascular diseases are older, present more frequently with comorbidities (diabetes, hypertension, renal insufficiency, inflammatory diseases), have more physical and cardiac dysfunction as well as a lower overall quality of life.

In most cardiovascular diseases there are anatomical end/or physiopathological differences that need to be considered to ensure that treatment is successful.

This book provides valuable insights into gender-related differences and similarities and, as a consequence, can help practitioners to improve their approaches and outcomes.

Rozzano, Italy | Patrizia Presbitero
München, Germany | Julinda Mehilli
Pisa, Italy | Anna Sonia Petronio

Contents

Part I

Coronary Artery Disease

Women and Invasive Diagnostic Procedures

1

Yolande Appelman and Monique ten Haaf

1.1 Introduction

Cardiovascular disease (CVD) is the leading cause of death among women in Europe causing almost 2.1 million deaths each year. According to the European Heart Network, CVD accounts for 42 % of mortality in women under 75 years of age [1]. One of the main forms of CVD is coronary artery disease (CAD).

There are significant differences between men and women in the epidemiology, diagnosis, treatment, and prognosis of CAD that should be taken into account in the care of women with known or suspected disease. Unfortunately, data from clinical trials are limited, since women are generally underrepresented in randomized controlled studies [2]. This underrepresentation is partially related to the age when women develop symptomatic CAD – many studies have an age limit for patients' inclusion – and to a higher coexistence of comorbidities in women with CAD.

The prevalence of CAD is lower in women than in men at any given age. Women appear to develop symptomatic CAD about 10 years later than men, presumably because of higher estrogen levels in premenopausal period that slow the progression of atherosclerosis.

Angina is the most common symptom in patients with CAD. The complaints are mostly presented as a typical chest pain or pressure that results from the imbalance between a rise in oxygen demand of the myocardium, while the blood flow increase is insufficient. Women seem to present with more atypical features of CAD, which makes the evaluation more challenging.

Coronary angiography is the gold standard for the evaluation of CAD in both women and men and provides information on the location and extent of atherosclerotic lesions. However, coronary angiography alone may not be sufficient to make

Y. Appelman (✉) • M. ten Haaf
Department of Cardiology, VU Medical Center – VUMC,
de Boelelaan 1117, Amsterdam 1081, The Netherlands
e-mail: Y.Appelman@vumc.nl

P. Presbitero et al. (eds.), *Percutaneous Treatment of Cardiovascular Diseases in Women*,
DOI 10.1007/978-3-319-39611-8_1

the right diagnosis in women as they more often have angina related to nonobstructive CAD. Additional invasive and noninvasive diagnostic tools can provide information about other causes of angina, like microvascular disease (MVD) and spasm. According to this, Shaw et al. introduced the term ischemic heart disease (IHD) as being more appropriate for women instead of CAD [3]. In this chapter, we will review the indications for coronary angiography, anatomical features, and technical issues during angiography in women, therapeutic options, and complications after invasive assessment in women.

1.2 Clinical Presentation

Many clinical presentations lead to the suspicion of CAD. Angina pectoris is the most common initial presentation of CAD in women (47 vs. 32 %), whereas myocardial infarction is the most common initial manifestation in men (6 vs. 10 %) [4].

The distinction between a stable and unstable presentation can be made upon the clinical assessment of the nature of symptoms, the clinical risk profile, the presence of abnormalities on the surface electrocardiogram suggestive of CAD, and cardiac biomarker measurements. This chapter is separated into a stable pattern presentation, symptomatic or asymptomatic, and an acute unstable presentation highly suggestive of CAD, i.e., acute coronary syndromes (ACS).

1.2.1 Stable Coronary Artery Disease

Classical stable angina pectoris is the most common form of angina and is usually caused by a stenosis of a large epicardial artery. Other mechanisms are also likely to contribute to the genesis of anginal symptoms, though more often less typical, including microvascular dysfunction (microvascular angina), angina caused by vasospasm (vasospastic angina), and symptomatic ischemic cardiomyopathy [5]. The prevalence of these different forms of angina differs between women and men.

Women have a 20 % higher prevalence of angina than men [6]. Many studies classify chest pain into three groups of typical angina, atypical angina, and nonspecific or noncardiac angina. Typical angina pectoris is characterized by a substernal chest pain, sometimes accompanied by other symptoms like shortness of breath, nausea, or fatigue that occurs after exertion and diminishes in rest or upon nitroglycerine use. Atypical angina is characterized by two of these features and aspecific angina by at most one of these features. The probability of epicardial artery obstructions increases in aging women, and symptoms become more typical with advancing age [7]. Women more often present with atypical symptoms and have more concomitant other symptoms, like shortness of breath, nausea, vomiting, and back pain, and also report a higher number of symptoms compared to men.

Microvascular and vasospastic angina are also more often reported in women. There is a lack of reliable prevalence numbers, due to referral and selection bias in current studies. Previous studies showed a prevalence of 20–50 % of myocardial ischemia and/or microvascular dysfunction (MVD) in women with chest pain and normal coronary arteries. Moreover, patients might share a combination of different forms of angina, so these numbers can be underestimated. Finally, women appear to have more silent ischemia than men.

1.2.2 Acute Coronary Syndrome

Acute coronary syndrome (ACS) refers to a spectrum of clinical conditions ranging from unstable angina or non-ST-segment elevation myocardial infarction (NSTEMI) to ST-segment elevation myocardial infarction (STEMI). The conditions are associated with acute myocardial ischemia and/or infarction, which are usually due to an abrupt reduction in coronary blood flow.

In the setting of ACS, women have different clinical profiles and presentation as compared to men, with fewer women than men presenting with STEMI (68 vs. 77 %) but more presenting with unstable angina (21 vs. 12 %) [8]. Although women experience atypical angina more frequently than men, chest pain is the most predominant symptom of ACS in women, regardless of ACS type [9, 10]. Sex differences in ECG findings and cardiac biomarker measurements should be taken into account in the interpretation of ACS type.

1.2.3 ECG Findings

Unstable angina is characterized by new-onset angina or a recent destabilization of previously stable angina. There is no release of cardiac biomarkers (i.e., troponin I or T); however, ST-segment depression and T-wave changes can be present. In premenopausal women, the influence of changing endogenous estrogen levels during the menstrual cycle on ECG results must be taken into account. Lower midcycle estradiol levels are associated with more ischemia-related ECG findings and can influence the accuracy of chest pain and the inducibility of ST-segment abnormalities [7].

The characteristic ECG findings of STEMI slightly differ according to sex and age. Typically, ST-segment elevation in acute myocardial infarction (AMI), measured at the J point, is present in two contiguous leads and is ≥0.25 mV in men <40 years, ≥0.2 mV in men >40 years, and ≥0.15 mV in women in leads V2–V3 or ≥0.1 mV in other leads (in the absence of left ventricular (LV) hypertrophy or left bundle branch block (LBBB)) [11].

1.2.4 Cardiac Biomarker Measurements

In both NSTEMI and STEMI, a rise and/or fall of cardiac specific myocardial necrosis markers is detected, which define them clinically as AMI, and distinguishes them from unstable angina [12]. Cardiac troponins have become the cardiac markers of choice for patients with ACS in the guidelines from the European Society of Cardiology (ESC). The recommended cutoff value for cardiac biomarker values is the 99th percentile upper reference limit of a healthy reference population [13]. However, there is no universal consensus of how to define a reference population according to age, sex, ethnicity, race, or the number of study participants needed in each category for a total reference population. The analytical quality of troponin T and troponin I assays has been repeatedly improved during the last decade, making it possible to detect lower enzyme release. Highly sensitive troponin assays have identified differences in the normal reference range between women and men with 99th percentiles twofold higher in men. In the High-STEACS study, a randomized controlled trial in patients with suspected ACS, the diagnostic accuracy of a high-sensitivity assay with sex-specific diagnostic thresholds was compared to the contemporary assay. The high sensitivity troponin I assay doubled the diagnosis of myocardial infarction in women (from 11 % to 22 %; $P<0.001$) but had a minimal effect in men (from 19 % to 21 %, $P=0.002$) [14]. In a study of Slagman et al., the influence of sex on the diagnostic performance of cardiac troponin in chest pain patients was investigated [15]. Especially in patients that presented more than four hours after the onset of symptoms, sex differences in the predictive value of cardiac troponin were found. Women with a NSTEMI were less likely to have an initially elevated troponin value as compared to men. Also, the sensitivity and positive predictive value were lower in women as compared to men, while specificity and negative predictive value as well as diagnostic accuracy are slightly higher. Current diagnostic thresholds may lead to under diagnosis of AMI in women and contribute to sex inequalities in treatment and outcome. The implementation of sex-dependent cutoff values for cardiac troponin assays might be recommended in the future; however, further studies are needed to evaluate possible cutoff values in order to optimize diagnostic accuracy of cardiac troponin for women and men and to confirm the consequences on clinical outcome.

1.3 Pretest Probability of Coronary Artery Disease

The possibility that physicians underestimate the risk of disease in women cannot be ruled out. Therefore, the clinical assessment and prediction of the pretest risk for CAD in women is very important.

1.3.1 Gender, Age, and Clinical Presentation

The pretest likelihood of CAD in symptomatic patients depends on gender, age, and type of symptoms. Advancing age, male gender, and typical angina are associated with obstructive CAD. Women usually present at older age and with more atypical symptoms as compared to men and therefore have lower probability of CAD on catheterization per age category. For example, when a man of 35 years presents with typical angina, he has a pretest probability of 59 % for having CAD, compared with 28 % in women. Sex differences in pretest probability diminish with advancing age. In patients who have a high pretest probability and severe symptoms or a clinical condition indicating high risk, early invasive intracoronary angiography without previous noninvasive risk stratification is a good strategy to identify lesions potentially amenable to revascularization. Women less frequently reach a pretest probability of 85 % or higher, which implies that women should always undergo exercise stress testing or noninvasive imaging before being referred to the catheterization laboratory [5].

1.3.2 Risk Factors

Especially when the clinical presentation is not completely clear, it is also important to take risk factors into account. Age is the most important risk factor for CAD. From menopause, when the relative protection of estrogen has diminished, the burden of CAD increases significantly. Furthermore, most of the burden of CAD can be explained by a set of traditional risk factors (RFs) that affect both women and men, including elevated blood pressure, smoking, overweight and obesity, diabetes, and elevated cholesterol. Although these RFs do not differ between both genders, the impact of these RFs might be different for women and men. In a recent review by Appelman et al., it has been demonstrated, for instance, that prolonged smoking and diabetes are significantly more hazardous for women than for men [16]. However, these differences between women and men are not implemented in current guidelines yet. In addition, several female-specific RFs like pregnancy-induced hypertension and gestational diabetes have been identified with a high lifetime risk of cardiovascular disease. Attention for female-specific RF may enable early detection of CAD and subsequent early disease detection in apparently healthy women. Studies are needed to assess if and how the added RFs should be implemented in current risk assessment and management strategies to maximize benefit and cost-effectiveness specific in women.

1.3.3 Noninvasive Testing

The development and widespread use of noninvasive tests have contributed to the improvement in evaluation of patients with known or suspected CAD. Unfortunately, all available tests have advantages and drawbacks, and no single imaging modality has been proven to be superior overall. With coronary computed tomography angiography (CCTA) or magnetic resonance imaging (MRI) angiography, the coronary anatomy can be visualized, and additional information about the plaque composites can be obtained. Cardiac MRI also offers the possibility of functional imaging. Functional tests can add important information with respect to the causal relationship between ischemia and the occurrence of the patient's symptoms. Other functional imaging techniques include dobutamine stress echocardiography, single-photon computed tomography (SPECT), and positron emission tomography (PET) imaging.

The sensitivity and specificity of all tests are lower in women compared to men, partly due to the lower prevalence of obstructive CAD (Table 1.1) [18]. The choice

Table 1.1 Accuracy of noninvasive testing compared with coronary angiography for diagnosing CAD in women

Modality	Population	Quality of included studies	Number of studies	Number of women	Summary sensitivity (95 % CI)	Summary specificity (95 % CI)
Exercise/stress ECG	No known	All	29	3,392	62 % (55–68 %)	68 % (63–73 %)
	CAD	Good	10	1,410	70 % (58–79 %)	62 % (53–69 %)
	Mixed population	All	41	4,879	61 % (54–67 %)	65 % (58–72 %)
		Good	13	1,679	65 % (52–76 %)	60 % (52–68 %)
ECHO	No known	All	14	1,286	79 % (74–83 %)	83 % (74–89 %)
	CAD	Good	5	561	79 % (69–87 %)	85 % (68–94 %)
	Mixed population	All	22	1,873	78 % (73–83 %)	86 % (79–91 %)
		Good	8	807	77 % (65–85 %)	89 % (76–95 %)
SPECT	No known	All	14	1,000	81 % (76–86 %)	78 % (69–84 %)
	CAD	Good	4	394	83 % (52–95 %)	72 % (37–92 %)
	Mixed population	All	30	2,146	82 % (77–87 %)	81 % (74–86 %)
		Good	10	982	82 % (72–88 %)	79 % (66–87 %)
CMR	No known	All	5	501	72 % (55–85 %)	84 % (69–93 %)
	CAD	Good	5	501	72 % (55–85 %)	84 % (69–93 %)
	Mixed population	All	6	778	78 % (61–89 %)	84 % (74–90 %)
		Good	5	610	76 % (55–89 %)	84 % (72–91 %)
Coronary CTA	No known	All	53	474	93 % (69–99 %)	77 % (54–91 %)
	CAD	Good		124	85 % (26–99 %)	73 % (17–97 %)
	Mixed population	All	8	690	94 % (81–98 %)	87 % (68–96 %)
		Good	4	201	83 % (58–94 %)	77 % (40–94 %)

Adapted with permission from [17]

CAD coronary artery disease, *CI* confidence interval, *CMR* cardio magnetic resonance, *CTA* computed tomography angiography, *ECG* electrocardiogram, *ECHO* echocardiogram, *SPECT* single-proton emission computed tomography

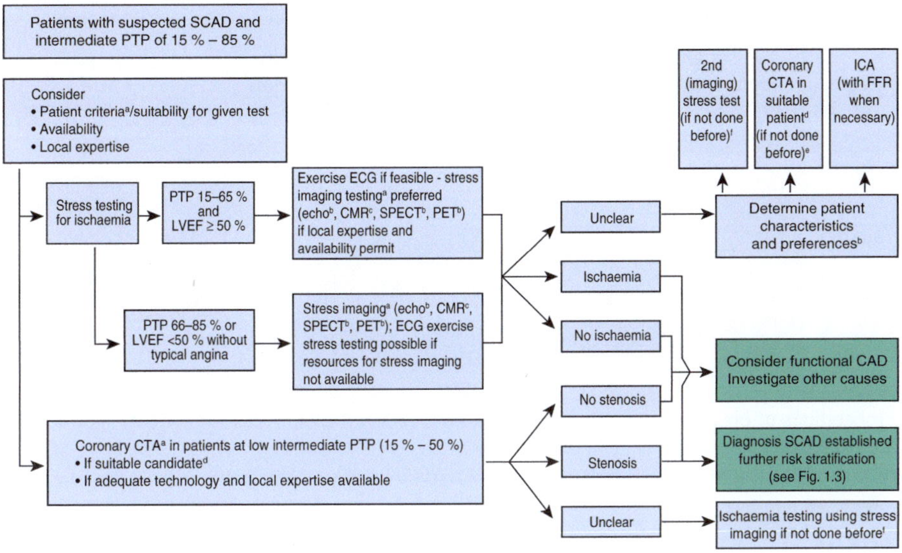

Fig. 1.1 Noninvasive testing in patients with suspected SCAD and an intermediate pretest probability. *CAD* coronary artery disease, *CTA* computed tomography angiography, *CMR* cardiac magnetic resonance, *ECG* electrocardiogram, *ICA* invasive coronary angiography, *LVEF* left ventricular ejection fraction, *PET* positron emission tomography, *PTP* pretest probability, *SCAD* stable coronary artery disease, *SPECT* single-photon emission computed tomography. (a) Consider age of patient versus radiation exposure. (b) In patients unable to exercise use echo or SPECT/PET with pharmacologic stress instead. (c) CMR is only performed using pharmacologic stress. (d) Patient characteristics should make a fully diagnostic coronary CTA scan highly probable consider result to be unclear in patients with severe diffuse or focal calcification. (e) Proceed as in lower left coronary CTA box. (f) Proceed as in stress testing for ischemia box (Adapted with permission from the ESC guidelines stable CAD [5])

of the imaging method should be tailored to each person based on the pretest probability of CAD, clinical history, and local expertise (Fig. 1.1) [5]. If noninvasive testing demonstrates myocardial ischemia, women should undergo cardiac catheterization to confirm the presence or absence of obstructive CAD.

1.4 Indications for Invasive Coronary Angiography

Despite the advances in noninvasive testing over recent years for the investigation of chest pain in women, invasive coronary angiography remains the gold standard in the diagnosis and assessment of CAD [5]. With invasive angiography, a two-dimensional outline of the coronary artery anatomy and of the luminal changes can be visualized.

Indications for the use of catheterization and coronary intervention have been described in the guidelines of the ESC and are focused on stable angina pectoris and

Table 1.2 Clinical pretest probabilities in men and women with stable chest pain symptoms

	Typical angina		Atypical angina		Non-anginal pain	
Age	Men	Women	Men	Women	Men	Women
30–39	59	28	29	10	18	5
40–49	69	37	38	14	25	8
50–59	77	47	49	20	34	12
60–69	84	58	59	28	44	17
70–79	89	68	69	37	54	24
>80	93	76	78	47	65	32

PTP < 15 %: no further testing (low probability of SCAD)
PTP 15–65%: exercise ECG or non-invasive imaging based test for ischaemia as initial test
PTP 66–85%: non-invasive imaging functional test
PTP>85%: only risk stratification (high probability of SCAD)

Adapted with permission from ESC guidelines [5]

Probabilities of obstructive coronary disease shown reflect the estimates for patients aged 35, 45, 55, 65, 75, and 85 years

ECG electrocardiogram, *PTP* pretest probability, *SCAD* stable coronary artery disease

ACS [5, 11, 13]. Currently these recommendations do not make a distinction between women and men with regard to these indications. However, since the prevalence of significant obstructive CAD is generally lower in women, a careful estimation of the pretest probability is necessary to avoid unnecessary invasive procedures (Table 1.2) [5].

Coronary angiography is valuable when the pretest probability of obstructive CAD is intermediate or high. Douglas et al. proposed an algorithm for the assessment of the need of coronary angiography in women already 20 years ago (Table 1.3) [19].

1.4.1 Referral Bias

A delay in the referral for coronary angiography and subsequent diagnosis of CAD may lead to a higher morbidity and mortality. As women more often present with atypical symptoms, misinterpretation of symptoms and underdiagnosis cannot be ruled out.

There is conflicting evidence as to whether there is a bias against women in the referral for cardiac catheterization and likelihood for revascularization. Rates of coronary angiography and PCI increased among both women and men over time. Although there seems equal access to cardiac invasive procedures in Europe, there are still sex-related differences in the use of these procedures and subsequent revascularizations (Fig. 1.2) [20].

Several studies have examined the gender-related difference in the referral rate for coronary angiography with or without prior noninvasive testing. Tobin et al. documented the highest estimated male–female odds ratios for relative risks of referral, reporting that women were much less likely than men to be referred for coronary angiography after an abnormal nuclear exercise test, even when important covariates that could influence the referral decision had been considered [21]. However, more recent studies concluded that lower crude referral rates for coronary

Table 1.3 Assessment need for coronary angiography in women

Likelihood of CAD	Initial test	Subsequent test
Low (<20 %) No major and ≤1 intermediate or ≤2 minor determinants	→ None indicated	→ None indicated
Moderate (20–80 %) 1 Major or multiple intermediate and minor determinants	→ Routine ETT:	
	Negative	→ None indicated
	Inconclusive	→ Further testing indicated; selection must be individualized
	Positive	→ Imaging test for catheterization
	→ Imaging ETT:	
	Negative	→ None indicated
	Inconclusive	→ Catheterization
	Positive	→ Catheterization
High (>80 %) ≤2 Major or 1 major plus >1 intermediate and minor determinants	→ Routine ETT:	
	Negative	→ None indicated, observe patient carefully
	Inconclusive	→ Catheterization
	Positive	→ Catheterization
	→ Imaging ETT:	→ None indicated

Determinants of CAD in women with chest pain
Major - *Typical angina pectoris* - *Postmenopausal status – without hormone replacement* - *Diabetes mellitus* - *Peripheral vascular disease*
Intermediate - *Hypertension* - *Smoking* - *Lipoprotein abnormalities, especially low HDL cholesterol levels*
Minor - *Age > 65* - *Obesity, especially central obesity* - *Sedentary lifestyle* - *Family history of coronary heart disease* - *Other risk factors for coronary heart disease (e.g. psychological or hemostatic)*

Adapted with permission from Douglas et al. [19]
CAD coronary artery disease, *ETT* exercise tolerance test, *HDL* high density lipoprotein

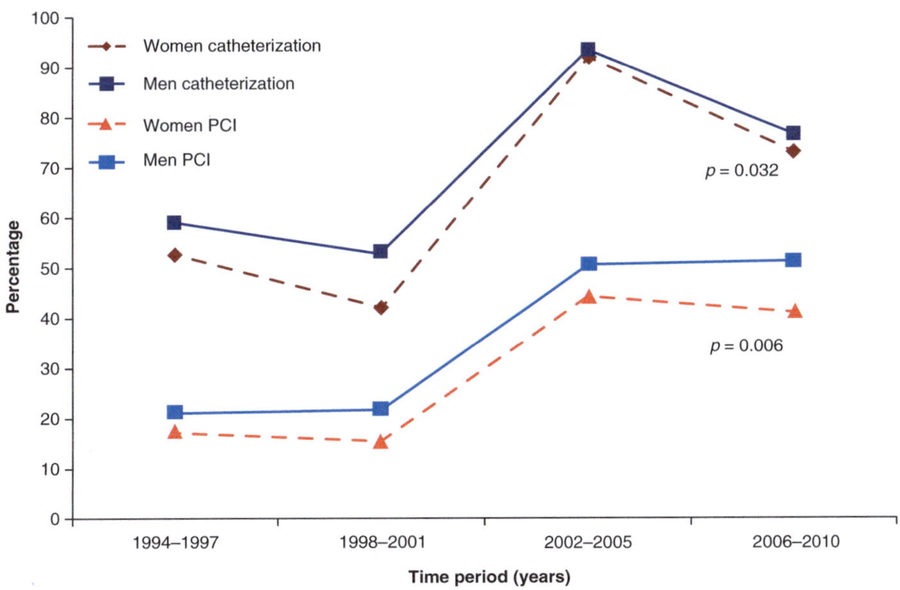

Fig. 1.2 Sex-stratified trends in use of catheterization and PCI. P values are from sex and time interaction term with trial as random effect. Significant P values indicate a significant change in rates of use between women (*dashed line*) and men (*blue*) over time. *PCI* percutaneous coronary intervention (Adapted with permission from Kragholm et al. [20])

angiography in women no longer persisted after adjustment for confounding variables or appropriateness of its use. Nguyen et al. reported similar referral rates for revascularization procedures, once significant CAD was elucidated [22]. Interestingly, since women appear to have more nonobstructive CAD, sex differences in referral and revascularization can also be interpreted as overuse of angiography in women or under-referral in men. In a German registry study of Heer et al., women with NSTEMI and stable CAD had even higher rates of PCI as compared to men and similar rates in case of STEMI [23].

1.5 Anatomical Features

The anatomy of the heart differs slightly between women and men. The size of a woman's heart is two-thirds that of a man's and a woman's coronary arteries are smaller. The chance of having obstructive coronary lesions increases also in aging women. Women have less calcification of coronary plaques, smaller intramedial plaques and lower atheroma volume within the intima and media of the coronary arteries. Women who undergo catheterization are less likely to have multivessel disease and more likely to have nonobstructive disease compared with men.

The link between myocardial ischemia and obstructive atherosclerosis of the epicardial coronary arteries is well established, and coronary angiography has demonstrated a relationship between the severity and extent of CAD and survival. However, women have a higher prevalence of nonobstructive CAD, and symptoms seem to be more frequently related to abnormal coronary reactivity, microvascular dysfunction, and plaque erosion. This reinforces the fact that a description of the coronary anatomy alone is not enough in women without obstructive CAD [3].

1.5.1 Rationale for Revascularization

Clinical guidelines do not differentiate between women and men regarding revascularization recommendations. If despite medical treatment, flow-limiting coronary stenoses are present, revascularization, by either PCI or coronary artery bypass graft (CABG) surgery, may be indicated to reduce myocardial ischemia and its adverse clinical manifestations and to relieve symptoms. Revascularization of nonischemic lesions not only increases the treatment costs but also poses an increased risk for the CAD patient rather than offering any benefit. Since women have less severe CAD with less obstruction, revascularization strategies will be applied less frequently. At present, 15–38 % of patients treated with revascularization techniques are women [17]. Modern stent implantation with new generation drug eluting stents (DES) have shown to be effective and safe in women and are recommended as the standard of care for PCI in women [24].

1.5.2 Women and Nonobstructive CAD

The Women's Ischemia Syndrome Evaluation (WISE) studies have demonstrated that up to 50 % of women undergoing coronary angiography do not have obstructive CAD [25]. While women compared to men have a higher incidence of angina-like symptoms of IHD, these women are often reassured and frequently not treated or further investigated although this finding is not benign and is associated with an adverse cardiovascular outcome compared to asymptomatic women. This syndrome of angina-like symptoms and evidence of ischemia but without obstructive epicardial CAD is attributed to functional disorders of the larger and smaller coronary arteries, spasm and microvascular disease (MVD), and is associated with 3.5 times greater risk of MACE (hospitalization for heart failure, MI, and stroke rate or all-cause mortality) and worse quality of life compared to women with no CAD (hazard ratio [HR] 3.58; 95 % CI 1.87–6.86), whereas for men with nonobstructive CAD, there was no difference in MACE compared to men with no CAD (HR, 0.82; 95 % CI, 0.35–1.93) [26].

Although the prevalence of nonobstructive CAD is higher in women, it is not only a women's disease. A recent publication by Murthy et al. demonstrated no difference in the prevalence of MVD (documented by PET) and showed that the severity of MVD was associated with older age and cardiovascular RF [27]. Furthermore, they found that the presence of MVD increased adverse cardiovascular outcomes irrespective of gender. It can be concluded that these findings establish the importance to consider the diagnosis of MVD in both sexes. Further studies are needed to establish the role of the particular higher prevalence of MVD in women compared to men.

Therefore, after obstructive CAD has been ruled out by invasive coronary angiography, other etiologic mechanisms for angina-like complaints should be investigated by noninvasive (Doppler echocardiography, MRI, or PET) or invasive tests as demonstrated in Table 1.4 [28]. The golden standard for the diagnosis of spasm and MVD is invasive coronary reactivity testing by using adenosine, acetylcholine, ergonovine, or nitroglycerine. Measurement such as coronary flow reserve (CFR), fractional flow reserve (FFR), instantaneous wave-free ratio (iFR), and index myocardial resistance (IMR) will help to understand the pathophysiology in patients presenting with angina without obstructive CAD. However, there is still concern about the safety of using acetylcholine, like the occurrence of arrhythmias reported with acetylcholine (9.3 %), and also transient atrioventricular blocks have been reported. Chapter 2 will provide more details with respect to these invasive measurements.

1.5.3 Treatment of Angina in Women with Nonobstructive CAD

There have been several pharmacological and non-pharmacological therapies tested in women with MVD; however, there is still lack of evidence-based studies that have evaluated the impact on CV outcome. Therefore, treatment of these symptomatic patients can be frustrating for both patient and their physicians and leads to a high economic burden of healthcare costs. Women with angina and nonobstructive CAD should be screened for CVD risk factors and treated according to risk stratification as described

Table 1.4 Diagnosis and management of women with angina and nonobstructive CAD

Diagnostic test	Diagnosis
Intracoronary ergonovine	Epicardial coronary spasm
Acetylcholine	Epicardial coronary spasm Microvascular spasm
Adenosine test	Coronary microvascular endothelium-independent dysfunction
Intracoronary nicorandil	Coronary microvascular endothelium-independent dysfunction
Management	**Treatment**
A. Microvascular coronary dysfunction	
Coronary endothelial dysfunction	ACE inhibitors
	Angiotensin receptor blockers (if ACE inhibitor intolerant)
	HMG CoA reductase inhibitors (statins)
	Antiplatelet agent (aspirin)
	Enhanced external counterpulsation
Diminished coronary blood flow reserve	Beta-blockers
	L-Arginine supplementation
Coronary smooth muscle dysfunction	Calcium channel blockers
	Nitrates
Antianginal medication	Ranolazine
	Cognitive behavioral therapy
	Tricyclic medication
	Spinal cord stimulation (TENS unit)
B. Coronary vasospasm (prinzmetal angina)	Calcium channel blockers
C. Abnormal cardiac nociception	Tricyclic medication
	Spinal cord stimulation (TENS unit)

CAD coronary artery disease, *ECG* electrocardiogram, *ACE* angiotensin-converting enzyme, *HMG-CoA* 3-hydroxy-3-methylglutaryl-coenzyme A, *TENS* transcutaneous electrical nerve stimulation [28, 29]

in CVD prevention guidelines [30], supplemented by individualized symptomatic treatment for angina (Table 1.4). One can consider starting with the following medication: aspirin, statin, beta-blocker, ACE inhibitor, calcium blocker, or nitrate which is comparable with the treatment of obstructive CAD. Lifestyle interventions are also very important to lower the CV risk in patients with nonobstructive CAD as CV RFs play an important role in the pathophysiology of this disease. For instance, correction of endothelial dysfunction in postmenopausal hypertensive women may lower IHD events 7.3-fold [31].

1.6 Technical Issues and Complications of Invasive Coronary Angiography

As always, patients must be fully informed of the purpose of the procedure as well as its risks and limitations. Major complications, though rare in experienced hands, include death, stroke, coronary artery dissection, and arterial access complications.

Risks depend on the individual patient, and predictors include age, coronary anatomy, impaired left ventricular function, valvular heart disease, the clinical setting, and non-cardiac disease. The most common complications are transient or minor and include arterial access bleeding and hematoma, pseudoaneurysm, arrhythmias, reactions to the contrast medium, and vagal reactions.

Higher rates of procedural complications have been reported in women after both coronary angiography and PCI. In particular, women are prone to more vascular and bleeding complications than men. From 1994 to 1998, a national database from the United States reported twice as many complications in women for stroke (0.4 vs. 0.2 %, $P<0.001$) and vascular complications (5.4 vs. 2.7 %, $P<0.001$) [32]. Factors that are also associated with vascular complication are more prevalent in women, like advanced age, chronic kidney disease, low BMI, use of anticoagulation, and small vessel size. Lower BMI increases the risk of bleeding in patients undergoing PCI. As women are smaller than men, they have a higher PCI-related bleeding risk [33]. Several studies confirm the relationship between higher bleeding risk and low BMI. This might be explained via a higher platelet reactivity found in PCI patients using antiplatelet therapy and having high BMI. Barker et al. found that BMI was negatively associated with platelet reactivity in patients on antiplatelet therapy [34]. Thus women, having a lower BMI, might have enhanced platelet suppression.

1.6.1 Vascular Access

A mixture of patient-related, anatomical, and technical factors usually influences the choice of vascular access. Key considerations for all percutaneous approaches are the antithrombotic environment, the Seldinger technique, and the potential need for interventions. Until recent years, the femoral approach was the most commonly used vascular access. In the last decade, there has been an increase in the uptake of radial access for angiography and PCI for both elective and emergency cases in Europe and North America driven by the higher bleeding complications rate using the femoral approach.

In general, women undergoing coronary angiography and PCI are at higher risk of vascular complications after diagnostic and interventional procedures compared with men. The femoral approach is still the most performed procedure in both men and women, but the radial approach gains in popularity in both genders during the last few years and seems preferred due to the reduction in vascular complications after PCI [35]. It seems that a safe femoral artery puncture is more challenging in women compared to men as women have smaller and shorter common femoral artery [36]. However, although there is a higher risk of access site bleeding in women compared to men, there is has been no relationship demonstrated with these anatomic differences using the femoral approach. The reason for this higher access site bleeding in women therefore remains unclear. The study by Pandie et al. showed that major vascular complications were significantly reduced with the use of radial access in both sexes, but this effect was more prominent among women, irrespective of whether PCI was performed. The number of patients needed to treat with radial access instead of femoral access to prevent 1 vascular complication was 33 in women and 49 in men. These data suggest that women undergoing coronary angiography for ACS may particularly benefit from the radial approach. However, the SAFE-PCI for women trial compared radial and femoral artery access in women undergoing procedures either electively or for non-STEMI and was terminated early because of lower than expected rates of bleeding and vascular complications. There was no significant difference in access site complication rates in the PCI subgroup, although there was a significant decrease in bleeding and vascular complications using the radial approach in the entire cohort of PCIs and diagnostic coronary angiography [37].

Furthermore, there are concerns that radial access may be technically more challenging in women due to smaller caliber radial arteries (2.43 ± 38 versus 2.69 ± 0.40 mm), greater tortuosity, and increased rates of radial artery spasm, potentially leading to lower procedural success rates. This was demonstrated in several studies.

Women with a radial access approach are more likely to cross over to femoral access than men (11.1 % in women vs. 6.3 % in men). This is related to higher rates of radial spasm (9.5 % in women vs. 3.3 % in men). Technical skill and the use of 5-F catheters help to extend the benefits of radial access to women. A recent study suggested the greater need for pre-selecting adequate access arteries in women to reduce radial artery spasm rates [35]. Chugh et al. showed that women have more commonly only a single adequate forearm artery of the four available forearm arteries as compared with men, who more commonly have multiple adequately sized access arteries [38]. So, proactive measures to decrease access site complications, such as fluoroscopy of the groin before catheterization, smaller sheath size, and increased attention to access management, should be considered routinely in women [32].

In terms of patient preference for subsequent procedures, both women and men would prefer radial access, especially because of mobility reasons. However, in conclusion, at present, the most important reasons for the radial access preference are the reduction in bleeding risk in both women and men.

1.6.2 Vascular Closure in Femoral Approach

Already several years ago, vascular closure devices were introduced to the clinic. Tavris et al. studied the association of gender, sheath size, and closure techniques and found that large sheath size and both manual compression and collagen plug devices to control femoral artery bleeding increased the relative risk of vascular complications for women [36]. This is surprising as the target vessels are supposed to be smaller in diameter. Therefore, these increased complications persist even in the era of closure devices.

1.6.3 Radiation Exposure

The catheterization laboratory is a place where the use of ionizing radiation is high every day. Personnel and patients are at risk to radiation exposure, and procedures such as performing PCI are considered as highest radiation dose for patients and staff. The exposure of a diagnostic coronary angiogram for a patient lies in the range of 350 X-rays, while that of a coronary intervention lies in a range of 750 X-rays. Every day we expose ourselves to radiation from natural cosmic rays in our environment (gamma radiation). However, it is proven that radiation is carcinogenic and that medical exposure to radiation may increase the risk of developing cancer in patients as well as in medical staff. Furthermore, it can lead to skin injuries and damage to the eye especially the formation of cataract. The number of diagnostic and interventional coronary procedures has increased during the last decades and contributes for 10 % to the collective dose in patients. Therefore, it is of highest importance to minimize the risk of radiation exposure, and this can be achieved by following an intensive training program. In this program, the key methods for the reduction of radiation reduction are focused on the following items and can be generalized to all patients and staff members who work with radiation:

1. Time: minimizing the fluoroscopy time decreases radiation damage for patients and staff.
2. Distance: the risk of radiation exposure decreases exponential by increasing the distance from the radiation beam.
3. Shielding: protection using lead shields (mobile shielding, thyroid collar, lead apron, lead glasses) decreases the risk of radiation exposure.

With the increasing use of the radial approach, there was a concern if this might lead to higher radiation exposure for the operator and patient. Recently, a randomized trial demonstrated that radiation exposure for the patient during diagnostic coronary angiography using femoral approach was similar compared to radial approach using either right or left radial artery (LRA). However, using the LRA led to a higher operator radiation exposure than using the FA or RRA. Unfortunately, there were no data reported with respect to gender differences as it might be that even in female patients the risk for the operator, due to the smaller size of the patient, might even be higher [33].

For any given radiation exposure, the cancer risk is higher in women compared to men at all ages (about 38 %). Next to that, it is important to know if a female patient is pregnant as the ionizing radiation can be both teratogenic and carcinogenic for the fetus (particularly leading to leukemia). This is due to the fact that the sensitivity of a tissue to radiation is related to its rate of proliferation that is high in fetal cells. Therefore, prior to the investigation, it is necessary to ask a female of reproductive age if she might be pregnant, and if so, the examinations needing radiation should be postponed (if possible) until the organogenesis is completed (>12-week pregnancy). Consequently, it is of special importance for medical staff to take gender into account when a cardiac radiation procedure is performed in female patients and that a women's pregnancy is acknowledged. Furthermore, women are strongly encouraged to declare their pregnancy as early as possible.

1.6.4 Contrast-Induced Nephropathy

Contrast-induced nephropathy is a complication which is associated with increased in-hospital and long-term morbidity and mortality [34]. At present, there are no approved diagnostic tests or preventive therapies for contrast-induced nephropathy.

Women are at a greater risk for the development of renal complications in the period after angiography than men. The significantly higher incidence of contrast-induced nephropathy in women seems largely due to their less favorable baseline characteristics, including lower glomerular filtration rate (GFR), more anemia, higher incidence of arterial hypertension, and advanced age. However, in a STEMI study of Lucreziotti et al., female gender and a left ventricular ejection fraction (LVEF) of lower than 40 % were independent predictors of contrast-induced nephropathy [39]. A reduced glomerular volume in women might be a possible mechanism to explain a greater susceptibility to acute renal failure.

1.7 Therapeutic Options

Coronary angiography was performed in 1958 by Sones as he tried to perform a selective aortic root injection. He noticed that the catheter tip accidently had entered the right coronary artery when the contrast dye was injected. Since then, the technique has been developed and has proven to be of great importance in patients with CAD. Years later, the first coronary angioplasty, generally known as percutaneous coronary intervention (PCI), was performed in September 1979 by Andreas Gruntzig. Of the first fifty patients reported, only four patients were female with stenotic lesions of 75 % or more [40]. At that time, it was thought that especially patients with an accessible stenosis of less than 1 cm length based on coronary angiography and a short history of pain (less than 1 year) were most suitable for the procedure. It is unknown if differences in the outcome of the angiography or the symptoms clarify the small proportion women in these early reports. Nowadays the indications for coronary intervention have been broadened, and the proportion of women undergoing PCI has increased.

The therapeutic response of women, both to revascularization procedures and pharmacological treatment, presents certain peculiarities. Details of the (invasive) coronary treatment in subsequently stable angina, NSTEMI, and STEMI and anti-thrombotic treatment will be discussed in paragraph three to six.

Take-Home Messages

- Women are more likely to present with atypical angina at older age with a high coexistence of comorbidities when they develop symptomatic CAD.
- Women less frequently reach a pretest probability for CAD of 85 % or higher which suggests an obligatory noninvasive testing prior to invasive diagnostics in case the cardiac biomarkers are negative.
- Invasive coronary angiography is the gold standard for diagnosis of CAD in women.
- Women more often present with nonobstructive CAD, which urges investigation of other causes of angina with additional (non)invasive testing.
- Radial access approach for invasive coronary angiography is preferable particularly in women since they are at increased risk of bleeding and vascular complications during invasive procedures.

References

1. Nichols M, Townsend N, Luengo-Fernandez R, et al. European Cardiovascular Disease Statistics 2012. European Heart Network. Brussels: European Society of Cardiology, Sophia Antipolis.
2. Safdar B, Nagurney JT, Anise A, et al. Gender-specific research for emergency diagnosis and management of ischemic heart disease: proceedings from the 2014 Academic Emergency Medicine Consensus Conference Cardiovascular Research Workgroup. Acad Emerg Med. 2014;21(12):1350–60.
3. Shaw LJ, Bugiardini R, Merz CN. Women and ischemic heart disease: evolving knowledge. J Am Coll Cardiol. 2009;54(17):1561–75.
4. Murabito JM, Evans JC, Larson MG, et al. Prognosis after the onset of coronary heart disease. An investigation of differences in outcome between the sexes according to initial coronary disease presentation. Circulation. 1993;88(6):2548–55.
5. Montalescot G, Sechtem U, Achenbach S, et al. 2013 ESC guidelines on the management of stable coronary artery disease: the Task Force on the management of stable coronary artery disease of the European Society of Cardiology. Eur Heart J. 2013;34(38):2949–3003.
6. Hemingway H, Langenberg C, Damant J, et al. Prevalence of angina in women versus men: a systematic review and meta-analysis of international variations across 31 countries. Circulation. 2008;117(12):1526–36.
7. Shaw LJ, Bairey Merz CN, Pepine CJ, et al. Insights from the NHLBI-Sponsored Women's Ischemia Syndrome Evaluation (WISE) Study: part I: gender differences in traditional and novel risk factors, symptom evaluation, and gender-optimized diagnostic strategies. J Am Coll Cardiol. 2006;47(3 Suppl):S4–20.
8. Berger JS, Elliott L, Gallup D, et al. Sex differences in mortality following acute coronary syndromes. JAMA. 2009;302(8):874–82.
9. Patel H, Rosengren A, Ekman I. Symptoms in acute coronary syndromes: does sex make a difference? Am Heart J. 2004;148(1):27–33.

10. Khan NA, Daskalopoulou SS, Karp I, et al. Sex differences in acute coronary syndrome symptom presentation in young patients. JAMA Intern Med. 2013;173(20):1863–71.
11. Steg PG, James SK, Atar D, et al. ESC Guidelines for the management of acute myocardial infarction in patients presenting with ST-segment elevation. Eur Heart J. 2012;33(20):2569–619.
12. Thygesen K, Alpert JS, Jaffe AS, et al. Third universal definition of myocardial infarction. Eur Heart J. 2012;33(20):2551–67.
13. Roffi M, Patrono C, Collet JP, et al. 2015 ESC Guidelines for the management of acute coronary syndromes in patients presenting without persistent ST-segment elevation: task force for the management of acute coronary syndromes in patients presenting without persistent ST-segment elevation of the European Society of Cardiology (ESC). Eur Heart J. 2016;37(3):267–315.
14. Shah AS, Griffiths M, Lee KK et al. High sensitivity cardiac troponin and the under-diagnosis of myocardial infarction in women: prospective cohort study. BMJ. 2015;350:g7873.
15. Slagman A, Searle J, Vollert JO, et al. Sex differences of troponin test performance in chest pain patients. Int J Cardiol. 2015;187:246–51.
16. Appelman Y, van Rijn BB, Ten Haaf ME, et al. Sex differences in cardiovascular risk factors and disease prevention. Atherosclerosis. 2015;241(1):211–8.
17. Dolor RJ, Patel MR, Melloni C. Noninvasive technologies for the diagnosis of coronary artery disease in women [Internet]. Rockville: Agency for Healthcare Research and Quality (US); (Comparative Effectiveness Reviews, No. 58.). 2012.
18. Douglas PS, Ginsburg GS. The evaluation of chest pain in women. N Engl J Med. 1996;334(20):1311–5.
19. Kragholm K, Halim SA, Yang Q, et al. Sex-stratified trends in enrollment, patient characteristics, treatment, and outcomes among non-ST-segment elevation acute coronary syndrome patients: insights from clinical trials over 17 Years. Circ Cardiovasc Qual Outcomes. 2015;8(4):357–67.
20. Tobin JN, Wassertheil-Smoller S, Wexler JP, et al. Sex bias in considering coronary bypass surgery. Ann Intern Med. 1987;107(1):19–25.
21. Nguyen HL, Goldberg RJ, Gore JM, et al. Age and sex differences, and changing trends, in the use of evidence-based therapies in acute coronary syndromes: perspectives from a multinational registry. Coron Artery Dis. 2010;21(6):336–44.
22. Heer T, Hochadel M, Schmidt K, et al. Gender differences in therapeutic recommendation after diagnostic coronary angiography: insights from the coronary angiography and PCI registry of the German Society of Cardiology. Clin Res Cardiol. 2015;104(6):507–17.
23. Lansky AJ, Hochman JS, Ward PA, et al. Percutaneous coronary intervention and adjunctive pharmacotherapy in women: a statement for healthcare professionals from the American Heart Association. Circulation. 2005;111(7):940–53.
24. Stefanini GG, Baber U, Windecker S, et al. Safety and efficacy of drug-eluting stents in women: a patient-level pooled analysis of randomised trials. Lancet. 2013;382(9908):1879–88.
25. Gulati M, Cooper-Dehoff RM, McClure C, et al. Adverse cardiovascular outcomes in women with nonobstructive coronary artery disease: a report from the Women's Ischemia Syndrome Evaluation Study and the St James Women Take Heart Project. Arch Intern Med. 2009;169(9):843–50.
26. Sedlak TL, Lee M, Izadnegahdar M, et al. Sex differences in clinical outcomes in patients with stable angina and no obstructive coronary artery disease. Am Heart J. 2013;166(1):38–44.
27. Murthy VL, Naya M, Taqueti VR, et al. Effects of sex on coronary microvascular dysfunction and cardiac outcomes. Circulation. 2014;129(24):2518–27.
28. Radico F, Cicchitti V, Zimarino M, et al. Angina pectoris and myocardial ischemia in the absence of obstructive coronary artery disease: practical considerations for diagnostic tests. JACC Cardiovasc Interv. 2014;7(5):453–63.
29. Mehta PK, Merz CB. Treatment of angina in patients with evidence of myocardial ischemia and no obstructive coronary artery disease. In: Braunwald's heart disease: a textbook of cardiovascular medicine. 9th ed. Philadelphia: Elsevier; 2012.
30. Perk J, De BG, Gohlke H, et al. European guidelines on cardiovascular disease prevention in clinical practice (version 2012). The fifth joint task force of the European Society of Cardiology

and other societies on cardiovascular disease prevention in clinical practice (constituted by representatives of nine societies and by invited experts). Eur Heart J. 2012;33(13):1635–701.
31. Modena MG, Bonetti L, Coppi F, et al. Prognostic role of reversible endothelial dysfunction in hypertensive postmenopausal women. J Am Coll Cardiol. 2002;40(3):505–10.
32. Akhter N, Milford-Beland S, Roe MT, et al. Gender differences among patients with acute coronary syndromes undergoing percutaneous coronary intervention in the American College of Cardiology-National Cardiovascular Data Registry (ACC-NCDR). Am Heart J. 2009; 157(1):141–8.
33. Pancholy SB, Joshi P, Shah S, et al. Effect of vascular access site choice on radiation exposure during coronary angiography: the REVERE Trial (Randomized Evaluation of Vascular Entry Site and Radiation Exposure). JACC Cardiovasc Interv. 2015;8(9):1189–96.
34. Marenzi G, Lauri G, Assanelli E, et al. Contrast-induced nephropathy in patients undergoing primary angioplasty for acute myocardial infarction. J Am Coll Cardiol. 2004;44(9):1780–5.
35. Pandie S, Mehta SR, Cantor WJ, et al. Radial versus femoral access for coronary angiography/intervention in women with acute coronary syndromes: insights from the RIVAL Trial (Radial Vs femorAL access for coronary intervention). JACC Cardiovasc Interv. 2015;8(4):505–12.
36. Tavris DR, Wang Y, Jacobs S, et al. Bleeding and vascular complications at the femoral access site following percutaneous coronary intervention (PCI): an evaluation of hemostasis strategies. J Invasive Cardiol. 2012;24(7):328–34.
37. Rao SV, Hess CN, Barham B, et al. A registry-based randomized trial comparing radial and femoral approaches in women undergoing percutaneous coronary intervention: the SAFE-PCI for Women (Study of Access Site for Enhancement of PCI for Women) trial. JACC Cardiovasc Interv. 2014;7(8):857–67.
38. Chugh SK, Chugh Y, Chugh S. Overcoming the challenge of transradial interventions in women: insights from a color doppler study [Abstract TCT-822]. J Am Coll Cardiol. 2014;64:B240.
39. Lucreziotti S, Centola M, Salerno-Uriarte D, et al. Female gender and contrast-induced nephropathy in primary percutaneous intervention for ST-segment elevation myocardial infarction. Int J Cardiol. 2014;174(1):37–42.
40. Gruntzig AR, Senning A, Siegenthaler WE. Nonoperative dilatation of coronary-artery stenosis: percutaneous transluminal coronary angioplasty. N Engl J Med. 1979;301(2):61–8.

Intracoronary Imaging and Intracoronary Functional Tests

2

Maria D. Radu and Lene Holmvang

2.1 Introduction

Coronary artery disease is the leading cause of morbidity and mortality worldwide and embodies the effect of atherosclerosis – a condition caused by the accumulation of cholesterol in the coronary arterial intima leading to chronic inflammation with endothelial dysfunction, luminal narrowing, and eventually plaque rupture and thrombosis. Understanding the pathophysiology of atherosclerosis and the processes taking place after coronary stent implantation is crucial for improving cardiovascular outcomes. This chapter presents the most commonly used diagnostic intracoronary imaging techniques and functional tests, with an emphasis on technical issues and specific findings related to the female gender.

2.2 Intracoronary Imaging

Coronary angiography remains the reference modality to assess the severity of coronary lesions and guide stent implantation. The technique is, however, limited by its lumenographic nature preventing the visualization of processes taking place at the level of the vessel wall. These include (1) atherosclerosis, which is often diffuse with remodeling, where it is well known that angiography underestimates the extent and severity of disease, and (2) the healing and failure of coronary stents.

Traditional intracoronary imaging modalities such as intravascular ultrasound (IVUS) and optical coherence tomography (OCT) overcome these limitations by enabling a pathology-like cross-sectional view of the vessel wall and implanted devices. Other intracoronary imaging techniques are also available, although the target is different, such that angioscopy, which offers a forward-looking view of the

---

M.D. Radu (✉) • L. Holmvang
Department of Cardiology, The Heart Center, Rigshospitalet, Copenhagen, Denmark
e-mail: maria_d_radu@yahoo.com

P. Presbitero et al. (eds.), *Percutaneous Treatment of Cardiovascular Diseases in Women*,
DOI 10.1007/978-3-319-39611-8_2

luminal surface of the coronary vessel, whereas near-infrared spectroscopy (NIRS) provides a chemogram specifically of the cholesterol presence in the vessel wall. With IVUS and OCT providing the basis of most of our experience so far and since available data on gender differences primarily are derived using these techniques, they will be the focus of this section.

2.2.1 IVUS

Intravascular ultrasound (IVUS) imaging was introduced in the 1990s and allows a real-time, tomographic assessment of the lumen area, plaque burden, composition, longitudinal distribution, and remodeling as well as stent size, apposition, and expansion (Table 2.1). The standard ultrasonic catheters apply frequencies in the range 20–45 MHz, providing an axial resolution of 100–250 μm, and a tissue penetration up to 10 mm [1].

Conventional gray-scale (GS)-IVUS characterizes atheroma based on tissue echogenicity in relation to the surrounding adventitia, not necessarily reflecting

Table 2.1 Features assessable with optical coherence tomography (OCT) and intravascular ultrasound (IVUS) in comparison with gold-standard histology

Feature	Histology	OCT	IVUS
In general			
Resolution	1 μm	10–20 μm	100–250 μm
Imaging depth	∞	1–2.5 mm	8–10 mm
Detailed surface morphology	+	+	–
Vessel remodeling	+	–	+
In vivo and serial imaging	–	+	+
Imaging longitudinal segments	–	+	+
Atherosclerosis			
Lumen area	±	+	+
Plaque burden	+	–	+
Thin fibrous caps (TCFA)	+	+	–
Superficial calcification	+	+	–
Differentiation between deep lipid and calcification	+	–	+
Macrophage accumulation	+	+	–
Cholesterol crystals	+	±	–
Microvessels	+	±	–
Stent implantation			
Stent area	+	+	+
Apposition/malapposition	+	+	+
Stent expansion	[a]	+	+
Vessel injury	+	+	+
Thin neointima	+	+	+
Vessel remodeling	+	+	+
Other			
Red vs. white thrombi	+	+	+

histological composition. Due to a poor reproducibility, GS-IVUS cannot be recommended for characterization of tissue composition. This can, however, be improved by analysis of the radiofrequency signal together with the application of different diagnostic algorithms. Several such methods exist, of which virtual histology (VH)-IVUS has been most commonly used to study gender differences in plaque composition. VH-IVUS differentiates between fibrous, fibrofatty, dense calcium, and necrotic core composition with satisfactory histological correlation and reproducibility [1].

2.2.2 OCT

Optical coherence tomography (OCT) is a near-infrared (frequency: 1310 nm) light-based technology with an ultrahigh resolution of 10–20 μm: 10–20 times higher than IVUS [2]. Accordingly, OCT offers a significantly improved visualization of plaque characteristics by identifying fibroatheromas, fibrocalcific, and fibrous plaques with a high sensitivity and specificity. Of note, OCT is the only modality capable of providing accurate measurements of the thickness of the fibrous cap and can detect minor cap disruptions as well as accumulations of macrophages, microvessels, cholesterol crystals, and even differentiate between red and white thrombi. Compared with IVUS, OCT is associated with a noticeably reduced number of artifacts making the imaging of metallic stents and the evaluation at the strut level more feasible: these include small degrees of strut malapposition, thin strut coverage, intra-stent dissections, and other acute and long-term effects of stent implantation. Since the introduction of newer-generation Fourier-domain OCT systems in 2009, which provide ultrafast image acquisition in a user-friendly manner, OCT has emerged as the modality of choice in a majority of clinical scenarios. Nevertheless, at the cost of the high resolution is a relatively low tissue penetration (4–6 mm), rendering the assessment of plaque burden and remodeling in stented segments impossible [2].

2.2.2.1 Technical Issues

Current IVUS and OCT catheters range from 2.6 to 3.2 French in size and can be introduced through conventional six French guide catheters. Following the administration of nitroglycerine to avoid coronary spasm, the catheters are advanced over standard 0.014 in. guide wires, distal to the region of interest. Image acquisition with both IVUS and OCT is associated with high success rates (92–97 %), even with three-vessel imaging during ST-elevation myocardial infarction [3]. Technical issues are generally related to handling the catheters through diseased and/or tortuous segments, which might be more challenging in women due to smaller vessels. Care should particularly be taken when crossing coronary stents (both metallic and bioresorbable scaffolds) to avoid device displacement and fracture, for the interrogation of thrombosed lesions due to risk of distal embolization, and for assessment of edge dissections after device implantation. Serious complications in terms of coronary artery dissection/perforation or malignant arrhythmias are rare, although slightly more frequent with OCT (~1 %) due to the need for vessel flushing with contrast during image acquisition [3]. Discomfort from ischemia due to catheter obstruction during assessment of tight stenoses may be seen with increasing stenosis and acquisition time with IVUS (standard acquisition rate: 0.5 mm/s, meaning it takes 60 s to scan 30 mm vessel), whereas this is a decreasing issue with new-generation OCT systems with ultrafast acquisition (30 mm vessel in 1.5 s).

2.3 Findings from Clinical Studies

2.3.1 Intracoronary Imaging to Evaluate Atherosclerosis

Considering the morphometric similarity with pathology, data from intracoronary imaging studies represent an important continuation of the results from autopsy reports. One should, however, keep in mind that findings derived with these techniques need to be interpreted in view of their specific strengths and limitations (Table 2.1).

In general, female cardiac patients are often older and have more risk factors and comorbidities than their male counterparts, frequently resulting in their exclusion from clinical trials. In addition to this selection bias, available studies of atherosclerosis using intracoronary imaging are limited and heterogeneous making comparison and confident conclusion drawing somewhat difficult.

For both genders, VH-IVUS indicates that plaque burden, necrotic core, and calcium content increase significantly with aging [4, 5]. Several studies suggest that women compared to men, at any age, exhibit less extensive coronary artery disease by angiography [6], and smaller plaque burden by IVUS in stable as well as unstable clinical settings [4, 5, 7]. With respect to plaque composition, gender-specific differences have been reported in patients <65 years such that women by VH-IVUS seem to exhibit less necrotic core and dense calcium than men – a difference that is attenuated in patients ≥65 years of age [4, 7].

According to the current paradigm, the thin-cap fibroatheroma (TCFA) is the proposed precursor lesion of ruptured plaques responsible for the majority (60 %) of acute coronary syndromes (ACS) as defined by autopsy [8]. The TCFA is histologically characterized by a large necrotic core, covered by a thin fibrous cap (<65 μm) infiltrated with macrophages. Regions with histology-defined TCFA and VH-IVUS-defined TCFA typically exhibit a large plaque burden with positive remodeling, with a predilection for the proximal coronary arteries [2, 9]. OCT has confirmed that TCFAs are regularly found in culprit lesions of ST-elevation myocardial infarction (STEMI) (51–85 %), are relatively frequent in non-STEMI (22–50 %), and are fairly prevalent in patients with stable angina (SAP) (13–29 %) [2]. Guagliumi et al. recently found in a prospective study of gender differences in culprit plaques in STEMI that the rate of plaque rupture (~50 %) and eroded plaques (~25 %) were similar between genders, as was the composition of aspirated thrombus and inflammatory biomarkers [10].

In the study of the natural history of non-culprit lesions, the PROSPECT trial demonstrated that 51 % of lesions associated with clinical events at 3.4 years exhibited a TCFA by VH-IVUS ("VH-TCFA") at baseline, while the estimated rate for a VH-TCFA to cause a clinical event was only 4.9 %. Instead, a plaque burden >70 % was found to be the best predictor of events during the follow-up [11]. Among the possible explanations of the absence of a stronger TCFA-signal is the fact that the VH-TCFA definition relies on a composite of criteria, namely the presence of a plaque burden ≥40 % and confluent necrotic core >10 % in direct contact with the lumen [12] – thus representing a surrogate of the histological TCFA. Whether the direct visualization by OCT of the thin fibrous cap of TCFA (Fig. 2.1) may improve the prediction of future coronary events is currently being investigated.

In a gender-specific subanalysis of the PROSPECT trial, vulnerable features such as plaque rupture and total necrotic core volume by VH-IVUS were, as opposed to above, less common in women despite their older age, while the plaque burden and presence of TCFA were similar between genders. At the same time, there were no difference in major adverse cardiac events related to non-culprit lesions up to 3 years. Whereas, the predictors of MACE in men included a minimal lumen area ≤4 mm, plaque burden ≥70 %, and TCFA, only the two latter were predictive in women, and authors suggest that VH-IVUS-defined TCFA may be a stronger marker of vulnerability in women than men [6]. These findings should be interpreted in view of an expected underestimation of VH-IVUS to detect plaque rupture, due to the relatively low resolution.

In the assessment of the influence of different drugs on plaque progression or regression, IVUS has provided inconsistent results in spite of the unequivocal

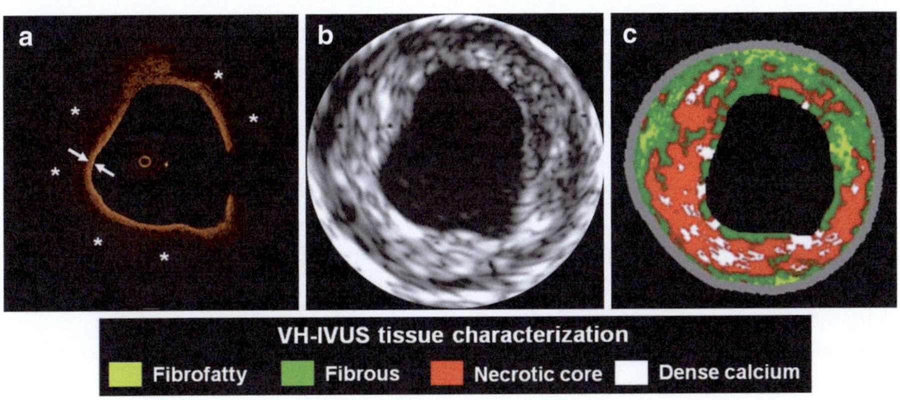

Fig. 2.1 The appearance of thin-cap fibroatheroma (TCFA) by optical coherence tomography (OCT) (panel **a**), gray-scale intravascular ultrasound (GS-IVUS) (panel **b**), and virtual histology (VH)-IVUS (panel **c**), in corresponding cross sections from the same patient. By OCT, TCFA is recognized as a signal-poor diffusely delineated region (*) covered by a signal-rich layer close to the lumen, here seen from 1 to 10 o'clock along the circumference, where the thin fibrous cap measures <65 μm (indicated by *two arrows*). GS-IVUS (panel **b**) shows a good correlation in luminal contours; however, no fibrous cap can be identified. Using radiofrequency analysis with tissue characterization according to the color-coding as below, VH-IVUS shows at the corresponding site a plaque burden >40 % and confluent necrotic core >10 % in direct contact with the lumen at 5-, 8-, and 9 o'clock (Reprinted with permission from [33])

effects of e.g., statins with many possible explanations [2]. In a study of 978 patients (26 % women), there was no difference in the rate of change in plaque burden between genders during treatment with combined statins and ACE-inhibitors, suggestively supporting the use of established medical therapies in women [13]. In a recent report, however, women appeared to have greater plaque regression than men on rosuvastatin, with the benefit appearing in the setting of lower on-treatment LDL-cholesterol levels [14]. Studies using serial evaluation with OCT and/or IVUS/NIRS to assess the medical (IBIS 4: Rosuvastatin) and interventional (PROSPECT 2: bioresorbable vascular scaffolds) effect on plaque burden and vulnerability are currently undergoing and are expected to provide important information that will eventually help us improve cardiovascular outcomes.

2.3.2 Intracoronary Imaging to Evaluate Coronary Stents

Following the introduction of coronary stents, IVUS demonstrated that the majority of these were inadequately expanded despite the appearance of a satisfactory angiographic result, and subsequent data demonstrated that IVUS-guided optimization of stent implantation by high-pressure dilatation is able to reduce the rates of early stent thrombosis, establishing postdilatation as a routine procedure [15]. Accordingly, a threshold of stent expansion of 5.0–5.5 mm^2 was proposed to predict the occurrence of events. The application of IVUS-guided PCI has subsequently been associated both with reduced rates of stent thrombosis and improved survival in the long term – results that should be interpreted in view of their lack of randomization and prespecified guidelines for performing and acting on IVUS findings [16]. Specific evaluation of gender differences remains to be performed.

With the advent of DES, IVUS confirmed the correlation between reduced restenosis and inhibition of neointimal hyperplasia; and that vascular responses after DES implantation are diverse and may include large numbers of unevenly covered and uncovered segments of IVUS-detected neointimal hyperplasia. These uncovered stent regions have together with varying degrees of late-acquired stent malapposition been frequently observed in cases of late stent thrombosis [2]. Limited by the resolution, IVUS has gradually been replaced by OCT which is diligently used in the preclinical testing and clinical evaluation of the healing responses following coronary device implantation, notably, to evaluate stent tissue coverage, apposition, the natural history of dissections and other acute effects of stent implantation, and extent and composition of neoatherosclerosis but also with the purpose of revealing the underlying mechanisms in patients with stent failure. With respect to edge dissections, these were in a study found to be more common in women only for proximal dissections (31 vs. 16 %), where they exhibited more complex features (longer and thicker) than in men [17]. Predictors included a combination of clinical (diabetes, hypertension) and procedural characteristics (stent oversizing) and gender, where it would have been interesting to know whether this was related to vessel size. Short- and long-term clinical and healing outcomes were not evaluated.

As for the healing following stent implantation, Guagliumi et al. reported that women at 9 months following implantation of everolimus-eluting stents in the setting of STEMI had similar strut coverage (~91 %) and amount of in-stent neointimal obstruction (10 %) as men, without differences in clinical outcomes at 30-day and 1-year follow-up [10]. Until additional reports emerge, these data suggest a similar vascular healing response irrespective of gender, supporting for the time being the use of established, same interventional treatment in both men and women.

2.4 Conclusions and Indications

Overall, available data from studies using diagnostic imaging tools such as IVUS and OCT to assess gender differences in the setting of atherothrombosis and prevention of stent failure are scarce and not entirely consistent, emphasizing the necessity of additional studies. Based on the above reviewed and other data, recent revascularization guidelines recommend the use of IVUS (evidence IIa, B) and OCT (evidence IIa, C) in selected patients to optimize stent implantation, and particularly with IVUS to assess the severity and optimize treatment of unprotected left main lesions (IIa, B). As for the mechanisms of stent failure, these can be evaluated with both IVUS and OCT (IIa, C) [16], and future studies to determine how to individualize treatment based on these findings, as well as the clinical value of using OCT, VH-IVUS, and other intracoronary imaging techniques to identify supposedly vulnerable lesions, are eagerly awaited.

2.5 Functional Tests

2.5.1 Fractional Flow Reserve

2.5.1.1 Indication

Percutaneous coronary intervention (PCI) guided by measurements of the fractional flow reserve (FFR) has proven superior to PCI guided by angiography alone in patients with stable coronary artery disease [18], and deferral of revascularization in patients with FFR > 0.80 is recommended. Current ESC/EACTS guidelines on revascularization recommend FFR as a decision-making tool in stable patients with borderline stenosis (>50, <90 %) and no previous documentation of ischemia [19]. Several studies found a higher visual-functional mismatch between angiographically significant stenosis and measured FFR values, in particular among women, probably due to smaller body size, left ventricular mass, vessel size, and smaller myocardial territory Table 2.2 [20, 21].

2.5.1.2 Technical Issues

Before resting measurements, adequate nitrates should be administrated. In addition to nitrates, adenosine administrated as intravenous infusion (140 μg/kg/min) is the most widely used method of obtaining hyperemia during FFR measurements.

Table 2.2 Diagnostic and clinical utility of fractional flow reserve (FFR), coronary flow reserve (CFR), and index of myocardial resistance (IMR)

Modality	Diagnostic and clinical utility
FFR	Moderate coronary artery stenosis and no previous evidence of ischemia
	Serial coronary stenoses (for "spot stenting")
	Intermediate left main stenosis
	Evaluation of residual ischemia post PCI
	Side branch lesion severity in bifurcations
	Saphenous vein grafts stenosis severity
	Nonculprit lesions in ACS
CFR	Assessment of coronary vascular function
	Diagnosis of microvascular angina
IMR	Assessment of coronary vascular function
	Prognostic assessment in acute myocardial infarction

Adapted from Colin Berry, *RadcliffeCardiology.com*

Serious side effects are rare, but discomfort related to flushing and dyspnea is frequently reported. A single bolus regadenoson, seems to be as efficient as adenosine infusion for inducing hyperemia, and FFR values are comparable [22]. Gender differences have not been reported regarding the tolerance of adenosine or regadenoson, but blunted vasodilator response may be seen in patients with endothelial impairment or increased vasoconstrictor activity. This microvascular dysfunction may be more prevalent in (postmenopausal) women [23]. Further technical issues of the procedure are primarily related to handling of the FFR wire which may be a little more challenging in smaller and/or more tortuous coronary arteries. In all wire-based methods, manipulation of wire or pressure manifolds during readings should be avoided.

2.5.1.3 Outcomes in Women

In general, several studies have found that FFR values are higher in women than in men – also after correction for visually assessed stenosis severity. A substudy of the FAME study found that an FFR-guided PCI strategy is equally beneficial in women as in men [20]; however, a registry-based study found a higher risk of death/myocardial infarction among women undergoing FFR-based PCI compared with men, and also a higher event rate among women with so-called "gray zone" FFR values of 0.75–0.8 where revascularization was deferred [24]. In general, current guidelines on revascularization do not differentiate their treatment recommendations based on gender, and the study may, as many other register-based and randomized trials, have suffered from poor representation of women [16]. The discussion, however, of the optimal cutoff values for identifying lesions for revascularization in women is very relevant. In guidelines, FFR values <0.80 is recommended for treatment decision; however, many consider values between 0.75 and 0.80 to be "gray zone." Since women are more likely to have impaired coronary microvascular reactivity as a consequence of more microvascular disease, this may explain the poorer reactivity to adenosine and the higher FFR values. The Women's Ischemia Syndrome Evaluation study demonstrated that a poor microvascular response to adenosine was associated with increased risk for major adverse events [25].Whether optimal medical therapy aiming at vasodilatation before performing FFR could reduce the problem has not been investigated.

Conclusively, the risk of "false-negative," above-threshold FFR values may be higher in women, since microvascular dysfunction can influence adenosine-induced hyperemia. Still, FFR is highly recommended for evaluation of borderline stenoses in all patients with stable coronary artery disease, but especially in women, the treatment threshold of FFR <0.8 should be used.

2.5.2 Instantaneous Wave-Free Ratio

Instantaneous wave-free ratio (iFR) is, like FFR, measured using a pressure wire that is placed distal to the suspected stenotic area. Peak coronary flow (pressure) is measured during diastolic wave-free period and does not require vasodilatation. The theory behind is that coronary artery blood flow occurs almost entirely during diastole when the cardiac muscle relaxes allowing the capillaries to dilate. Resistance at this time is constant. A normal value is 1.0, and values below 0.9 are suggesting a flow-limiting stenosis [26]. Discrepancies between stenosis classification between FFR and iFR have been reported, and a recent study suggests an iFR-FFR hybrid approach where a traditional adenosine-based FFR is performed in patients with iFR values <0.9 [27].

2.5.3 Coronary Flow Reserve

Whereas fractional flow reserve addresses the blood flow through a specific stenosis in an epicardial artery, the coronary flow reserve represents the maximum increase in all blood flow through the coronary arteries above the normal resting value. Coronary flow reserve (CFR) can be detected noninvasively by positron emission tomography as well as invasively using a pressure- and temperature-sensitive coronary guidewire.

2.5.3.1 Indication and Technical Issues

The indication for CFR is assessment of coronary vascular function and diagnosis of microvascular angina which can be helpful in patients with atypical chest pain and no lesion-level ischemia determined by FFR. CFR measurements are based on the thermodilution principle and performed using a dedicated wire. Adenosine infusion is used as in the FFR procedure, and the technical considerations are the same.

2.5.3.2 Outcomes in Women

In both genders, a normal CFR is >2.0, and lower values may explain angina symptoms due to microvascular dysfunction, especially when FFR >0.80. A decreased CFR in patients with an otherwise normal stress test is associated with a markedly increased risk among both men and women [28].

2.6 Index of Microvascular Resistance

The index of microvascular resistance (IMR) may be indicated for assessment of coronary microvascular function [29], and smaller studies have also shown that impaired IMR is associated with poorer prognosis after an acute myocardial infarction [30].

2.6.1 Technical Issues

Several FFR wire systems allow for measuring the FFR, CFR, as well as IMR. As CMR, IMR measurements are based on the thermodilution principle and performed using a dedicated wire during maximal hyperemia. Wedge and venous pressure are needed, but if these variables are not available, the variable FFR_{cor} are calculated as $FFR_{cor} = 1.34 \times FFR - 0.32$, and then, $IMR = P_a \times Tmn \times FFR_{cor}$, where P_a is proximal artery pressure and Tmn is transit time during hyperemia [31]. $IMR < 20$ is considered normal, whereas $IMR > 30$ is elevated and $IMR > 40$ has been related to impaired prognosis after STEMI [30].

2.6.2 Outcomes in Women

A recent study found IMR to be abnormal in 29 of 139 (21 %) patients (mostly women) with angina and apparently normal coronary arteries [32]. Whether prognosis can be improved by reducing IMR, for example, by using vasodilators, has not been proved.

Conclusion

Taken together, FFR is the most validated method for functional evaluation of borderline stenosis in both men and women. CFR may be valuable for diagnosing microvascular dysfunction in patients with atypical chest pain and no obvious obstructive coronary artery disease.

References

1. Garcia-Garcia HM, Gogas BD, Serruys PW, Bruining N. IVUS-based imaging modalities for tissue characterization: similarities and differences. Int J Cardiovasc Imaging. 2011; 27(2):215–24.
2. Radu MD, Kelbaek H, Jørgensen E, Helqvist S, Løjmand B, Engstrom T, Saunamaki K. Intracoronary optical coherence tomography: insights from clinical research – what do we need to learn? Curr Cardiovasc Imaging Rep. 2014;7:9286–302.
3. Taniwaki M, Radu MD, Garcia-Garcia HM, Heg D, Kelbaek H, Holmvang L, Moschovitis A, Noble S, Pedrazzini G, Saunamaki K, Dijkstra J, Landmesser U, Wenaweser P, Meier B, Stefanini GG, Roffi M, Luscher TF, Windecker S, Raber L. Long-term safety and feasibility of three-vessel multimodality intravascular imaging in patients with ST-elevation myocardial infarction: the IBIS-4 (integrated biomarker and imaging study) substudy. Int J Cardiovasc Imaging. 2015;31(5):915–26.

4. Ruiz-Garcia J, Lerman A, Weisz G, Maehara A, Mintz GS, Fahy M, Xu K, Lansky AJ, Cristea E, Farah TG, Teles R, Botker HE, Templin B, Zhang Z, de Bruyne B, Serruys PW, Stone GW. Age- and gender-related changes in plaque composition in patients with acute coronary syndrome: the PROSPECT study. EuroIntervention. 2012;8(8):929–38.
5. Qian J, Maehara A, Mintz GS, Margolis MP, Lerman A, Rogers J, Banai S, Kazziha S, Castellanos C, Dani L, Fahy M, Stone GW, Leon MB. Impact of gender and age on in vivo virtual histology-intravascular ultrasound imaging plaque characterization (from the global Virtual Histology Intravascular Ultrasound [VH-IVUS] registry). Am J Cardiol. 2009;103(9):1210–4.
6. Lansky AJ, Ng VG, Maehara A, Weisz G, Lerman A, Mintz GS, De Bruyne B, Farhat N, Niess G, Jankovic I, Lazar D, Xu K, Fahy M, Serruys PW, Stone GW. Gender and the extent of coronary atherosclerosis, plaque composition, and clinical outcomes in acute coronary syndromes. JACC Cardiovasc Imaging. 2012;5(3 Suppl):S62–72.
7. Pundziute G, Schuijf JD, van Velzen JE, Jukema JW, van Werkhoven JM, Nucifora G, van der Kley F, Kroft LJ, de Roos A, Boersma E, Reiber JH, Schalij MJ, van der Wall EE, Bax JJ. Assessment with multi-slice computed tomography and gray-scale and virtual histology intravascular ultrasound of gender-specific differences in extent and composition of coronary atherosclerotic plaques in relation to age. Am J Cardiol. 2010;105(4):480–6.
8. Burke AP, Farb A, Malcom GT, Liang Y, Smialek JE, Virmani R. Plaque rupture and sudden death related to exertion in men with coronary artery disease. JAMA. 1999;281(10):921–6.
9. Cheruvu PK, Finn AV, Gardner C, Caplan J, Goldstein J, Stone GW, Virmani R, Muller JE. Frequency and distribution of thin-cap fibroatheroma and ruptured plaques in human coronary arteries: a pathologic study. J Am Coll Cardiol. 2007;50(10):940–9.
10. Guagliumi G, Capodanno D, Saia F, Musumeci G, Tarantini G, Garbo R, Tumminello G, Sirbu V, Coccato M, Fineschi M, Trani C, De Benedictis M, Limbruno U, De Luca L, Niccoli G, Bezerra H, Ladich E, Costa M, Biondi Zoccai G, Virmani R. Mechanisms of atherothrombosis and vascular response to primary percutaneous coronary intervention in women versus men with acute myocardial infarction: results of the OCTAVIA study. JACC Cardiovasc Interv. 2014;7(9):958–68.
11. Stone GW, Maehara A, Lansky AJ, de Bruyne B, Cristea E, Mintz GS, Mehran R, McPherson J, Farhat N, Marso SP, Parise H, Templin B, White R, Zhang Z, Serruys PW. A prospective natural-history study of coronary atherosclerosis. N Engl J Med. 2011;364(3):226–35.
12. Garcia-Garcia HM, Costa MA, Serruys PW. Imaging of coronary atherosclerosis: intravascular ultrasound. Eur Heart J. 2010;31(20):2456–69.
13. Nicholls SJ, Wolski K, Sipahi I, Schoenhagen P, Crowe T, Kapadia SR, Hazen SL, Tuzcu EM, Nissen SE. Rate of progression of coronary atherosclerotic plaque in women. J Am Coll Cardiol. 2007;49(14):1546–51.
14. Puri R, Nissen SE, Shao M, Ballantyne CM, Barter PJ, Chapman MJ, Erbel R, Libby P, Raichlen JS, Uno K, Kataoka Y, Nicholls SJ. Sex-related differences of coronary atherosclerosis regression following maximally intensive statin therapy: insights from SATURN. JACC Cardiovasc Imaging. 2014;7(10):1013–22.
15. Radu MD, Räber L, Gomez-Lara J, Kelbaek H, Stefanini GG, Jørgensen E, Helqvist S, Tellez A, Granada JF, Saunamaki K, Serruys PW, Windecker S. Optical coherence tomography for the assessment of intracoronary stents. In: Radu MD, Räber L, Garcia-Garcia HM, Serruys PW, editors. The clinical atlas of intravascular optical coherence tomography. Toulouse: Europa Edition; 2012.
16. Windecker S, Kolh P, Alfonso F, Collet JP, Cremer J, Falk V, Filippatos G, Hamm C, Head SJ, Juni P, Kappetein AP, Kastrati A, Knuuti J, Landmesser U, Laufer G, Neumann FJ, Richter DJ, Schauerte P, Sousa Uva M, Stefanini GG, Taggart DP, Torracca L, Valgimigli M, Wijns W, Witkowski A. 2014 ESC/EACTS Guidelines on myocardial revascularization: the task force on Myocardial Revascularization of the European Society of Cardiology (ESC) and the European Association for Cardio-Thoracic Surgery (EACTS) developed with the special contribution of the European Association of Percutaneous Cardiovascular Interventions (EAPCI). Eur Heart J. 2014;35(37):2541–619.

17. Zeglin-Sawczuk M, Jang IK, Kato K, Yonetsu T, Kim S, Choi SY, Kratlian C, Lee H, Dauerman HL. Lipid rich plaque, female gender and proximal coronary stent edge dissections. J Thromb Thrombolysis. 2013;36(4):507–13.
18. Tonino PA, De Bruyne B, Pijls NH, Siebert U, Ikeno F, van' t Veer M, Klauss V, Manoharan G, Engstrom T, Oldroyd KG, Ver Lee PN, MacCarthy PA, Fearon WF. Fractional flow reserve versus angiography for guiding percutaneous coronary intervention. N Engl J Med. 2009;360(3):213–24.
19. Palmerini T, Biondi-Zoccai G, Della Riva D, Stettler C, Sangiorgi D, D'Ascenzo F, Kimura T, Briguori C, Sabate M, Kim HS, De Waha A, Kedhi E, Smits PC, Kaiser C, Sardella G, Marullo A, Kirtane AJ, Leon MB, Stone GW. Stent thrombosis with drug-eluting and bare-metal stents: evidence from a comprehensive network meta-analysis. Lancet. 2012;379(9824):1393–402.
20. Kim HS, Tonino PA, De Bruyne B, Yong AS, Tremmel JA, Pijls NH, Fearon WF. The impact of sex differences on fractional flow reserve-guided percutaneous coronary intervention: a FAME (Fractional Flow Reserve Versus Angiography for Multivessel Evaluation) substudy. JACC Cardiovasc Interv. 2012;5(10):1037–42.
21. Fineschi M, Guerrieri G, Orphal D, Palmerini E, Munzel T, Warnholtz A, Pierli C, Gori T. The impact of gender on fractional flow reserve measurements. EuroIntervention. 2013;9(3):360–6.
22. Nair PK, Marroquin OC, Mulukutla SR, Khandhar S, Gulati V, Schindler JT, Lee JS. Clinical utility of regadenoson for assessing fractional flow reserve. JACC Cardiovasc Interv. 2011;4(10):1085–92.
23. Sedlak T, Izadnegahdar M, Humphries KH, Bairey Merz CN. Sex-specific factors in microvascular angina. Can J Cardiol. 2014;30(7):747–55.
24. Li J, Rihal CS, Matsuo Y, Elrashidi MY, Flammer AJ, Lee MS, Cassar A, Lennon RJ, Herrmann J, Bell MR, Holmes DR, Bresnahan JF, Hua Q, Lerman LO, Lerman A. Sex-related differences in fractional flow reserve-guided treatment. Circ Cardiovasc Interv. 2013;6(6):662–70.
25. Pepine CJ, Anderson RD, Sharaf BL, Reis SE, Smith KM, Handberg EM, Johnson BD, Sopko G, Bairey Merz CN. Coronary microvascular reactivity to adenosine predicts adverse outcome in women evaluated for suspected ischemia results from the National Heart, Lung and Blood Institute WISE (Women's Ischemia Syndrome Evaluation) study. J Am Coll Cardiol. 2010;55(25):2825–32.
26. Sen S, Escaned J, Malik IS, Mikhail GW, Foale RA, Mila R, Tarkin J, Petraco R, Broyd C, Jabbour R, Sethi A, Baker CS, Bellamy M, Al-Bustami M, Hackett D, Khan M, Lefroy D, Parker KH, Hughes AD, Francis DP, Di Mario C, Mayet J, Davies JE. Development and validation of a new adenosine-independent index of stenosis severity from coronary wave-intensity analysis: results of the ADVISE (ADenosine Vasodilator Independent Stenosis Evaluation) study. J Am Coll Cardiol. 2012;59(15):1392–402.
27. Escaned J, Echavarria-Pinto M, Garcia-Garcia HM, van de Hoef TP, de Vries T, Kaul P, Raveendran G, Altman JD, Kurz HI, Brechtken J, Tulli M, Von Birgelen C, Schneider JE, Khashaba AA, Jeremias A, Baucum J, Moreno R, Meuwissen M, Mishkel G, van Geuns RJ, Levite H, Lopez-Palop R, Mayhew M, Serruys PW, Samady H, Piek JJ, Lerman A. Prospective assessment of the diagnostic accuracy of instantaneous wave-free ratio to assess coronary stenosis relevance: results of ADVISE II International, Multicenter Study (ADenosine Vasodilator Independent Stenosis Evaluation II). JACC Cardiovasc Interv. 2015;8(6):824–33.
28. Cortigiani L, Rigo F, Gherardi S, Galderisi M, Bovenzi F, Picano E, Sicari R. Prognostic effect of coronary flow reserve in women versus men with chest pain syndrome and normal dipyridamole stress echocardiography. Am J Cardiol. 2010;106(12):1703–8.
29. Melikian N, Vercauteren S, Fearon WF, Cuisset T, MacCarthy PA, Davidavicius G, Aarnoudse W, Bartunek J, Vanderheyden M, Wyffels E, Wijns W, Heyndrickx GR, Pijls NH, de Bruyne B. Quantitative assessment of coronary microvascular function in patients with and without epicardial atherosclerosis. EuroIntervention. 2010;5(8):939–45.
30. Fearon WF, Low AF, Yong AS, McGeoch R, Berry C, Shah MG, Ho MY, Kim HS, Loh JP, Oldroyd KG. Prognostic value of the index of microcirculatory resistance measured after primary percutaneous coronary intervention. Circulation. 2013;127(24):2436–41.

31. Yong AS, Layland J, Fearon WF, Ho M, Shah MG, Daniels D, Whitbourn R, Macisaac A, Kritharides L, Wilson A, Ng MK. Calculation of the index of microcirculatory resistance without coronary wedge pressure measurement in the presence of epicardial stenosis. JACC Cardiovasc Interv. 2013;6(1):53–8.
32. Lee BK, Lim HS, Fearon WF, Yong AS, Yamada R, Tanaka S, Lee DP, Yeung AC, Tremmel JA. Invasive evaluation of patients with angina in the absence of obstructive coronary artery disease. Circulation. 2015;131(12):1054–60.
33. Räber L, Radu MD, Garcia-Garcia HM, Akasaka T, Banz Y, Kume T, Windecker S, Serruys PW. Atherosclerosis. In: Radu MD, Räber L, Garcia-Garcia HM, Serruys PW, editors. The clinical atlas of intravascular optical coherence tomography. Toulouse: Europa Edition; 2012.

Interventional Treatment of Stable Coronary Artery Disease in Women

3

Ieva Briede and Marie-Claude Morice

3.1 Women in Cardiovascular Clinical Trials

It is well known that women with ischemic heart disease (IHD) are older and tend to have a greater burden of comorbidities and more functional disability than men; it is also established that IHD is less prevalent in premenopausal women, its incidence lagging 10–15 years behind that of men until approximately the seventh decade of life. In the Euro Heart Survey of Stable Angina, women with angina pain were less likely to undergo an exercise electrocardiogram and less likely to be referred for coronary angiography [1]. Melloni et al. (2010) found similarly low rates with sex-specific results discussed in only 31 % of the 156 primary trial publications cited by the American Heart Association's 2007 women's prevention guidelines [2].

The enrolment of women in cardiovascular clinical trials funded by the National Heart, Lung, and Blood Institute (NHLBI) was 38 % between 1965 and 1998 and 27 % between 1997 and 2006. Furthermore, only 13 of 19 studies reported gender-based outcomes. In the European cardiovascular clinical trials of the same period, the proportion of women enrolled varied between 16 and 25 %, although the female prevalence of clinical conditions under study in the general population was similar to that of men [3]. Usually, women present with heart disease later in life and older patients are often excluded from clinical trials, which may account for the fact that women are under-recruited. Of greater relevance is the finding that angina in women is less likely to be associated with angiographically significant coronary artery stenosis than in men. Moreover, studies reporting sex-specific analyses are often conducted post hoc without regard to whether the initial trial was adequately powered

I. Briede, MD • M.-C. Morice, MD, FESC, FACC (✉)
Ramsay Générale de Santé, Institut Cardiovasculaire Paris Sud,
Hôpital Privé Jacques Cartier, Massy, France

CERC (European Cardiovascular Research Center), Massy, France
e-mail: mc.morice@icps.com.fr

P. Presbitero et al. (eds.), *Percutaneous Treatment of Cardiovascular Diseases in Women*,
DOI 10.1007/978-3-319-39611-8_3

for such analyses. Underpowered subgroup analyses can produce false negatives and incorrect conclusions, which can lead to the institution of ineffective or even harmful treatment strategies in women.

3.2 Guidelines for Stable Coronary Disease Revascularization

3.2.1 American Heart Association (AHA) Guidelines for Stable Coronary Disease Revascularization 2012 (ACCF/AHA/SCAI)

Accumulating evidence suggests that vascular reactivity related to abnormalities in microvascular and endothelial function and possibly plaque erosion or distal microembolization contribute to ischemia to a greater extent in women than in men. Despite increasing recognition of the risks of worsening IHD and attendant complications in women, the frequency with which they are prescribed important risk-modifying therapies such as statins, aspirin, and beta-blockers after episodes of ACS remains significantly lower than among men. In various risk models, the odds of in-hospital death after PCI have ranged from 25 to 80 % higher for women than for men although this trend might have improved in recent years after the higher incidence of diabetes mellitus and hypertension in women is taken into account.

The risk of procedural complications also appears to be significantly higher in women. Although fewer data on the experience of women after coronary artery bypass grafting (CABG) are available, in the New York State registry, the odds of in-hospital death for women were twofold higher than for men. On the basis of these observations, the initial approach to therapy for women with SIHD should be to prescribe a full regimen of GDMT and to reserve consideration of revascularization for patients who do not obtain a satisfactory response or who experience unacceptable adverse effects. On the basis of the higher risk associated with PCI in women, it might be reasonable to adopt a more conservative approach in undertaking this procedure than in men, although the general principle of using revascularization in patients whose symptoms are refractory to medical therapy and who are not satisfied with their current level of angina persists.

The 2012 ACCF/AHA/SCAI PCI guidelines for SIHD give a class I indication for revascularization to improve survival compared with medical therapy alone only for survivors of sudden cardiac death with presumed ischemia-mediated ventricular tachycardia, CABG surgery in patients with unprotected left main disease, CABG for three-vessel disease with or without proximal left anterior descending (LAD) artery disease, and CABG for two-vessel disease with proximal LAD disease [4].

3.2.2 European Society of Cardiology (ECS) Guidelines for Revascularization 2014

Nevertheless, CVD is responsible for 42 % of premature deaths in women under the age of 75 and for a high proportion of lost disability-adjusted life years, in particular in low- and lower-middle income countries. CVD guidelines in general are based on research conducted primarily in men, the mean percentage of women enrolled in clinical trials since 2006 being 30%. In the future, objective demonstration of microvessel disease may identify a group at increased risk that requires more intensive pharmacological treatment to improve prognosis. Compared with men, women have higher rates of procedural complications, including mortality, stroke, and vascular complications. Women also have higher complication rates following CABG but, although the numbers of women included in trials are limited, results do not indicate gender-related differences in outcome. Pharmacological management recommendations are similar in men and women. The gender-based difference in revascularization complication rates seems to be greatest among younger women [5].

The 2007 ESC Guidelines on NSTE-ACS recommend that women be evaluated and treated similarly to men. The 2008 guidelines on acute myocardial infarction did not include specific gender-related recommendations [3]. According to AHA and ESC guidelines for stable coronary artery disease and revascularization, interventional treatment should be implemented similarly in women and men alike. However, operators should keep in mind that there may be a higher probability of complications associated with interventional treatment of coronary artery disease in women.

The heart team synergy is potentially even more important in women due to their age, comorbidities, and rate of complications.

The heart team is a multidisciplinary team composed of an interventional cardiologist and a cardiac surgeon who jointly (1) review the patient's medical condition and coronary anatomy, (2) determine that PCI and/or CABG are technically feasible and reasonable, and (3) discuss revascularization options with the patient before a treatment strategy is selected [6].

3.3 Management of Coronary Artery Disease in Woman

The treatment of stable angina has two major purposes. The first is to prevent myocardial infarction (MI) and death and thereby increase the quantity of life. The second is to reduce symptoms of angina and occurrence of ischemia, which should improve the quality of life. All patients with stable angina are candidates for optimal medical therapy and may be candidates for revascularization with PCI or CABG based on findings from coronary angiography and if symptoms persist despite optimal medical therapy. Among women with symptoms of myocardial ischemia who have been demonstrated to have angiographically nonobstructive CAD, the prognosis was initially felt to be benign. However, more recent data have shown that the prognosis is not benign and the risk of cardiovascular events is higher than it is for asymptomatic women [7]. Not only diagnostic evaluation of women may be misleading but also the appropriate treatment selection can be difficult. It was already recognized in 1991 that women suffering from CAD had less chances to be introduced either in coronary angiography or percutaneous coronary intervention (15.4% of women vs. 27.3% of men, $P<0.001$). Symptomatic women in the WISE study with nonobstructive CAD (lesion stenosis 1–49 %) had a CAD event rate of 16 % versus only 7.9 % in women with no CAD and only 2.4 % in asymptomatic age- and race-matched control subjects [8].

3.4 Coronary Artery Revascularization

The mortality risk associated with the procedure in SCAD is 0.5 %. The efficacy of PCI in SCAD in comparison to medical therapy and CABG has been the subject of extensive evaluation. Revascularization by PCI or CABG more effectively relieves angina, reduces the use of anti-angina drugs, and improves exercise capacity and quality of life, compared with a strategy of medical therapy alone. Usually female patients with CVD tend to have a higher risk profile by the time they are referred for PCI. They are often older with more comorbidity, including diabetes and hypertension. It is important to consider that the best current revascularization results achieved with PCI are with new-generation drug-eluting stents (DES) and for CABG with maximal use of arterial grafts. Revascularization, by either PCI or CABG, may be indicated in flow-limiting coronary stenosis to reduce myocardial ischemia and its adverse clinical manifestations [5]. Revascularization procedures improve outcomes in women with unstable angina, significant angina interfering with lifestyle despite maximal medical therapy, and those with high-risk findings on noninvasive testing. Coronary artery bypass surgery should be considered in patients with significant left main coronary artery stenosis; three-vessel disease, especially with left ventricular dysfunction; and two-vessel disease that includes a stenosis of more than 75 % in the proximal left anterior descending artery and is accompanied by abnormal left ventricular function. Women who undergo coronary artery bypass surgery have more cardiac risk factors than men and are also more likely to experience complications such as death, heart failure, bleeding, and infarction [9].

3.5 Percutaneous Coronary Intervention in Women

Bare-metal stents (BMS) are associated with a 20–30 % rate of recurrence of angiographic stenosis within 6–9 months after implantation. Drug-eluting stents (DES) reduce the incidence of angiographic restenosis and ischemia-driven repeat revascularization. DES is recommended in both gender SCAD patients undergoing stenting if there is no contraindication to prolonged dual antiplatelet therapy (DAPT) (Class A, Level I recommendation 2013) [10]. One of the first studies comparing the impact of PCI with BMS implantation between females and males revealed that women had 50 % more chance of death in comparison to men after adjustment for age, comorbidities, and extent of coronary atherosclerosis. However, in the same analysis, after final adjustment for body surface area, mortality rates were similar between the two genders, although a slightly increased rate of stroke, vascular complications, and repeat in-hospital revascularization was observed in women [11]. Similar results were reported in a retrospective analysis from Mayo Clinic investigating 18,885 consecutive patients who underwent PCI between 1979 and 1995 (early group) and between 1996 and 2004 (late group). The results indicated no difference in terms of 30-d and 1-year mortality, while after adjustment for baseline risk factors, again there was no difference observed in short- or long-term mortality between the two genders [12]. These were earlier first studies, but in latest trials gender gap has narrowed with time since the stenting era, and more recent studies have failed to show any differences in post-PCI outcomes between both genders [13]. Several recent trials have specifically examined drug-eluting stent placement in men and women and, overall, have found similar outcomes for genders after stent placement [14].

The risk of adverse events during and after PCI is greater in women than in men, although the success rate is similar, as well as the effects of antithrombotic agents. Despite less favorable baseline clinical and angiographic features in women compared with men, the angiographic and clinical benefits of PCI were more substantial when using DES. However, in European registries, fewer women than men are treated with percutaneous or surgical revascularization, clopidogrel, and GP IIb/IIIa inhibitors. More adverse events with GP IIb/IIIa inhibitors have been reported in women. Indeed, women experience more bleeding than men independently of the type of treatment. Bleeding complications at the point of vascular puncture, hematomas, and retroperitoneal bleedings are decreased in the current era. Data available in the literature have shown that women still continue to be at 1.5–4 times greater risk for bleeding in comparison to men. In addition, radial approach was related with a lower rate of minor bleeding. These favorable results indicate that the radial approach during PCI in women is safer in terms of bleeding, even though there are more difficulties to initiate the procedure through this particular access site. The latest (on) registry-based randomized trial SAFE-PCI for Women was carried out to compare radial vs. femoral approaches in women undergoing PCI. The aim of the study was to determine the effect of radial access on procedural outcomes (bleeding (Bleeding Academic Research Consortium BARC type 2, 3, or 5) or vascular complication rate). The trial was stopped early due to a lower than expected event rate. A total of 1787 women (691 undergoing PCI) were randomized at 60 sites. There was no significant difference in the primary efficacy endpoint between radial or femoral access among women undergoing PCI (radial 1.2 vs. 2.9 % femoral, odds ratio [OR]: 0.39; 95 % confidence interval [CI]: 0.12–1.27). In this pragmatic trial, which was terminated early, the radial approach did not significantly reduce bleeding or vascular complications in women undergoing PCI. This is mainly due to introduction of less aggressive anticoagulant regimens, adjustment of heparin dose according to body mass index, smaller size catheters, and better closure devices [15].

Once the indication to interventional treatment is established, and when more information is needed, intravascular ultrasound (IVUS) is far superior to fractional flow reserve (FFR) because it provides an anatomical characterization of the lesion in terms of vessel size and plaque composition and can control stent expansion and strut apposition. We suggest that IVUS should be used more frequently for percutaneous revascularization in women, because of different plaque characteristics, vessel sizes, and anatomy. IVUS can provide additional information enabling operators to choose correct stent diameters and lengths, but it should be used cautiously because women's coronary arteries are usually more calcified and tortuous. A retrospective cohort study from Rotterdam, that analyzed RESEARCH and T-SEARCH registries with 4936 patients (28.2 % woman) who underwent PCIs between 2000 and 2004 before and after introduction of DES, investigated the outcomes of sirolimus-eluting stents, paclitaxel-eluting stents, and BMS in women. In this study, even though women had worse baseline characteristics compared to men, no differences in 3-year outcomes were detected between males and females. The procedural complexity was higher in the DES era; nevertheless, risks for target vessel revascularization and major adverse cardiac event at 3 years were significantly lower in women treated with DES than in women treated with BMS [16].

Abbott et al. [17] published data from NHLBI registry data and analyzed gender-specific in-hospital and 1-year outcomes after PCI with DES. There were no gender-related differences in in-hospital myocardial infarction, coronary artery bypass grafting, and death in those treated with BMSs or DESs. Antiplatelet use and stent thrombosis (1.3 % of women vs. 1.2 % of men, $p=0.85$) were similar at 1 year with DESs. At 1 year, patients with DESs had a lower rate of repeat PCI (14.1 % in women vs. 9.5 %, $p=0.02$; 12.0 % in men vs. 8.8 %, $p=0.02$). Adjusted 1-year outcomes in patients with BMSs and DESs, including death and myocardial infarction, were independent of gender. Use of DESs was the only factor, other than age, that conferred a lower risk for the need for repeat PCI in women (relative risk 0.61, 95 % confidence interval 0.41–0.89, $p=0.01$) and men (relative risk 0.68, 95 % confidence interval 0.51–0.91, $p=0.001$) This study shows that women with stable angina receiving interventional treatment with stents have better results with DES.

New-generation DES, with thin strut stent platforms, biocompatible durable or biodegradable polymers and limus-based antiproliferative agents, have further advanced efficacy and safety compared with early-generation DES and BMS. Compared with early-generation DES, repeat revascularization was reduced by 10–20 % A recent meta-analysis published in The Lancet by Stefanini et al. [18] included 43,904 patients (26.3 % women) from 26 randomized trials and assessed the safety and efficacy of DES compared with BMS in women. The use of DES was associated with a significant reduction in the 3-year rates of target lesion revascularization (197 [18.6 %] women in the bare-metal stent group, 294 [7.8 %] in the early-generation DES group, and 330 [6.3 %] in the newer-generation DES group, $p<0.0001$) (Fig. 3.1). The study showed that DES implantation in women was more effective and safe than BMS implantation during long-term follow-up. Furthermore, it was observed that second- and third-generation DES were associated with an improved safety profile compared with early-generation DES. These results suggest that women undergoing PCI may benefit more when DES and especially newer-generation DES are used. This meta-analysis showed that newer-generation DES should be selected as the standard of care for women undergoing coronary revascularization.

According to the 2012 guidelines of the American College of Cardiology–American Heart Association for percutaneous coronary interventions, use of

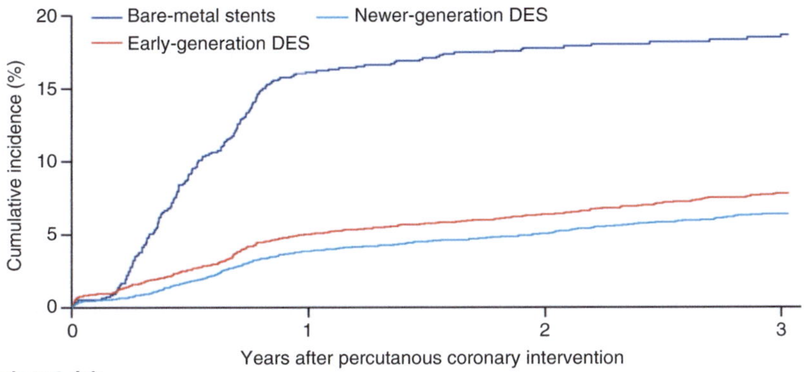

Number at risk

	0	1	2	3
Bare-metal stents	1108	898	710	457
Early-generation DES	4171	3764	3113	1955
Newer-generation DES	6278	5217	3307	1951

Fig. 3.1 Cumulative event rates of target lesion revascularization during 3-years of follow-up (From Stefanini et al. [18])

drug-eluting stents has a class IA recommendation for patients undergoing elective percutaneous revascularization who are able to adhere to a prolonged regimen of dual antiplatelet therapy (DAPT). However, the 2014 ESC guidelines for revascularization recommend DAPT for 6 months after DES implantation (class IB). More details in this regard are given in Chap. 6 of this book. The risk of stent thrombosis has become exceedingly low and no longer represents a limitation to the use of drug-eluting stents [19].

Lesion length remains a predictor of target lesion revascularization and results of long lesion stenting remain poor. The ADVANCE study was the first to demonstrate that stenting in long lesions (>40 mm) was associated with higher MACE rates. Sirolimus-eluting stents (SES) have been shown to yield superior results to paclitaxel-eluting stents in most, but not all studies. At 9-months and 1-year, outcomes of Biolimus biodegradable polymer (BES) and sirolimus permanent polymer stents (SES) in long lesions (>20 mm) appear similar with respect to MACE in long lesions in this "all-comer" patient population (1707 patients) included in the LEADERS sub-study. However, long lesions tended to have a higher rate of binary in-segment restenosis and target lesion revascularization (TLR) following BES than SES treatment. Similar results for BES and SES have been observed in small diameter vessels (<2.75 mm). There were no differences in MACE and TLR rates for both stent types [20].

The Clinical Outcomes Utilizing Revascularization and Aggressive Drug Evaluation (COURAGE) trial published in 2007 and the Bypass Angioplasty Revascularization Investigation 2 Diabetes (BARI 2D) trial published in 2009 failed to show a benefit of PCI over optimal medical therapy for the prevention of death or MI in patients with SIHD. Data from the COURAGE trial suggest that the benefits of optimal medicament therapy (OMT) alone in comparison with OMT plus PCI were similar for men and women. Moreover, the outcomes of revascularization appeared to be less favorable among women than men although very few women were enrolled in COURAGE (15 % of patients).

3.6 Coronary Artery Bypass Grafting

Women who undergo coronary artery bypass grafting (CABG) are less likely to receive a mammary graft and have more incomplete revascularization, greater bleeding, and mortality compared with men. Regarding endovascular and surgical treatment of CAD, intervention in women has some distinct features. Fisher LD et al. in 1982 published data from the Coronary Artery Surgery Study (CASS). They studied association of sex, physical size, and operative mortality after coronary artery bypass in the Coronary Artery Surgery Study (CASS). The study showed that women after coronary artery bypass surgery (CABG) had a 4.5 % mortality compared with 1.9 % in men with shorter graft durability, lesser degree of symptom improvement in the postoperative period, frequent postoperative myocardial infarction, more frequent heart failure occurrence, and were more likely to require reoperation within 5 years after CABG. The study investigators concluded that physical size of the patient, including coronary artery diameter, helps predict operative mortality even after adjusting for differences in risk predicted by the basic variables and gender. However, patient's gender is not statistically significantly related to the risk of surgical death given the information available from clinical and angiographic variables and from knowledge of patient size. The explanation for the excess risk associated with coronary artery operations in women in this study was the smaller stature and the smaller diameter of the coronary arteries in this group of patients [21]. Abramov et al. [22] published data showing that women have a higher risk of morbidity and mortality and experience less relief from angina than do men after CABG, despite accounting for less than 30 % of the CABG population. Interestingly, this sex discrepancy appears to be reduced when an off-pump CABG is performed [23].

These first trial results raised the issue of CABG safety in women and initiated the conduction of several newer trials. Studies were carried out to evaluate short- and long-term mortality in women who undergo coronary artery bypass grafting (CABG). Results for these were conflicting. Recently, investigators conducted a meta-analysis of all existing studies to evaluate the impact of female gender on mortality in patients who undergo isolated CABG. A comprehensive search of studies published through May 31, 2012 identified 20 studies comparing men and women who underwent isolated CABG. All-cause mortality was evaluated at short-term (postoperative period and/or at 30 days), midterm (1-year), and long-term (5-year) follow-up. A total of 966,492 patients (688,709 men [71 %] and 277,783 women [29 %]) were included in this meta-analysis. Women were more likely to be older; had significantly greater comorbidities, including hypertension, diabetes mellitus, hyperlipidemia, unstable angina, congestive heart failure, and peripheral vascular disease; and were more likely to undergo urgent CABG (51 vs. 44 %, p <0.01). Short-term mortality (OR 1.77, 95 % CI 1.67–1.88) was significantly higher in women (Fig. 3.2).

Study or Subgroup	Female Events	Female Total	Male Events	Male Total	Weight	Odds ratio M-H, Random, 95 % CI	Year
Fisher 1982	52	1153	119	6258	2.9 %	2.44 [1.75, 3.40]	1982
O' Connor 1993	58	819	67	2236	2.5 %	2.47 [1.72, 3.54]	1993
Christakis 1995	47	1331	102	5694	2.6 %	2.01 [1.41, 2.85]	1995
Hammar 1997	18	607	56	3326	1.2 %	1.78 [1.04, 3.06]	1997
Edwards 1998	4388	97153	6465	247760	21.5 %	1.77 [1.70, 1.84]	1998
Aldea 1999	8	523	12	1220	0.4 %	1.56 [0.64, 3.85]	1999
Hogue 2001	5729	133231	7644	283116	21.9 %	1.62 [1.56, 1.68]	2001
Abramov 2002	25	932	70	3891	1.6 %	1.50 [0.95, 2.39]	2002
Woods 2003	55	1742	70	3582	2.6 %	1.64 [1.14, 2.34]	2003
Koch 2003	87	3596	170	12001	4.4 %	1.73 [1.33, 2.24]	2003
Hassan 2005	26	893	55	2511	1.5 %	1.34 [0.83, 2.15]	2005
Humphries 2007	179	4983	404	20229	7.7 %	1.83 [1.53, 2.19]	2007
Ennker 2009	65	3079	122	9527	3.4 %	1.66 [1.23, 2.25]	2009
Fukui 2010	2	188	8	766	0.2 %	1.02 [0.21, 4.84]	2010
Emmert 2010	6	176	14	807	0.4 %	2.00 [0.76, 5.28]	2010
Bukkapatnam 2010	493	10708	751	29669	12.7 %	1.86 [1.66, 2.09]	2010
Alam 2012	184	3267	264	9848	7.0 %	2.17 [1.79, 2.63]	2012
Saxena 2012	112	4780	272	16754	5.6 %	1.45 [1.16, 1.82]	2012
Total (95% CI)		**269161**		**659195**	**100.0 %**	**1.77 [1.67, 1.88]**	
Total events	11534		16665				

Hetergeneity: Tau² = 0.00, Chi² = 33.34, df = 17 (P = 0.01); I² = 49 %
Test for overall effect: Z = 18.47 (P < 0.00001)

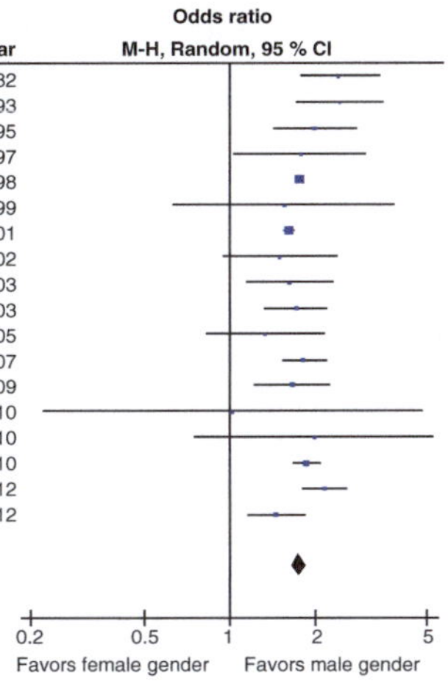

Fig. 3.2 Association of female gender with short-term mortality (composite of postoperative or 30-day mortality) (From Alam et al. [24])

Study or subgroup	Female Events	Female Total	Male Events	Male Total	Weight	Odds ratio M-H, Random, 95 % CI	Year
Hammar 1997	13	607	59	3326	2.9 %	1.21 [0.66, 2.22]	1997
Guru 2006	295	14393	858	52800	59.6 %	1.27 [1.11, 1.45]	2006
Saxena 2012	196	4780	503	16754	37.5 %	1.38 [1.17, 1.63]	2012
Total (95 % CI)		**19780**		**72880**	**100.0 %**	**1.31 [1.18, 1.45]**	
Total events	504		1420				

Hetergeneity: Tau² = 0.00, Chi² = 0.69, df=2 (P = 0.71); I²=0 %
Test for overall effect: Z = 5.09 (P < 0.00001)

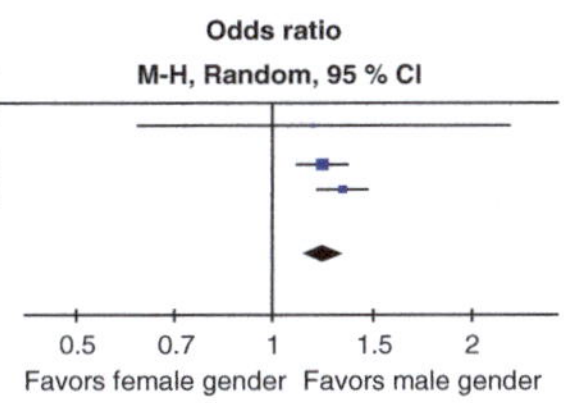

Fig. 3.3 Association of female gender with midterm (1-year) mortality (From Alam et al. [24])

Study or subgroup	Female Events	Female Total	Male Events	Male Total	Weight	Odds ratio M-H, Random, 95% CI	Year
Hammar 1997	35	607	196	3326	2.2 %	0.98 [0.67, 1.42]	1997
Guru 2006	1233	14393	3940	52800	67.8 %	1.16 [1.09, 1.24]	2006
Saxena 2012	564	4780	1809	16754	30.0 %	1.11 [1.00, 1.22]	2012
Total (95 % CI)		**19780**		**72880**	**100.0 %**	**1.14 [1.08, 1.20]**	
Total events	1832		5945				

Hetergeneity: Tau² = 0.00, Chi² = 1.34, df = 2 (P = 0.51); I²=0 %
Test for overall effect: Z = 4.68 (P < 0.00001)

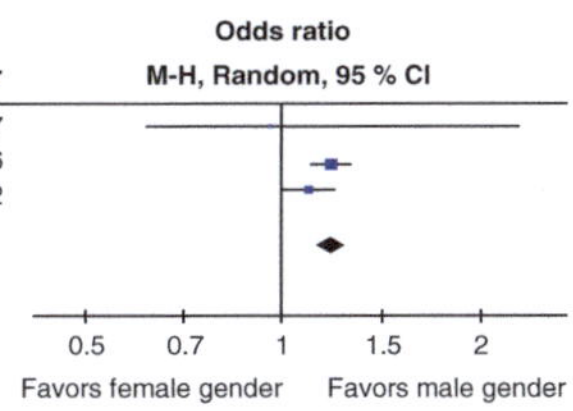

Fig. 3.4 Association of female gender with long-term follow-up 5-year mortality after isolated CABG (From Alam et al. [24])

At midterm and long-term follow-up, mortality remained high in women compared with men (Figs. 3.3 and 3.4).

Women remained at increased risk for short-term mortality in two subgroup analyses including prospective studies (n=41,500, OR 1.83, 95 % CI 1.59–2.12) and propensity score-matched studies (n=11,522, OR 1.36, 95 % CI 1.04–1.78). In conclusion, investigators observed that women who underwent isolated CABG experienced higher mortality at short-term, midterm, and long-term follow-up compared with men. Mortality remained independently associated with female gender despite propensity score-matched analysis of outcomes [24]. Several explanations for this observation have been proposed such as the delayed reference of women to CABG when CAD extends to a greater degree, the smaller size of women coronary vessels that creates technical issues to the surgeon, or finally the limited use of left internal mammary artery in women [11].

Arterial Revascularization Therapies Study Part I (ARTS I) was one of the studies which compared gender-related differences following coronary revascularization procedures (CABG and PCI with BMS). The study demonstrated that for a total of $n=1205$ patients included in time from 1997 to 1998, there was no significant difference in terms of death, stroke, or myocardial infarction between the two genders. However, stenting was associated to a greater need for repeated revascularization. There was a similar early- and long-term outcome between female and male subjects. The only difference observed was an increased risk of bleeding complications in women treated with PCI. In both genders of the ARTS I population, treatment with CABG was associated with a lower incidence of MACCE (death, CVA, MI, CABG, RPCI) compared to PCI at 5 years. Vaina et al. [25] published data of a multicenter nonrandomized open label study, Arterial Revascularization Therapies Study Part II (ARTS II), that was designed to evaluate the outcomes of sirolimus-eluting stent implantation in comparison to BMS implantation and CABG in patients with multivessel CAD from ARTS I. In ARTS II were included a total of $n=605$ patients during year 2003. The study showed that the overall MACCE rate at 1 year was similar to that of the ARTS I – CABG arm and significantly reduced when compared to the ARTS I – PCI arm (Fig. 3.5). Additionally, it was observed that both genders had a more favorable clinical outcome with sirolimus-eluting stents compared with BMS but similar to CABG. These results could potentially institute PCI as the first choice treatment in women with multivessel disease.

Mansur et al. [26] published another study – a post hoc analysis from randomized MASS II study with 10 years follow-up data for 188 women with chronic stable multivessel coronary artery disease who underwent medical treatment, percutaneous coronary intervention, or coronary artery bypass graft surgery. Patients were enrolled between May 1995 and May 2000. The primary end points of the study were the incidence of total mortality, Q-wave myocardial infarction, or refractory angina. Sub-study results showed that women treated with percutaneous coronary intervention and medical treatment had more primary events than those treated with coronary artery bypass graft surgery: 34 %, 44 %, and 22 %, respectively ($P=0.003$). Survival rates at 10 years were 72 % for coronary artery bypass graft surgery, 72 % for percutaneous coronary intervention, and 56 % for medical treatment ($P=0.156$). Regarding death, a protective effect was observed with percutaneous coronary intervention compared with medical treatment [HR = 0.44 (95 % CI: 0.21–0.90); $P=0.025$] but no differences between coronary artery bypass graft surgery and percutaneous coronary intervention. In conclusion, PCI and CABG compared with medical treatment had better results after 10 years of follow-up. Nevertheless, recent studies have shown that this gender gap of higher mortality after PCI and CAGB is narrowing. The latest meta-analysis, however, showed, that there are still differences between genders in

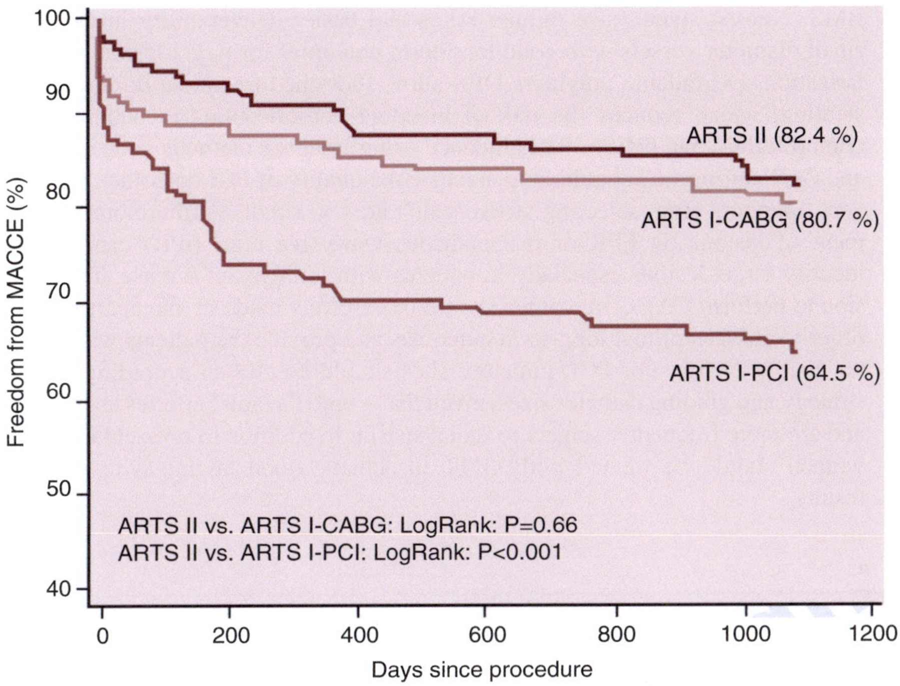

Fig. 3.5 Kaplan-Meier curves out to 3 years in female patients in ARTS I and ARTS II population (From Vaina et al. [25])

CABG revascularization and that we should not treat all patients according to a uniform standard of care, especially women with CAD and comorbidities. We recommend that this patient group with angiographically proven CAD should be managed very carefully and we believe that probably one of the best treatments could be coronary angioplasty with implantation of newest-generation DES and intravascular imaging guided procedure. The coronary revascularization technique, either PCI or CABG in three-vessel disease with low ejection fraction, should be discussed jointly by the heart team.

Conclusion

Ischemic heart disease is a different disease in women and is strongly dependent upon stage of life. Dedicated randomized control data on women with chest pain and CAD are currently lacking; further research in this area is needed. Women are undertreated both medically and procedurally with respect to current guidelines. They are less likely to receive referrals to cardiologists by primary care providers. When medically treated, women have more disability, lower quality of life, and poorer outcomes. This is partially due to bias in evaluation and treatment but, to an even greater extent, because of innate biological differences between men and women not yet fully appreciated [27]. Women undergoing percutaneous revascularization benefit more from newest-generation DES than

BMS. Newest stents have thinner struts and easier deliverability in tortuous, small diameter vessels with good long-term outcomes for target lesion revascularization. Degradable polymers DES allow shortened treatment duration after stenting, which reduces the risk of bleeding complications in patients with comorbidities. We believe that guidance using imaging methods such as IVUS and OCT during PCI should help enhance the quality of PCI outcomes and prevent operators from selecting stents which are too small. Furthermore, assessment of lesions by FFR or instantaneous wave-free ratio (iFR) can help to identify target lesions especially in patients with multivessel disease. The decision to perform CABG in women should be carefully made by the heart team in order to ensure optimal long-term outcomes and provide the patients with a better quality of life. For PCI, puncture sites should be chosen according to PCI strategy and guiding catheter sizes, given that women's radial arteries are smaller and are more frequently subject to radial spasm. In addition to revascularization, women should be treated with OMT to achieve good angina-symptom-free results.

References

1. Daly C, et al. Gender differences in the management and clinical outcome of stable angina. Circulation. 2006;113:490–8.
2. Melloni C, et al. Representation of women in randomized clinical trials of cardiovascular disease prevention. Circ Cardiovasc Qual Outcomes. 2010;3(2):135–42.
3. Stramba-Badiale M. Women and research on cardiovascular diseases in Europe: a report from the European Heart Health Strategy (EuroHeart) project. Eur Heart J. 2010;31:1677–85.
4. Fihn SD, Gardin JM, Abrams J, et al. American College of Cardiology Foundation/American Heart Association Task Force. 2012 ACCF/AHA/ACP/AATS/PCNA/SCAI/STS guideline for the diagnosis and management of patients with stable ischemic heart disease: a report of the American College of Cardiology Foundation/American Heart Association task force on practice guidelines, and the American College of Physicians, American Association for Thoracic Surgery, Preventive Cardiovascular Nurses Association, Society for Cardiovascular Angiography and Interventions, and Society of Thoracic Surgeons. Circulation. 2012;126:e354–471.
5. ECS Guidelines for revascularization 2014. Eur Heart J. 2014;35:2541–619.
6. Stephan DF. 2014 ACC/AHA/AATS/PCNA/SCAI/STS focused update of the guideline for the diagnosis and management of patients with stable ischemic heart disease. Circulation. 2014;130:1749–67.
7. Diver DJ, Bier JD, Ferreira PE, et al. Clinical and arteriographic characterization of patients with unstable angina without critical coronary arterial narrowing (from the TIMI-IIIA Trial). Am J Cardiol. 1994;74:531–7.
8. Gulati M, et al. Adverse cardiovascular outcomes in women with nonobstructive coronary artery disease: a report from the Women's Ischemia Syndrome Evaluation Study and the St. James Women Take Heart Project. Arch Intern Med. 2009;169:843–50.
9. Lori M, et al. Evidence-based guidelines for cardiovascular disease prevention in women: 2007 update. Circulation. 2007;115:1481–501.
10. 2013 ESC guidelines on the management of stable coronary artery disease. Eur Heart J 2013;34:2949–3003.

11. Vaina S, et al. Coronary artery disease in women: from the yentl syndrome to contemporary treatment. World J Cardiol. 2015;7(1):10–8.
12. Peterson ED, et al. Effect of gender on the outcomes of contemporary percutaneous coronary intervention. Am J Cardiol. 2001;88:359–64.
13. Parikh PB, Gruberg L. Forget Mars and Venus, men and women are from the same planet after all. J Invasive Cardiol. 2012;24(6):261–2.
14. Lansky AJ, et al. Gender-based outcomes after paclitaxel-eluting stent implantation in patients with coronary artery disease. J Am Coll Cardiol. 2005;45:1180–5.
15. Rao SV, et al. A registry-based randomized trial comparing radial and femoral approaches in women undergoing percutaneous coronary intervention: the SAFE-PCI for Women (Study of Access Site for Enhancement of PCI for Women) trial. JACC Cardiovasc Interv. 2014;7(8):857–67.
16. Onuma Y, et al. Impact of sex on 3-year outcome after percutaneous coronary intervention using bare-metal and drug-eluting stents in previously untreated coronary artery disease: insights from the RESEARCH (Rapamycin-Eluting Stent Evaluated at Rotterdam Cardiology Hospital) and T-SEARCH (Taxus-Stent Evaluated at Rotterdam Cardiology Hospital) Registries. JACC Cardiovasc Interv. 2009;2:603–10.
17. Abbott JD, et al. Gender-based outcomes in percutaneous coronary intervention with drug-eluting stents (from the National Heart, Lung, and Blood Institute Dynamic Registry). Am J Cardiol. 2007;99:626–31.
18. Stefanini GG, et al. Safety and efficacy of drug-eluting stents in women: a patient-level pooled analysis of randomised trials. Lancet. 2013;382:1879–88.
19. Stefanini GG, et al. Drug-eluting coronary-artery stents. N Engl J Med. 2013;368:254–65.
20. Wykrzykowska JJ, et al. Biolimus-eluting biodegradable polymer versus sirolimus-eluting permanent polymer stent performance in long lesions: results from the LEADERS multicentre trial substudy. EuroIntervention. 2009;5:310–7.
21. Fisher LD, et al. Association of sex, physical size, and operative mortality after coronary artery bypass in the Coronary Artery Surgery Study (CASS). J Thorac Cardiovasc Surg. 1982;84(3):334–41.
22. Abramov D, et al. The influence of gender on the outcome of coronary artery bypass surgery. Ann Thorac Surg. 2000;70:800–5; discussion 806.
23. Puskas JD, et al. Off-pump techniques benefit men and women and narrow the disparity in mortality after coronary bypass grafting. Ann Thorac Surg. 2007;84:1447–54; discussion 1454e6.
24. Alam M, et al. Comparison by meta-analysis of mortality after isolated coronary artery bypass grafting in women versus men. Am J Cardiol. 2013;112(3):309–17.
25. Vaina S, et al. Effect of gender differences on early and mid-term clinical outcome after percutaneous or surgical coronary revascularisation in patients with multivessel coronary artery disease: insights from ARTS I and ARTS II. EuroIntervention. 2008;4:492–501.
26. Mansur AP, et al. Long-term follow-up of a randomized, controlled clinical trial of three therapeutic strategies for multivessel stable coronary artery disease in women. Interact Cardiovasc Thorac Surg. 2014;19:997–1001.
27. Kones R. Recent advances in the management of chronic stable angina I: approach to the patient, diagnosis, pathophysiology, risk stratification, and gender disparities. Vasc Health Risk Manag. 2010;6:635–56.

4 Interventional Treatment of Acute Coronary Syndrome (ACS): Non-ST Elevation ACS (NSTE-ACS)

Piera Capranzano

4.1 Introduction

Cardiovascular disease, of which coronary artery disease (CAD) is the prevalent manifestation, is the most common cause of death for both genders in industrialized countries; women develop CAD nearly a decade later in life. Across the entire spectrum of CAD, acute coronary syndromes (ACSs), characterized by acute plaque rupture or erosion with sudden coronary blood flow impairment, are associated with the highest rates of adverse clinical events. Among ACSs, the non-ST elevation ACS (NSTE-ACS), including non-ST elevation MI (NSTEMI) or unstable angina, is more frequent than ST elevation acute myocardial infarction (STEMI). While hospital mortality is higher in patients with STEMI than among those with NSTE-ACS, at 6 months, the mortality rates are similarly high in both clinical conditions and are higher among patients with NSTE-ACS at longer-term follow-up, most likely due to the more widely heterogeneous and worse overall risk profile of patients with NSTE-ACS. These latter epidemiological data suggest the need for defining optimal acute and chronic treatment strategies for NSTE-ACS.

Recent temporal trends show declining of short- and long-term mortality after an ACS, but some reports suggest less effective reduction in women [1]. In addition, previous studies demonstrated that women with ACSs have higher mortality compared with men. Ongoing debates are focusing on whether gender-specific differences exist in diagnosis, clinical course, management, and response to treatment of all spectrums of CAD presentations and the extent to which these differences can impact on overall clinical approach and on the relative prognosis of both genders.

P. Capranzano, MD
Cardiovascular Department, Ferrarotto Hospital, University of Catania, Catania, Italy
e-mail: pcapranzano@gmail.com

P. Presbitero et al. (eds.), *Percutaneous Treatment of Cardiovascular Diseases in Women*,
DOI 10.1007/978-3-319-39611-8_4

This chapter describes current recommended treatments for NSTE-ACS, with a special focus on issues regarding specific disease features, outcomes, and management of women.

4.2 Specific Features of Women with NSTE-ACS

Women present more frequently with NSTE-ACS and less frequently with STEMI compared with men. Atypical chest pain or presentations, including dyspnea, vasovagal symptoms, or symptoms of heart failure (HF), are more common in women presenting with NSTE-ACS. Absent or atypical chest pain leads to underrecognition and undertreatment of the disease [1], especially when the ECG is normal or nearly normal or when the ECG is abnormal at baseline. Of note, women around 55 years of age are an important subset with missed ACS diagnosis in the emergency department. Several studies have reported that men with ACS are more likely to have ruptured plaques, whereas women were more likely to present with plaque erosion, suggesting that the mechanism of ACS development in men and women may differ. Patients presenting with plaque erosions are more likely to have a longer indolent period of ischemia as opposed to those with ruptured plaques who present more suddenly. This may partly explain why women with ACS present later than men and with typical or atypical angina symptoms rather than a clear-cut ACS.

Women presenting with NSTE-ACS are older than men and have a higher frequency of diabetes, hypertension, HF, and other comorbidities. Despite being older and having higher prevalence of most CAD risk factors than men, women with NSTE-ACS are more likely than men to have nonobstructive CAD on angiography. There are many potential explanations for NSTEMI without evidence of obstructive CAD at angiography, including plaque rupture with angiographic underestimation of the true burden of CAD, microvascular dysfunction, or coronary spasm. Additional explanations may include noncoronary causes leading to symptoms and/or troponin elevation that may be confused with ACS, such as HF, uncontrolled hypertension, arrhythmias, and pulmonary embolism.

A sex-based analysis from the PROSPECT study demonstrated that women presenting with ACS have less extensive CAD by both angiographic and IVUS assessments, as evidenced by fewer and more focal non-culprit lesions and fewer vessels with angiographic non-culprit lesions compared with men even after multivariable adjustment for age and risk factors [2]. Moreover, this latter analysis showed that non-culprit lesions in women who have less necrotic core volume are less prone to rupture and have similar plaque burden per lesion; however, other observed higher-risk plaque characteristics of women including less calcium, smaller lumen areas, greater proportion of minimal lumen area $\leq 4\ mm^2$, and significantly less total fibrous volume may explain the similar cardiovascular event rates during 3 years of follow-up, despite women having less extensive coronary atherosclerosis. Of note, the between-sexes differences in the ACS pathophysiology, which were observed in the PROSPECT subanalysis, appeared to balance out with no impact on culprit- or non-culprit-related clinical outcomes [2].

4.3 Prognosis of Women with NSTE-ACS

A significant gender by type of ACS interaction has been demonstrated. Indeed, in STEMI, the 30-day mortality was higher among women, whereas in NSTEMI, mortality was lower among women [3]. In a recent analysis of trends in gender differences in cardiac care and outcome after an acute myocardial infarction (MI) from the RIKS-HIA (Register of Information and Knowledge About Swedish Heart Intensive Care Admissions) registry, women as a group have better-adjusted prognosis than men after acute MI; however, younger women and women with STEMI have disproportionately poor prognosis [1]. The lower mortality risk of women with NSTEMI may be due to the higher proportion of women with nonobstructive CAD regardless of ACS type, as demonstrated in a cohort of 35,128 patients with angiographic data. In this latter analysis, after additional adjustment for angiographic disease severity, 30-day mortality among women was not significantly different than men, regardless of ACS type [3]. Moreover, the relationship between sex and 30-day mortality was similar across the levels of angiographic disease severity [3].

Despite presenting with higher-risk characteristics and having higher in-hospital risk and similar mortality than men when adjusting for risk profile, women with NSTE-ACS are treated less aggressively than men [4]. One perceived obstacle in treating women, especially those older, might be related to an increased incidence of bleeding [5]. Indeed, despite reductions in bleeding events over time, female sex remained a strong independent predictor of bleeding and vascular complications. The risk of bleeding complications can be assessed using integer scoring systems involving clinical variables associated with a heightened risk. Although the use of scores goes beyond sex in providing an overall estimation of bleeding risk, common to all scores is the independent association between female sex and risk of bleeding complications. Clinical factors, such as older age, renal failure, cardiogenic shock, and use of larger sheaths, have been specifically identified as predictors of risk in women. However, the female propensity for bleeding persists beyond these risk factors. Indeed, while the sex-specific risk of increased cardiovascular events persists after adjustment for comorbidities, the association between bleeding and female sex persists after adjustment for confounding clinical factors. Sex-specific mechanisms surrounding body mass index, access vessel anatomy, platelet-vessel biology, and percutaneous coronary intervention (PCI)-related pharmacotherapy may play a role [5].

The observed higher rates of access site bleeding among women set the rationale for the Study of Access Site for Enhancement of PCI for Women (SAFE-PCI) trial, in which women were randomized to undergoing radial or femoral access coronary angiography and if required PCI [6]. The study was stopped early due to a lower-than-expected event rate. Among the 1787 women enrolled (>50 % presented with NSTE-ACS) and 691 undergoing PCI, there was no significant difference in bleeding or vascular complications (primary endpoint) between radial and femoral access among those undergoing PCI (radial 1.2 % vs. 2.9 % femoral, $p = 0.12$), while in the overall cohort of women undergoing coronary angiography, a benefit associated with the radial access was detected (0.6 % radial vs. 1.7 % femoral; $p = 0.03$).

4.4 Management of NSTE-ACS

The first step of NSTE-ACS management is assessment of acute risk, which drives the selection of the site of care and treatment, including antithrombotic treatment and timing of coronary angiography. The indication and optimal timing for an invasive approach are mostly based on overall clinical presentation and several risk factors. Indeed, a routine invasive strategy compared with a selective invasive strategy in NSTE-ACS has been shown to decrease mortality, recurrent ACS episodes, subsequent rehospitalization, and revascularization. Moreover, large meta-analyses have shown that the benefit of a routine invasive strategy was confined to biomarker-positive patients and was more pronounced in high-risk patients. Thus, the results of trials and meta-analyses support the broad implementation of a routine invasive strategy and highlight the role of risk stratification in the decision process. With regard to the optimal timing of the invasive approach in NSTE-ACS patients, available data indicate that an early as opposed to a delayed invasive strategy is safe and associated with a lower risk of refractory symptoms and a shorter hospitalization. Also the optimal timing of coronary angiography and revascularization should be guided by individualized risk stratification. Recommended indications for the invasive (urgent, early, or delayed) and conservative strategies for the treatment of NSTE-ACS according to risk stratification are illustrated in Fig. 4.1. It is recommended that patients at very high risk with at least one very high-risk criterion undergo an urgent invasive strategy (within 2 h). In patients at high risk with at least one high-risk criterion, an early invasive strategy (within 24 h) is recommended. In patients with at least one intermediate-risk criterion, the coronary angiography may be delayed up to 72 h from admission [7, 8]. Finally, in low-risk patients, a conservative is recommended, and decision for an invasive strategy is guided by a noninvasive stress test (preferably with imaging) for inducible ischemia. Besides risk factors indicated in Fig. 4.1, also comorbidities, frailty, cognitive status, and estimated life expectancy have to be assessed when deciding the invasive approach for NSTE-ACS.

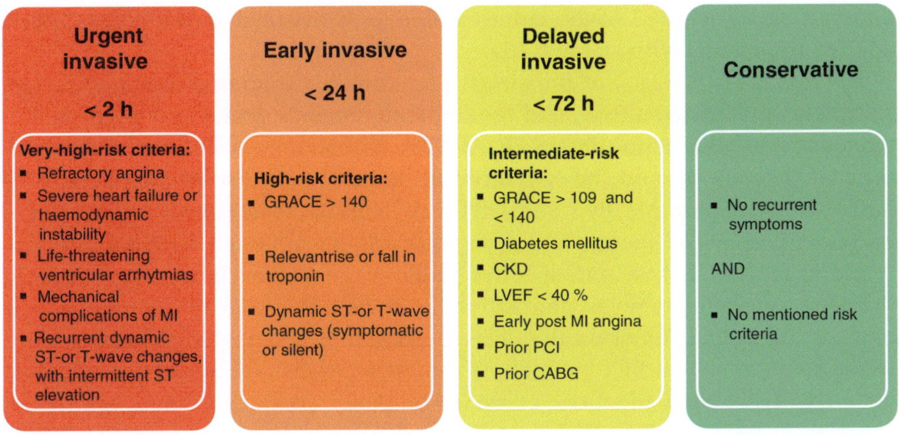

Fig. 4.1 Recommended indications for the invasive and conservative strategies for the treatment of NSTE-ACS according to risk stratification (*MI* myocardial infarction, *CKD* chronic kidney disease, *LVEF* left ventricular ejection fraction, *PCI* percutaneous coronary intervention, *CABG* coronary artery bypass grafting)

Coronary angiography has a central role in the management of patients with NSTE-ACS, as it helps clinicians in the diagnosis of ACS related to obstructive epicardial CAD and thus stratifying the patient's short- and long-term risk and guiding the long-term medical treatment, avoiding, for instance, unnecessary exposure to antithrombotic agents. Angiographic patterns of CAD in NSTE-ACS patients are widely heterogeneous, ranging from normal epicardial coronary arteries to a severely and diffusely diseased coronary artery tree. Up to 20 % of patients with NSTE-ACS have no lesions or nonobstructive lesions of epicardial coronary arteries, while among patients with obstructive CAD, half to two thirds of patients have multivessel disease.

The indication and timing of myocardial revascularization are based on the same factors, which drive also the selection of an invasive approach, and on the functional and anatomic severity of CAD. The selection of the revascularization modality, PCI, or coronary artery bypass grafting (CABG) is based on the assessment of risk features specific to each revascularization strategy and on the angiographic pattern of CAD. No contemporary trials comparing PCI with CABG in patients with NSTE-ACS and multivessel CAD are available. Moreover, in NSTE-ACS trials comparing an early with a delayed invasive strategy, or a routine invasive with a selective invasive strategy, the decision to perform PCI or CABG was left to the discretion of the operator. Retrospective subanalysis and meta-analysis comparing CABG versus PCI for the treatment of NSTE-ACS have shown similar long-term mortality, lower stroke, and higher need for repeat revascularization with PCI. To guide the choice of revascularization modality among stabilized patients with NSTE-ACS, including those undergoing ad hoc PCI of the culprit lesion, it is reasonable to use the criteria applied in patients with stable CAD.

Finally, there is a lack of prospective randomized studies assessing the type, complete versus incomplete, and timing, simultaneous versus staged, of percutaneous revascularization in NSTE-ACS. A complete revascularization of significant lesions should be pursued in multivessel disease patients with NSTE-ACS as multiple PCI and NSTE-ACS trials have shown a detrimental prognostic effect of incomplete revascularization, although unmeasured confounding factors in these retrospective studies cannot be excluded. Nevertheless, the need for complete revascularization has to be tailored to age, overall patient clinical status, and comorbidities. The decision to treat all the significant lesions in the same or staged PCI procedures should be based on clinical presentation, comorbidities, renal function, coronary anatomy complexity, and ventricular function. Indeed, a staged PCI in multivessel disease may be associated to lower periprocedural complications, especially in high-risk settings (i.e., low ejection fraction, chronic renal insufficiency).

4.5 Management of NSTE-ACS: Gender Issues

There is conflicting evidence regarding the benefit of an early invasive strategy in women with NSTE-ACS [7]. Indeed, while post hoc analysis of the FRISC II and RITA 3 trials showed no benefit of an invasive strategy in women, in contrast to its beneficial effect in men, the TACTICS-TIMI 18 indicated similar benefits of a routine early invasive versus a conservative (ischemia-guided) strategy in men and women. Caution is needed in interpreting the findings of these subgroup analyses, as differences in clinical and angiographic risk profile between women and men, and the markedly lower number of women included in those trials may explain the observed interaction of sex subgroup with the treatment effect of an invasive strategy in NSTE-ACS. Moreover, several important differences between the latter randomized trials may explain the discordant findings and the lack of benefits from a routine invasive strategy compared with a conservative strategy. For instance, in the FRISC II trial, the excess of risk with the invasive strategy group among women was driven by a particularly high CABG-related mortality; the RITA 3 trial included a cohort of women at lower risk, with no or single-vessel disease in the majority of cases (67 %) and lower rates of death and MI at 1 year in women in both the invasive (8.6 %) and conservative groups (5.1 %) than those of patients enrolled in the FRISC II and TACTICS-TIMI 18 trials. Importantly, in the TACTICS-TIMI 18 trial, the benefit of an early invasive therapy, in terms of significant reduction in death and MI at 1 year, was further enhanced in women with elevated troponin T levels [7]. Differently, women with NSTE-ACS and no elevation in troponin who underwent an early invasive strategy had a nonsignificant increase in events, as did women with a low-risk TIMI score. The meta-analysis by the Cochrane Collaboration pointed out that women derive a significant reduction in death or MI for a routine invasive versus a conservative strategy, although with an early hazard due to an increase in procedure-related events, including periprocedural MI and bleeding, suggesting the adoption of strategies minimizing these events especially in women (i.e., optimization of stenting strategies, staged PCI procedures, accurate selection of upstream and periprocedural medical therapy, and antithrombotic regimens and radial access). It has been shown that when bleeding avoidance strategies are not used, women have significantly higher rates of bleeding than men. Both genders have similar adjusted risk reductions of bleeding when any of those strategies are used. Thus, overall available data suggest that a routine early invasive strategy should be considered in women on the same principles as in men, that is, after careful risk stratification for both ischemic and bleeding risks including clinical and ECG evaluations, analysis of biomarkers, comorbidities, and use of risk scores. Indeed, as stated above in the paragraph on prognosis, sex-based differences in 30-day mortality observed among ACS patients are markedly attenuated after adjustment for baseline characteristics, angiographic disease severity, and treatment strategies in a cohort of 35,128 patients with angiographic data, taken from a pooled analysis of 11 trials [3]. Based on these overall evidences, according to the NSTE-ACS guidelines, both genders should be evaluated and treated in the same way for acute care and for secondary prevention. Women with NSTE-ACS and low-risk features should not undergo early invasive treatment because of the lack of benefit and the possibility of harm. The guidelines point out that particular attention to weight and/or renally calculated doses of antiplatelet and anticoagulant agents has to be placed to reduce bleeding risk among women. Despite the higher number of risk factors, the lack of gender differences in treatment guidelines, and no observed sex-specific treatment effect for most therapeutic agents, women with NSTE-ACS compared with men are less likely to receive evidence-based therapies including both invasive coronary angiography and revascularization [4]. Of interest, even after adjusting for age, cardiovascular risk factors, and extent of disease, myocardial revascularization (PCI or CABG) in patients with significant CAD was less frequently used in women. This has an important prognostic impact as it has been shown that elderly women who are not revascularized have a threefold higher in-hospital and 1-year mortality rate compared with revascularized women with no increased severe bleeding in this latter group undergoing revascularization [9]. Therefore, elderly women with an NSTEACS should not be denied an evidence-based diagnostic and therapeutic approach because of presumptive excess in risks.

Conclusions

A routine invasive strategy compared with a conservative therapy has been associated with better outcomes for women at higher risk and those with positive biomarkers. Thus, in NSTE-ACS, the choice of an invasive versus a conservative strategy, the optimal timing of catheterization, and the type and completeness of coronary revascularization should be based on objective risk stratification and not be influenced by the sex of patients, because of a presumption on an increased risk or frailty of women. Strategies to minimize possible complications (i.e., bleeding and periprocedural MI), that could be more frequent among women with NSTE-ACS managed invasively, should be implemented. Moreover, women should receive the guideline-recommended medical therapy as men.

References

1. Redfors B, Angerås O, Råmunddal T, Petursson P, Haraldsson I, Dworeck C, Odenstedt J, Ioaness D, Ravn-Fischer A, Wellin P, Sjöland H, Tokgozoglu L, Tygesen H, Frick E, Roupe R, Albertsson P, Omerovic E. Trends in gender differences in cardiac care and outcome after acute myocardial infarction in Western Sweden: a report from the Swedish Web System for Enhancement of Evidence-Based Care in Heart Disease Evaluated According to Recommended Therapies (SWEDEHEART). J Am Heart Assoc. 2015;4(7).
2. Lansky AJ, Ng VG, Maehara A, Weisz G, Lerman A, Mintz GS, De Bruyne B, Farhat N, Niess G, Jankovic I, Lazar D, Xu K, Fahy M, Serruys PW, Stone GW. Gender and the extent of coronary atherosclerosis, plaque composition, and clinical outcomes in acute coronary syndromes. JACC Cardiovasc Imaging. 2012;5:S62–72.
3. Berger JS, Elliott L, Gallup D, Roe M, Granger CB, Armstrong PW, Simes RJ, White HD, Van de Werf F, Topol EJ, Hochman JS, Newby LK, Harrington RA, Califf RM, Becker RC, Douglas PS. Sex differences in mortality following acute coronary syndromes. JAMA. 2009;302: 874–82.
4. Blomkalns AL, Chen AY, Hochman JS, Peterson ED, Trynosky K, Diercks DB, Brogan GX Jr, Boden WE, Roe MT, Ohman EM, Gibler WB, Newby LK. CRUSADE Investigators. Gender disparities in the diagnosis and treatment of non-ST-segment elevation acute coronary syndromes: large-scale observations from the CRUSADE (Can rapid risk stratification of unstable angina patients suppress adverse outcomes with early implementation of the American College of Cardiology/American Heart Association Guidelines) National quality improvement initiative. J Am Coll Cardiol. 2005;45:832–37.
5. Ahmed B, Dauerman HL. Women, bleeding, and coronary intervention. Circulation. 2013;127: 641–9.
6. Rao SV, Hess CN, Barham B, Aberle LH, Anstrom KJ, Patel TB, Jorgensen JP, Mazzaferri Jr EL, Jolly SS, Jacobs A, Newby LK, Gibson CM, Kong DF, Mehran R, Waksman R, Gilchrist IC, McCourt BJ, Messenger JC, Peterson ED, Harrington RA, Krucoff MW. A registry-based randomized trial comparing radial and femoral approaches in women undergoing percutaneous coronary intervention: the SAFE-PCI for Women (Study of Access Site for Enhancement of PCI for Women) trial. JACC Cardiovasc Interv. 2014;7:857–67.
7. Roffi M, Patrono C, Collet JP, Mueller C, Valgimigli M, Andreotti F, Bax JJ, Borger MA, Brotons C, Chew DP, Gencer B, Hasenfuss G, Kjeldsen K, Lancellotti P, Landmesser U, Mehilli J, Mukherjee D, Storey RF, Windecker S. 2015 ESC Guidelines for the management of acute coronary syndromes in patients presenting without persistent ST-segment elevation: task force for the management of acute coronary syndromes in patients presenting without persistent ST-segment elevation of the European Society of Cardiology (ESC). Eur Heart J. 2016;37:267–315.
8. Amsterdam EA, Wenger NK, Brindis RG, Casey DE Jr, Ganiats TG, Holmes DR Jr, Jaffe AS, Jneid H, Kelly RF, Kontos MC, Levine GN, Liebson PR, Mukherjee D, Peterson ED, Sabatine

MS, Smalling RW, Zieman SJ, ACC/AHA Task Force Members. 2014 AHA/ACC guideline for the management of patients with non-ST-elevation acute coronary syndromes: a report of the American College of Cardiology/American Heart Association Task Force on Practice Guidelines. Circulation. 2014;130:e344–426.

9. De Carlo M, Morici N, Savonitto S, Grassia V, Sbarzaglia P, Tamburrini P, Cavallini C, Galvani M, Ortolani P, De Servi S, Petronio AS. Sex-related outcomes in elderly patients presenting with non-ST-segment elevation acute coronary syndrome: insights from the Italian Elderly ACS Study. JACC Cardiovasc Interv. 2015;8:791–6.

Interventional Treatment of Acute Coronary Syndrome: ST-Segment Elevation Myocardial Infarction (STEMI)

5

Giulio G. Stefanini, Margherita Soldi, and Bindu Kalesan

5.1 Introduction

Cardiovascular diseases represent the most frequent cause of mortality in women, and the mortality from cardiovascular disease remained higher in women than men during the last three decades [1, 2]. Since the year 2000, however, there has been a marked reduction in cardiovascular mortality in both men and women [2]. This has been associated with improved therapeutic strategies for the treatment of cardiovascular diseases and particularly coronary artery disease (CAD) and ST-segment elevation myocardial infarction (STEMI) – the principal determinant of death from cardiovascular causes. Despite these advancements, STEMI remains as the leading cause of morbidity and mortality for millions of women worldwide.

5.2 Epidemiology of Acute Myocardial Infarction in Women

Over 7 million people die due to CAD every year, accounting for almost 15 % of all deaths globally [3]. As a matter of fact, almost three million of American women have a history of acute myocardial infarction, over 50,000 American women died of acute myocardial infarction, and one of every seven European woman will die from acute myocardial infarction [1, 4]. Notably, women are more likely to die than men during the first year after a STEMI (26 % women vs. 19 % men), and this trend is maintained during the following 5 years, irrespective of age [1, 2]. The worse long-term prognosis of women as compared with men after STEMI has been explained,

G.G. Stefanini, MD, PhD (✉) • M. Soldi, MD
Cardio Center, Humanitas Research Hospital, Rozzano, Milan, Italy
e-mail: giulio.stefanini@humanitas.it

B. Kalesan, PhD
Department of Medicine, Boston University School of Medicine, Boston, MA, USA

P. Presbitero et al. (eds.), *Percutaneous Treatment of Cardiovascular Diseases in Women*,
DOI 10.1007/978-3-319-39611-8_5

at least in part, by differences in age, cardiovascular risk factors, clinical presentation, and treatment [5].

Available evidence indicated that baseline risk profiles of women with STEMI differ from those of men. Specifically, women have higher prevalence of diabetes mellitus, hypertension, heart failure, and renal dysfunction compared with men [6–8]. In addition, women present with a first STEMI at an older age (mean 72 years) than men (mean 65 years) [1]. This has been attributed to the protective role of circulating estrogens on the vascular endothelium, determining a delayed onset of CAD in women compared with men [9]. The substantial increase in incidence of STEMI among postmenopausal women corroborates the hypothesis of a protective role of estrogens on CAD. Notwithstanding, it is hard to exclude that age may play confounding effect. Moreover, trials evaluating exogenous estrogen hormone therapy for the primary prevention of STEMI in postmenopausal women have been convincingly negative [10].

5.3 Clinical Presentation of STEMI in Women

Available evidence suggests that women are more likely to present without chest pain or with atypical symptoms – such as dyspnea, weakness, fatigue, and indigestion – as compared with men [2, 11–13]. Typical and atypical symptoms in STEMI patients are summarized in Table 5.1. Gender-based differences in STEMI clinical presentation may have consequences for timely identification of ischemic symptoms, appropriate triage, and judicious diagnostic testing and management. In the variations in recovery: role of gender on outcomes of young AMI patients (VIRGO) study, young women with STEMI were more likely to present with atypical chest pain or no symptoms (16% versus 10%; $p=0.008$) and more likely to present >6 h

Table 5.1 Features of typical and atypical symptoms in women with STEMI

	Typical symptoms	Atypical symptoms
Chest pain	Pressure Tightness Squeezing	Sharp Pleuritic Burning Aching Soreness Reproducible
Additional symptoms	Irradiation of pain to neck, jaw, shoulders, arms, and back Dyspnea Nausea and vomit Profused diaphoresis	Unusual shortness of breath Neck, jaw, arm, and/or shoulder pain Back pain Flu-like symptoms Dizziness Anxiety Generalized weakness Indigestion symptoms Palpitations

after symptom onset (35 % versus 23 %; $p=0.002$) as compared to young men with STEMI [14]. The detrimental consequences for women are the delay in seeking for treatment as well as misdiagnosis, resulting in an accumulation of prehospital and emergency department delays that leads to delayed reperfusion strategies with prolonged ischemic time, a greater degree of myocardial damage, and impaired short- and long-term clinical outcomes.

Multiple studies have shown that women with STEMI are less likely to be treated with guideline-directed medical therapies, less likely to undergo cardiac catheterization, and less likely to receive timely reperfusion [14–18].

A recently published analysis of the VIRGO study showed that young women presenting with STEMI are less likely to receive reperfusion and more prone to experience delays in receiving reperfusion as compared with similarly aged men [19]. Furthermore, women with >50 % coronary stenosis documented at cardiac catheterization were less likely to receive revascularization as compared with men. After adjustment for confounders, female gender persisted as an independent factor in the delay of reperfusion therapy. In addition, a differential access to treatment has been observed, with young women being less likely to receive revascularization than young men with subsequently higher in-hospital mortality as well as longer in-hospital stay [20].

Notably, previous data have indicated that when women are given effective reperfusion therapy with primary percutaneous coronary intervention (PCI), they experience the same risk of death as men [21]. A prompt diagnosis of STEMI and an adequate strategy to provide prompt myocardial reperfusion is crucial for women as for men. Therefore, it is important to maintain a high degree of awareness for STEMI in women with potential symptoms of ischemia. It must be underscored that delays in the timely implementation of reperfusion strategies represent key issues in the management of STEMI, since the greatest benefit achieved with reperfusion occurs within the first 2–3 h after symptoms onset. Optimal management of patients with STEMI – irrespective of sex – including pre- and in-hospital pathways and reperfusion strategies within 12 h of first medical contact with ideal time interval for interventions as recommended by the current European guidelines are depicted in Fig. 5.1 [22].

5.4 Reperfusion in Women with STEMI

A prompt restoration of coronary flow and myocardial tissue perfusion has been consistently shown to improve survival in women and men with STEMI [22]. According to the European and American guidelines, for women and men with STEMI within 12 h of symptom onset and with persistent electrocardiographic changes (ECG), early mechanical (PCI) or pharmacological reperfusion should be performed as early as possible [23]. There is general agreement that reperfusion strategies should be implemented also among patients with symptoms onset >12 h in case of clinical and/or electrocardiographic evidence of ongoing ischemia. Overall, as reflected by current guidelines, available evidence consistently indicates that patients with STEMI should be timely treated with reperfusion therapy irrespective of sex.

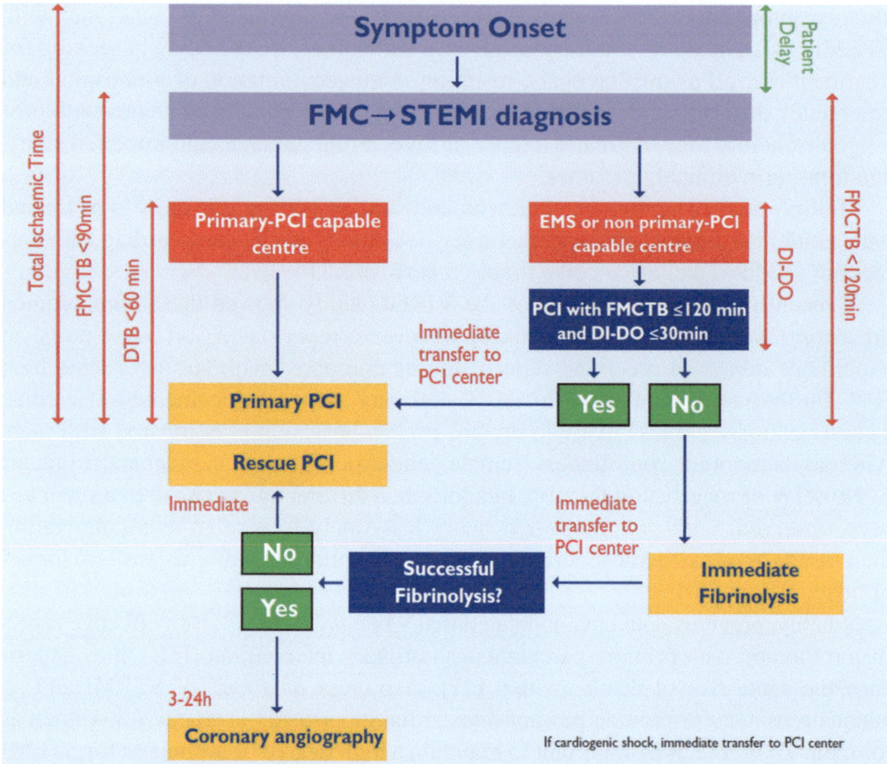

Fig. 5.1 Optimal management and reperfusion strategies in patients with STEMI within 12 h of first medical contact with ideal time interval for interventions. *DI-DO* door-in to door-out time, *DTB* door-to-balloon time, *EMS* emergency medical service, *FMC* first medical contact, *FMCTB* first-medical-contact-to-balloon time, *PCI* percutaneous coronary intervention, *STEMI* ST-segment elevation myocardial infarction (Reproduced with permission from [22])

5.5 Mechanical Reperfusion: Primary PCI in Women

Primary PCI is the preferred reperfusion strategy in patients with STEMI, provided that it can be performed expeditiously by experienced operators [4, 22]. During the last 15 years, primary PCI has become established as the dominant reperfusion therapy across the great majority of the European countries.

Since female patients represent a group at high risk of complications from pharmacological reperfusion with fibrinolysis, it is not unsurprising that they benefit the most from primary PCI – mainly due to the near elimination of the risk of major bleeding. In a pooled analysis of 22 randomized trials, women with STEMI had a lower risk of mortality with primary PCI as compared to fibrinolysis, irrespective of whether they presented within the first 2 h of symptom onset (7.7 % vs. 9.6 %) or

>2-h delay (8.5 % vs. 14.4 %) [24]. It must be underscored that primary PCI resulted as an independent predictor of survival in women. The favorable treatment effect of primary PCI over fibrinolysis in women with STEMI was corroborated by a substudy of the GUSTO IIB, with primary PCI preventing 56 deaths per 1000 treated women as compared with 42 deaths per 1000 treated men [25].

However, despite the improvement in clinical outcomes among women treated with primary PCI, a meta-analysis of observational studies found that women have a higher risk of in-hospital mortality as compared with men after adjustment for baseline risk differences (RR 1.48; 95 % CI 1.07–2.05) [26]. Moreover, while primary PCI has eliminated the risk of intracranial bleeding as compared to fibrinolysis, female patients remain at higher risk of bleeding events and vascular complications as compared to male patients [27]. These findings indicate the need for a further optimization in the treatment of women with STEMI.

5.5.1 Multivessel Treatment Strategies in Women with STEMI

The infarct-related artery should be systematically treated during the initial intervention. This strategy is valid for both men and women with the aim of a rapid and stable reperfusion. In case of multivessel disease, evidence supporting complete revascularization with PCI of non-infarct-related lesions is a matter of debate [28]. The presence of extensive multivessel CAD has been associated with a reduced success in reperfusion and impaired clinical outcomes following primary PCI, supporting the need for complete revascularization in women and men with STEMI. Along this line, in the preventative angioplasty in acute myocardial infarction (PRAMI) trial, 465 patients with STEMI and multivessel CAD were randomly allocated to preventive PCI in non-infarct-related coronary arteries with stenosis ≥50 % or PCI limited to the infarct artery [29]. During a mean follow-up of 23 months, preventive PCI was associated with a reduced risk of the composite of death, myocardial infarction, or refractory angina as compared with PCI limited to the infarct-related artery (HR 0.35; 95 % CI 0.21–0.58; $p<0.001$). A stratified analysis of the primary endpoint showed that the treatment effect of preventive PCI with respect to the primary endpoint was consistent among women (HR 0.24, 95 % CI 0.08–0.73) and men (HR 0.39, 95 % CI 0.22–0.68) with no evidence of statistical interaction [29]. With respect to timing, staged PCI in STEMI patients with multivessel disease and no hemodynamic compromise has been identified as an independent predictor of survival. Moreover, a higher risk of ischemic events has been associated with simultaneous PCI of multiple vessels (in addition to the culprit vessel) at the time of STEMI as compared with staged revascularization of STEMI patients with multivessel disease. Based on the available evidence, current guidelines recommend to consider multivessel PCI in STEMI patients with cardiogenic shock in the presence of multiple, critical stenoses or highly unstable lesions, and if there is persistent ischemia after PCI on the culprit lesion [4, 22].

5.5.2 Stent Selection

Stenting is the default strategy over balloon angioplasty in women and men with STEMI treated with primary PCI, since it has been shown to reduce the risk of abrupt vessel closure, reinfarction, and repeat revascularization [30, 31]. Although early-generation drug-eluting stents (DES) have not been associated with an increased risk of death, myocardial infarction, or stent thrombosis during long-term follow-up [32], there have been concerns of an increased risk of very late stent thrombosis owing to delayed arterial healing of stents implanted into unstable lesions underlying STEMI [33, 34]. Two randomized trials in STEMI patients undergoing primary PCI directly compared new-generation DES with bare-metal stents (BMS). In the EXAMINATION trial, everolimus-eluting stent implantation in STEMI patients resulted into lower risks of target lesion revascularization (2.1 % vs. 5.0 %, $p=0.003$) and definite stent thrombosis (0.5 % vs. 1.9 %, $p=0.02$) as compared to BMS [35]. Similarly, the COMFORTABLE AMI trial reported a lower risk of the composite primary endpoint of cardiac death, target-vessel myocardial infarction, and target lesion revascularization (4.3 % vs. 8.7 %; HR 0.49, 95 % CI 0.30–0.80, $p=0.004$) as well as a lower risk of target-vessel myocardial infarction (0.5 % vs. 2.7 %; HR 0.20, 95 % CI 0.06–0.69, $p=0.01$) and a trend towards a lower risk of definite stent thrombosis (0.9 % vs. 2.1 %; HR 0.42, 95 % CI 0.15–1.19, $p=0.10$) in patients assigned to treatment with biolimus-eluting stents with a biodegradable polymer compared with BMS [36]. Results were maintained throughout longer-term follow-up and a pooled analysis of both trials confirmed a lower risk of stent thrombosis and reinfarction with DES compared with BMS [37]. As a matter of fact, the improved safety and efficacy of new-generation DES over early-generation DES as well as BMS has been shown in a pooled analysis of 26 randomized trials including 11,557 women with no evidence of interaction between treatment effect and acute presentation at baseline (Fig. 5.2) [38]. Taken together, these findings suggest that new-generation DES are more effective and potentially safer than BMS as well as early-generation DES during primary PCI in women and men with STEMI.

5.5.3 Arterial Access Site Selection

Access site selection may be of particular relevance in women with STEMI. Radial strategy has been shown to reduce the incidence of acute bleeding events, particularly in acute coronary syndromes, and was associated with lower mortality in the subset of STEMI patients enrolled in the RIVAL trial [39–41]. However, the beneficial effect of radial over femoral access appears to be dependent upon the radial expertise of operators [42]. In a sex-based subanalysis of the RIVAL trial, female patients resulted to have a higher risk of vascular access site complications

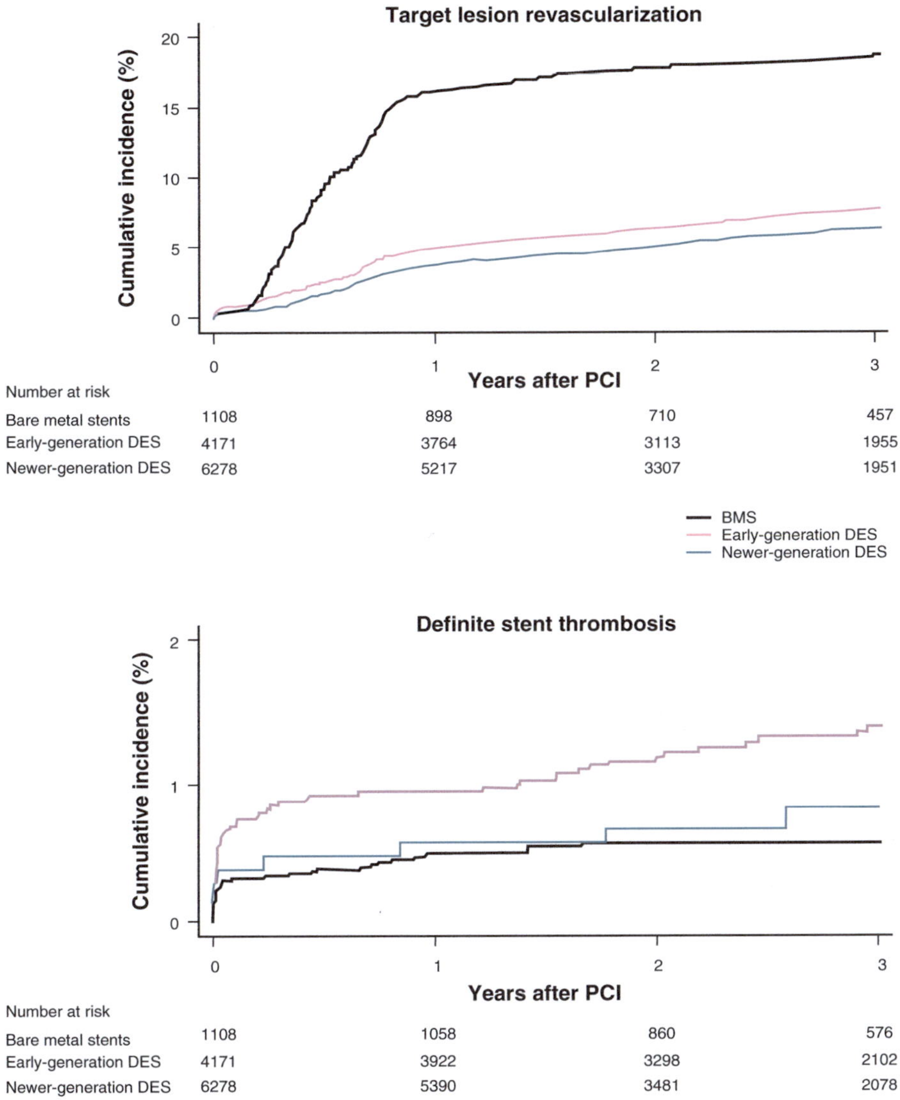

Fig. 5.2 Progressive improvements in safety and efficacy associated with coronary stent iterations in women. *DES* drug-eluting stents, *BMS* bare-metal stents (With permission from [38])

compared with male patients, and radial access emerged as an effective method to reduce these complications [43]. In the recently published MATRIX trial, 8,404 patients with acute coronary syndrome (with or without ST-segment elevation) were randomly allocated to radial (4197) or femoral (4207) access for coronary angiography and PCI [44]. At 30 days, radial access resulted in a reduced risk of the co-primary endpoints of major adverse cardiac events (MACE: death, myocardial infarction, or stroke; RR 0.85, 95% CI 0.74–0.99; $p=0.0307$) and net adverse clinical events (NACE: major adverse cardiovascular events or Bleeding Academic Research Consortium (BARC) major bleeding; *RR* 0.83, 95% *CI* 0.73–0.96; $p=0.0092$). A stratified analysis of the co-primary endpoints showed a more pronounced treatment effect in women (MACE: RR 0·73, 95% CI 0·56–0·95; NACE: RR 0·72, 95% CI 0·56–0·93) than men (MACE: RR 0·92, 95% CI 0·77–1·09; NACE: RR 0·89 95% CI 0·76–1·05) without formal statistical interaction. Overall, available evidence consistently indicate that radial access may improve the safety and efficacy outcomes of primary PCI in both sexes and might effectively reduce the gender difference in prognosis.

5.6 Future Outlook

Despite significant progresses in the treatment of STEMI with a marked improvement in patients' outcomes, the morbidity and mortality in female patients remain high. Based on available evidence, disease awareness, prevention, prompt diagnosis, and timely treatment of women with STEMI should be optimized to improve clinical outcomes. As a matter of fact, sex-specific attention in STEMI patients will need to represent the first step into personalized medicine in this setting. Of note, women tend to be underrepresented in clinical trials, generally making up only one-third of enrolled patients. Moreover, clinical trial findings are often not stratified by sex – limiting the available evidence-based information on the optimal treatment strategies for women with STEMI. Efforts will need to be made by clinical investigators, pharmaceutics, and device industry as well as regulators in order to increase the level of available evidence in women with STEMI.

References

1. Mozaffarian D, Benjamin EJ, Go AS, et al. Heart disease and stroke statistics – 2015 update: a report from the American Heart Association. Circulation. 2015;131:e29–322.
2. Mehta LS, Beckie TM, DeVon HA, et al. Acute myocardial infarction in women: a scientific statement from the American Heart Association. Circulation. 2016;133:916–47.
3. Widimsky P, Wijns W, Fajadet J, et al. Reperfusion therapy for ST elevation acute myocardial infarction in Europe: description of the current situation in 30 countries. Eur Heart J. 2010;31:943–57.
4. Steg PG, James SK, Atar D, et al. ESC Guidelines for the management of acute myocardial infarction in patients presenting with ST-segment elevation. Eur Heart J. 2012;33:2569–619.
5. Bucholz EM, Butala NM, Rathore SS, Dreyer RP, Lansky AJ, Krumholz HM. Sex differences in long-term mortality after myocardial infarction: a systematic review. Circulation. 2014;130:757–67.
6. Hochman JS, Tamis JE, Thompson TD, et al. Sex, clinical presentation, and outcome in patients with acute coronary syndromes. Global Use of Strategies to Open Occluded Coronary Arteries in Acute Coronary Syndromes IIb Investigators. N Engl J Med. 1999;341:226–32.

7. Hasdai D, Porter A, Rosengren A, Behar S, Boyko V, Battler A. Effect of gender on outcomes of acute coronary syndromes. Am J Cardiol. 2003;91:1466–9, A6.
8. Stefanini GG, Kalesan B, Pilgrim T, et al. Impact of sex on clinical and angiographic outcomes among patients undergoing revascularization with drug-eluting stents. JACC Cardiovasc Interv. 2012;5:301–10.
9. Chakrabarti S, Morton JS, Davidge ST. Mechanisms of estrogen effects on the endothelium: an overview. Can J Cardiol. 2014;30:705–12.
10. Mosca L, Benjamin EJ, Berra K, et al. Effectiveness-based guidelines for the prevention of cardiovascular disease in women—2011 update: a guideline from the american heart association. Circulation. 2011;123:1243–62.
11. Hemingway H, Langenberg C, Damant J, Frost C, Pyorala K, Barrett-Connor E. Prevalence of angina in women versus men: a systematic review and meta-analysis of international variations across 31 countries. Circulation. 2008;117:1526–36.
12. Khan NA, Daskalopoulou SS, Karp I, et al. Sex differences in acute coronary syndrome symptom presentation in young patients. JAMA Intern Med. 2013;173:1863–71.
13. Rubini Gimenez M, Reiter M, Twerenbold R, et al. Sex-specific chest pain characteristics in the early diagnosis of acute myocardial infarction. JAMA Intern Med. 2014;174:241–9.
14. D'Onofrio G, Safdar B, Lichtman JH, et al. Sex differences in reperfusion in young patients with ST-segment-elevation myocardial infarction: results from the VIRGO study. Circulation. 2015;131:1324–32.
15. Blomkalns AL, Chen AY, Hochman JS, et al. Gender disparities in the diagnosis and treatment of non-ST-segment elevation acute coronary syndromes: large-scale observations from the CRUSADE (Can Rapid Risk Stratification of Unstable Angina Patients Suppress Adverse Outcomes with Early Implementation of the American College of Cardiology/American Heart Association Guidelines) National Quality Improvement Initiative. J Am Coll Cardiol. 2005;45:832–7.
16. Radovanovic D, Erne P, Urban P, et al. Gender differences in management and outcomes in patients with acute coronary syndromes: results on 20,290 patients from the AMIS Plus Registry. Heart. 2007;93:1369–75.
17. Jneid H, Fonarow GC, Cannon CP, et al. Sex differences in medical care and early death after acute myocardial infarction. Circulation. 2008;118:2803–10.
18. Mehilli J, Ndrepepa G, Kastrati A, et al. Gender and myocardial salvage after reperfusion treatment in acute myocardial infarction. J Am Coll Cardiol. 2005;45:828–31.
19. Dreyer RP, Ranasinghe I, Wang Y, et al. Sex differences in the rate, timing, and principal diagnoses of 30-day readmissions in younger patients with acute myocardial infarction. Circulation. 2015;132:158–66.
20. Khera S, Kolte D, Gupta T, et al. Temporal trends and sex differences in revascularization and outcomes of ST-segment elevation myocardial infarction in younger adults in the United States. J Am Coll Cardiol. 2015;66:1961–72.
21. Mehilli J, Kastrati A, Dirschinger J, et al. Sex-based analysis of outcome in patients with acute myocardial infarction treated predominantly with percutaneous coronary intervention. JAMA. 2002;287:210–5.
22. Windecker S, Kolh P, Alfonso F, et al. 2014 ESC/EACTS Guidelines on myocardial revascularization: The Task Force on Myocardial Revascularization of the European Society of Cardiology (ESC) and the European Association for Cardio-Thoracic Surgery (EACTS). Developed with the special contribution of the European Association of Percutaneous Cardiovascular Interventions (EAPCI). Eur Heart J. 2014;35:2541–619.
23. Windecker S, Hernandez-Antolin RA, Stefanini GG, Wijns W, Zamorano JL. Management of ST-elevation myocardial infarction according to European and American guidelines. EuroIntervention 2014;10 Suppl T:T23–31.
24. Boersma E, Primary Coronary Angioplasty vs. Thrombolysis G. Does time matter? A pooled analysis of randomized clinical trials comparing primary percutaneous coronary intervention

and in-hospital fibrinolysis in acute myocardial infarction patients. Eur Heart J. 2006;27:779–88.
25. Tamis-Holland JE, Palazzo A, Stebbins AL, et al. Benefits of direct angioplasty for women and men with acute myocardial infarction: results of the Global Use of Strategies to Open Occluded Arteries in Acute Coronary Syndromes Angioplasty (GUSTO II-B) Angioplasty Substudy. Am Heart J. 2004;147:133–9.
26. Pancholy SB, Shantha GP, Patel T, Cheskin LJ. Sex differences in short-term and long-term all-cause mortality among patients with ST-segment elevation myocardial infarction treated by primary percutaneous intervention: a meta-analysis. JAMA Intern Med. 2014;174:1822–30.
27. Mehran R, Pocock SJ, Nikolsky E, et al. A risk score to predict bleeding in patients with acute coronary syndromes. J Am Coll Cardiol. 2010;55:2556–66.
28. Cavender MA, Milford-Beland S, Roe MT, Peterson ED, Weintraub WS, Rao SV. Prevalence, predictors, and in-hospital outcomes of non-infarct artery intervention during primary percutaneous coronary intervention for ST-segment elevation myocardial infarction (from the National Cardiovascular Data Registry). Am J Cardiol. 2009;104:507–13.
29. Wald DS, Morris JK, Wald NJ, et al. Randomized trial of preventive angioplasty in myocardial infarction. N Engl J Med. 2013;369:1115–23.
30. Nordmann AJ, Hengstler P, Harr T, Young J, Bucher HC. Clinical outcomes of primary stenting versus balloon angioplasty in patients with myocardial infarction: a meta-analysis of randomized controlled trials. Am J Med. 2004;116:253–62.
31. Stone GW, Grines CL, Cox DA, et al. Comparison of angioplasty with stenting, with or without abciximab, in acute myocardial infarction. N Engl J Med. 2002;346:957–66.
32. Stone GW, Witzenbichler B, Guagliumi G, et al. Heparin plus a glycoprotein IIb/IIIa inhibitor versus bivalirudin monotherapy and paclitaxel-eluting stents versus bare-metal stents in acute myocardial infarction (HORIZONS-AMI): final 3-year results from a multicentre, randomised controlled trial. Lancet. 2011;377:2193–204.
33. Kalesan B, Pilgrim T, Heinimann K, et al. Comparison of drug-eluting stents with bare metal stents in patients with ST-segment elevation myocardial infarction. Eur Heart J. 2012;33:977–87.
34. Nakazawa G, Finn AV, Vorpahl M, Ladich ER, Kolodgie FD, Virmani R. Coronary responses and differential mechanisms of late stent thrombosis attributed to first-generation sirolimus- and paclitaxel-eluting stents. J Am Coll Cardiol. 2011;57:390–8.
35. Sabate M, Cequier A, Iniguez A, et al. Everolimus-eluting stent versus bare-metal stent in ST-segment elevation myocardial infarction (EXAMINATION): 1 year results of a randomised controlled trial. Lancet. 2012;380:1482–90.
36. Raber L, Kelbaek H, Ostojic M, et al. Effect of biolimus-eluting stents with biodegradable polymer vs bare-metal stents on cardiovascular events among patients with acute myocardial infarction: the COMFORTABLE AMI randomized trial. JAMA. 2012;308:777–87.
37. Sabate M, Raber L, Heg D, et al. Comparison of newer-generation drug-eluting with bare-metal stents in patients with acute ST-segment elevation myocardial infarction: A pooled analysis of the EXAMINATION (Clinical Evaluation of the Xience-V stent in Acute Myocardial INfArcTION) and COMFORTABLE-AMI (Comparison of Biolimus Eluted From an Erodible Stent Coating With Bare Metal Stents in Acute ST-elevation Myocardial Infarction) trials. JACC Cardiovasc Interv. 2014;7:55–63.
38. Stefanini GG, Baber U, Windecker S, et al. Safety and efficacy of drug-eluting stents in women: a patient-level pooled analysis of randomised trials. Lancet. 2013;382:1879–88.
39. Jolly SS, Yusuf S, Cairns J, et al. Radial versus femoral access for coronary angiography and intervention in patients with acute coronary syndromes (RIVAL): a randomised, parallel group, multicentre trial. Lancet. 2011;377:1409–20.
40. Romagnoli E, Biondi-Zoccai G, Sciahbasi A, et al. Radial versus femoral randomized investigation in ST-segment elevation acute coronary syndrome: the RIFLE-STEACS (Radial Versus

Femoral Randomized Investigation in ST-elevation Acute Coronary Syndrome) study. J Am Coll Cardiol. 2012;60:2481–9.
41. Baklanov DV, Kaltenbach LA, Marso SP, et al. The prevalence and outcomes of transradial percutaneous coronary intervention for ST-segment elevation myocardial infarction: analysis from the National Cardiovascular Data Registry (2007 to 2011). J Am Coll Cardiol. 2013;61:420–6.
42. Hamon M, Pristipino C, Di Mario C, et al. Consensus document on the radial approach in percutaneous cardiovascular interventions: position paper by the European Association of Percutaneous Cardiovascular Interventions and Working Groups on Acute Cardiac Care** and Thrombosis of the European Society of Cardiology. EuroIntervention. 2013;8:1242–51.
43. Pandie S, Mehta SR, Cantor WJ, et al. Radial versus femoral access for coronary angiography/intervention in women with acute coronary syndromes: insights from the RIVAL trial (Radial Vs femorAL access for coronary intervention). JACC Cardiovasc Interv. 2015;8:505–12.
44. Valgimigli M, Gagnor A, Calabro P, et al. Radial versus femoral access in patients with acute coronary syndromes undergoing invasive management: a randomised multicentre trial. Lancet. 2015;385:2465–76.

6 Peri- and Post-procedural Antithrombotic Therapy in Women

Stefanie Schulz-Schüpke

Adjunct antithrombotic therapy is the prerequisite for the safe performance of percutaneous coronary interventions (PCI). Usually patients receive a combination of antiplatelet and anticoagulation therapy. Advances in antithrombotic therapy have significantly improved clinical outcome in patients undergoing PCI. However, the proportion of women enrolled in clinical trials of antithrombotic therapy usually ranges from 20 to 30 %. Consequently, clinical trials are not powered to assess the value of antithrombotics in women. Conclusions derived from men are often extrapolated to women. Moreover, women are less likely to receive evidence-based adjunct antithrombotic therapy [1]. The following reasons underlying low enrollment rates and underutilization of antithrombotics in women have been discussed.

Women incur coronary artery disease(CAD) at an older age (usually 6–10 years later) and have more comorbidities at their disease presentation (e.g., peripheral vascular disease, cerebrovascular disease, heart failure) including a more adverse cardiovascular risk profile (e.g. diabetes mellitus, arterial hypertension) compared to men [2]. This may prevent their enrolment in clinical trials which apply rigorous eligibility criteria. Unadjusted clinical outcome in women is worse compared to men, probably caused by differences in baseline risk and treatment biases. Worse outcome may be causative for less invasive treatment strategies in women, although high-risk patients typically have the most gain from aggressive therapy. Another important factor is the lack of awareness in both women and physicians [3]. Clinical symptoms in women with CAD are more often atypical (dyspnea, heart failure). Moreover, gender-specific differences in diagnostic tests including biomarkers

S. Schulz-Schüpke
Deutsches Herzzentrum München, Lazarettstr. 36, Munich 80636, Germany
e-mail: schuepke@dhm.mhn.de, schulzs@dhm.mhn.de, Stefanie-schulz@gmx.de

P. Presbitero et al. (eds.), *Percutaneous Treatment of Cardiovascular Diseases in Women*,
DOI 10.1007/978-3-319-39611-8_6

may hamper prompt and correct diagnosis in women, resulting in delayed and suboptimal treatment. Furthermore, women are less likely to receive invasive therapy and consequently adjunct antithrombotic therapy. Finally, the pathology underlying acute coronary syndrome (ACS) in women is less often obstructive CAD, but more frequently found to be microvascular dysfunction, spontaneous coronary artery dissection, and others [4], which may require different antithrombotic therapy compared to patients undergoing PCI for obstructive CAD.

The observed undertreatment in women is not supported by current evidence. Hitherto, no consistent gender-specific difference regarding the efficacy or safety of any antithrombotic therapy in patients undergoing PCI has been proven. The European Society of Cardiology therefore recommends in its guidelines on non-ST-segment elevation acute coronary syndrome (NSTE-ACS) that both genders should be treated in the same way (Class I, Level of Evidence B) [5]. Rigorous gender-specific analyses of mixed-gender trials and clinical trials enrolling women only remain unmet clinical needs. Moreover, appropriate dosing regimens in women have not yet been thoroughly investigated for many cardiovascular drugs routinely used in clinical practice.

6.1 Higher Bleeding Risk

A consistent finding across numerous trials with different antithrombotics is that women are at higher risk for vascular and bleeding complications. Female gender has been identified as an independent predictor for bleeding. In some studies, the risk of bleeding complications in women was increased more than fivefold [6]. On the other hand, bleeding is a strong and independent predictor for short- and long-term mortality [7, 8]. Thus, bleeding avoidance strategies receive particular attention in women.

The reasons underlying the increased bleeding risk in women are not completely understood. Factors like older age or smaller body weight have been suggested. Women are more vulnerable to overdosing if no dose adjustment according to body weight is performed. Overdosing in women has been suggested to account for 25 % of the gender-related difference in bleeding complications [9]. However, in an analysis of 3,351 women and 3,351 men, matched for age, body weight, and type of antithrombotic therapy, the bleeding risk in women remained significantly higher compared to men suggesting additional factors [10]. Interestingly, the difference in bleeding is driven by an excess in access site complications in women, whereas gastrointestinal bleeding is more common in men [11]. Differences in the local anatomy of the arterial access site including shorter and smaller common femoral arteries [12] and increased susceptibility to mechanical complications in women [13] have also been described.

6.2 Gender-Related Differences in Pharmacokinetics and Pharmacodynamics

Other reasons underlying the increased bleeding risk in women may be caused by gender-related differences in pharmacokinetics and pharmacodynamics of antithrombotic drugs. Numerous differences in the absorption, distribution, metabolization, and excretion of drugs between women and men have been described [14]. Women have a greater proportion of body fat and lower body water content. Thus, lipophilic drugs have a higher volume of distribution, whereas hydrophilic drugs have a smaller volume of distribution, resulting in higher initial plasma levels and greater effects compared to men [15]. The decreased proportion of muscles in women results in a lower creatinine level, while glomerular filtration rate is comparable. Thus, women are overdosed if dose adaption is based on serum creatinine only [9].

The following section aims to summarize current evidence of efficacy and safety for the most commonly used antithrombotic drugs in women undergoing PCI.

6.3 Antiplatelets (Table 6.1)

6.3.1 Acetylsalicylic Acid

Acetylsalicylic acid (ASA) continues to be the cornerstone of adjunct antithrombotic therapy in patients with CAD. ASA irreversibly inhibits platelet cyclooxygenase-1 (COX-1) thereby blocking the synthesis of thromboxane A2 (TXA2), a potent platelet activator. Other effects of ASA on platelet function have been described; however, their significance remains unclear.

Bioavailability of ASA is greater in women compared to men, owing to a slower clearance and prolonged half-life [16]. Platelet function studies on differential platelet reactivity to low-dose aspirin by gender have yielded controversial results:

In a registry of 326 stable cardiovascular patients on ASA (325 mg/day for 7 days), more women were found to be ASA resistant (47 % versus 21 %, $p=0.03$), defined as a mean aggregation of ≥70 % with 10 μM adenosine diphosphate (ADP) and ≥20 % with 0.5 mg/ml arachidonic acid [17].

Substudies of the HOPE [18] and CHARISMA [19] trial including 976 (16 % women) and 3,261 patients (28 % women) demonstrated higher levels of urinary 11-dehydrothromboxane B2 in ASA treated women. Eleven-dehydrothromboxane B2 is a stable metabolite of thromboxane A2 and a marker of in vivo thromboxane generation. Higher levels may indicate failure of ASA to suppress thromboxane generation and thereby ASA resistance, although it is not a specific measure of the antiplatelet effects of ASA [20].

In an ex vivo study of 571 men and 711 women with familiar disposition, women's platelets were significantly more reactive to multiple agonists at baseline [21], as it has been shown in several other studies. After ASA therapy, female platelets experienced a greater decrease in platelet reactivity compared to men, resulting in comparable results of platelet aggregation for direct COX-1 pathways (arachidonic acid) in women and men [21].

In a recent, large registry of 7,090 consecutive patients undergoing PCI after 500 mg i.v. ASA, women were less likely to incur high on aspirin platelet reactivity (HAPR), defined as the upper quintile of platelet aggregation measurements (assessed by impedance aggregometry using the Multiplate analyzer after trigger with arachidonic acid at the time of PCI) [22].

Yet, the clinical relevance of these findings remains uncertain. For the treatment of acute coronary syndrome (ACS) and for secondary prevention, no gender-specific difference in the efficacy and safety profile of ASA has been reported [23]. In a wide range of patients with established occlusive cardiovascular disease, there is a significant and profound relative risk reduction in the composite of cardiovascular death, nonfatal myocardial infarction (MI), or nonfatal stroke of about 25 %, outweighing the increased bleeding risk [24].

However, the value of ASA for primary prevention and the gender-specific benefit of ASA in primary prevention are more controversial.

In the Nurses' Health Study, a prospective cohort study of 87,678 apparently healthy women, there was a significant reduction in MI in women taking ASA 1–6 times per week [25].

In a gender-specific, aggregate data meta-analysis of 6 randomized controlled clinical trials (3 trials enrolled women) including 95,456 individuals (51,342 women) without established cardiovascular disease, the absolute risk reduction with ASA for the composite of cardiovascular death, nonfatal MI, or nonfatal stroke was lower compared to patients with established cardiovascular disease, yet the reduction was significant and comparable in women and men (relative risk reduction of 12 % in women and 14 % in men) [26]. However, gender-specific differences in the efficacy profile of ASA for the individual components were suggested: In women, the reduction was driven by a reduction in stroke but not MI, whereas in men, ASA was found to reduce the risk of MI but not to affect the risk of stroke [26].

In a later, patient-level meta-analysis of the same 6 trials, the Antithrombotic Trialists' (ATT) collaborators came to a different conclusion. The authors reported results of tests for heterogeneity of treatment effect in men and women, which were $p=0.03$ for major coronary events and $p=0.08$ for stroke. They argued that p values had to be adjusted due to multiple comparisons. After this adjustment, there was no more heterogeneity of treatment effect in women and men [23]. However, this approach has been criticized by others [27]. Of note, 78 % (39,876) of the women in these 2 meta-analyses were enrolled in the Women's Health Study [28]. In that study, 90 % of women were younger than 65 years. At that age, stroke is the predominant occlusive vascular disease in women [28]. In women aged >65 years, there was a significant reduction in MI comparable to that described in men. Thus, gender-specific differences in the efficacy profile of ASA for primary prevention are most likely related to differences in the baseline risk. No gender-specific differences in the increased bleeding risk with ASA have been reported [26].

Weighing the ischemic and bleeding risk, there is clear net clinical benefit with ASA for secondary prevention, whereas its value for primary prevention is of uncertain value. A growing body of evidence suggests that low-dose ASA may also have a role for primary prevention of cancer which should be taken into consideration when assessing the overall risk-to-benefit ratio of ASA for primary prevention [29].

6.4 Platelet ADP Receptor Blocker

6.4.1 Clopidogrel

About 2 decades ago, pivotal clinical trials showed that in patients undergoing PCI, the use of the $P2Y_{12}$ ADP receptor antagonist ticlopidin plus ASA significantly reduces the risk of stent thrombosis and also bleeding compared to a regimen of heparin and oral anticoagulation plus ASA [30]. Later, ticlopidin was replaced by its successor clopidogrel due to a faster onset of action and a more favorable hematological side effect profile (i.e., neutropenia, thrombotic thrombocytopenia, and aplastic anemia) [31]. Both drugs are thienopyridines and irreversible inhibitors of the platelet $P2Y_{12}$ ADP receptor. Dual antiplatelet therapy with ASA plus clopidogrel has been the standard antiplatelet regimen for patients undergoing PCI for many years and remains it for patients undergoing PCI for stable CAD [32].

Levels of clopidogrel's active metabolite are comparable in men and women [33]. Yet, ex vivo studies suggest higher clopidogrel platelet reactivity in women compared to men [33–35].

Clopidogrel has been tested in several large-scale, randomized clinical trials including a broad spectrum of CAD presentations. The value of clopidogrel in patients undergoing PCI has been assessed in the CREDO trial (enrolling patients with planned PCI) [36] and PCI-CURE trial of NSTE-ACS patients [37]. Both trials assessed the benefit of a loading dose of clopidogrel followed by long-term treatment compared with a strategy of no loading and short-term therapy. Although differences in the magnitude of treatment effect have been reported, there was no significant interaction for gender and treatment effect in any of these trials.

Accordingly, in a collaborative, gender-specific meta-analysis of 5 placebo-controlled, randomized trials including 79,613 patients (23,533 women) across a broad spectrum of cardiovascular disease, there was no significant gender-specific difference in the reduction of the composite endpoint of cardiovascular mortality, MI, or stroke with clopidogrel [38]. Point estimates favored clopidogrel in both genders, yet relative risk reduction with clopidogrel for the primary endpoint was numerically smaller and nonsignificant in women (OR 0.93, 95 % CI 0.86–1.01) compared to men (OR 0.84, 95 % CI 0.78–1.91). This may reflect play of chance since there was no significant heterogeneity (p interaction = 0.08) [38]. Both men and women are at increased risk of major bleeding with clopidogrel. The risk of major bleeding with clopidogrel was not significantly higher in women compared to men (OR women 1.43, 95 % CI 1.15–1.79 vs. OR men 1.22, 95 % CI 1.05–1.42; p interaction = 0.24). Another recent meta-analysis confirmed the finding of comparable efficacy and safety of clopidogrel in both genders [39].

For the treatment of acute coronary syndrome (ACS) patients, clopidogrel has been replaced by third-generation ADP receptor blockers prasugrel and ticagrelor. In ACS patients, clopidogrel is currently only recommended if prasugrel or ticagrelor are either contraindicated or not available [32].

6.4.2 Prasugrel

Prasugrel – like clopidogrel – is a thienopyridine and irreversible inhibitor of the platelet $P2Y_{12}$ ADP receptor, but more potent, with a faster onset of action and a more consistent antiplatelet effect.

Pharmacokinetics have shown a slight (<8 %) increase in exposure of the active metabolite in women, which was mainly driven by body weight and age [40].

In the TRITON-TIMI 38 trial of 13,608 patients (3,523 women) with ACS undergoing PCI, prasugrel compared to clopidogrel resulted in a significant 19 % relative risk reduction in the primary composite endpoint of cardiovascular death, MI, or stroke [41]. Although this increase in efficacy occurred at the expense of an increased risk of TIMI major bleeding, net clinical benefit was retained. In the TRITON-TIMI 38 trial, the relative risk reduction with prasugrel for the primary endpoint was smaller in women compared to men (12 % versus 21 %). Yet, there was no significant interaction for gender and treatment effect (*p* interaction = not significant, exact *p* value not reported) [41].

In a subsequent analysis, female gender was the strongest independent predictor for non-CABG-related serious bleeding in the overall population (HR 1.77, 95 % CI 1.44–2.18) [42]. A nonsignificant interaction between treatment group and gender for non-CAGB-related TIMI major or minor bleeding has been reported (HR women 1.38, 95 % CI 1.06–1.80, HR men 1.31, 95 % CI 1.05–1.64, *p* interaction = nonsignificant, exact *p* value not reported) [40].

There was also no significant interaction for gender and treatment effect in the TRILOGY trial which assessed the value of prasugrel against clopidogrel in 7,243 NSTE-ACS patients (2,599 women) without revascularization [43]. After a median of 17 months, there was no benefit with prasugrel regarding the composite of cardiovascular death, MI, or stroke (HR women 1.02, 95 % CI 0.80–1.29; HR men 0.86, 95 % CI 0.72–1.03; *p* interaction = 0.29) [43].

The ACCOAST trial evaluated prasugrel pretreatment in 4,033 patients (1,110 women) with NSTE-ACS. Prasugrel pretreatment with 30 mg before angiography followed by 30 mg in case of PCI compared with a strategy of deferred administration (60 mg prasugrel after angiography before PCI) did not reduce the composite of cardiovascular death, MI, stroke, urgent revascularization, or glycoprotein IIb/IIIa inhibitor rescue therapy after 7 days. There was no evidence of a differential efficacy according to gender (HR women 1.14, 95 % CI 0.76–1.70 versus HR men 0.99, 95 % CI 0.79–1.24; *p* interaction = 0.54). However, there was a significant increase in TIMI major bleeding with prasugrel pretreatment in the overall population (HR 1.90, 95 % CI 1.19–3.02). The increased bleeding risk was more pronounced in women; however, p values for interaction did not reach boundaries of significance (HR women 3.61, 95 % CI 1.46–8.95; HR men 1.43, 95 % CI 0.82–2.49, *p* interaction = 0.09) [44].

6.4.3 Ticagrelor

Ticagrelor is not a thienopyridine but a cyclopentyl triazolopyrimidine that reversibly blocks the ADP $P2Y_{12}$ platelet receptor in a noncompetitive manner by binding to a ligand binding site separate from that of ADP.

Gender-specific differences in pharmacokinetics and pharmacodynamics of ticagrelor were reported in a study of 40 healthy individuals. Ticagrelor exposure was higher, and elimination half-life was longer in women compared to men. However, platelet sensitivity (optical aggregometry after 20 μM ADP) was reported to be less in women compared to men [45].

In the PLATO trial of 18,624 ACS patients (5,288 women), there was a significant 16 % reduction in the composite ischemic endpoint of vascular death, MI, or stroke with ticagrelor compared to clopidogrel irrespective of revascularization strategy [46]. There was no increase in study-defined major bleeding, but in non-CABG-related TIMI major bleeding [46]. No significant interaction for gender and treatment effect regarding the primary endpoint (HR women 0.83, 95 % CI 0.71–0.97, HR men 0.85, 95 % CI 0.76–0.95; p interaction = 0.82) and bleeding was noted (HR women 1.01, 95 % CI 0.85–1.21, HR men 1.05, 95 % CI 0.94–1.16; p interaction = 0.76).

The ATLANTIC trial assessed the value of prehospital administration of ticagrelor compared to inhospital administration in the cath lab in 1,862 patients (369 women) with ongoing STEMI. The use of ticagrelor shortly before PCI neither improved reperfusion of the culprit artery nor ST-segment resolution before the procedure but was safe and may prevent post-procedural acute stent thrombosis. The treatment effect for the absence of ST-segment resolution was consistent in both genders. Regarding the co-primary endpoint of the absence of TIMI flow grade 3 before angiography, there were differences in the direction of treatment effect in both genders; however, the test for interaction did not show significant heterogeneity [47].

6.4.4 Cangrelor

Recently, the intravenous non-thienopyridine $P2Y_{12}$ ADP receptor blocker cangrelor has been approved by the European Medicines Agency for the reduction of thrombotic cardiovascular events in adult patients with CAD undergoing PCI who have not received an oral $P2Y_{12}$ inhibitor prior to the PCI procedure and in whom oral therapy with $P2Y_{12}$ inhibitors is not feasible or desirable. Compared to other platelet inhibitors, cangrelor provides reversible platelet inhibition with a very rapid onset and offset of action.

Cangrelor was tested in 3 large-scale, double-blind, randomized clinical trials against clopidogrel started either at the end of PCI [48], 30 min before PCI [49], or according to local standard [50]. Although in the CHAMPION-PCI [49] and CHAMPION-PLATFORM [48] trials cangrelor could not provide superiority regarding the composite of death, MI, or urgent target vessel revascularization (uTVR) at 48 h, there was a significant reduction in the composite of death, MI, uTVR, or stent thrombosis at 48 h with cangrelor over clopidogrel in the CHAMPION-PHOENIX trial [50]. A pooled analysis of these 3 trials, including 24,910 patients (6,905 women) confirmed increased efficacy of cangrelor over clopidogrel or placebo. This benefit was achieved at the expense of an increased bleeding risk according to GUSTO mild, TIMI minor, and any ACUITY definition. There was no significant increase in TIMI major or GUSTO moderate or severe bleeding [51]. Subgroup analysis confirmed consistency of efficacy irrespective of gender (composite of death, MI, or uTVR: HR women 0.71, 95 % CI 0.56–0.89; HR men 0.85, 95 % CI 0.74–0.99, *p* interaction = 0.18). There was an increase in GUSTO moderate/severe bleeding in women but not in men, which did not meet criteria for significant interaction: HR women 1.65, 95 % CI 1.11–2.46, HR men 0.97, 95 % CI 0.62–1.51, *p* interaction = 0.079.

6.5 Intravenous Glycoprotein IIb/IIIa Inhibitors

Glycoprotein IIb/IIIa inhibitors block the final common pathway of platelet aggregation by inhibiting the binding of platelets to fibrinogen. Commonly used agents are synthetic cyclic heptapeptides (eptifibatide), synthetic non-peptides (tirofiban), or chimeric Fab fragments of an immunoglobulin (abciximab) that target the glycoprotein IIb/IIIa receptor either reversibly (tirofiban, eptifibatide) or irreversibly (abciximab).

Glycoprotein IIb/IIIa inhibitors are the class of antithrombotics that has received most attention regarding gender-specific efficacy and safety.

In an ex vivo study, women's platelets were capable to convert a greater proportion of glycoprotein IIb/IIIa receptors to an activated state. After the administration of the same agonist, there was a 50–80 % increase in the number of activated receptor sites in women compared to men [52]. Based on these observations, it has been suggested that women would derive greater benefit from glycoprotein IIb/IIIa inhibitors compared to men.

The placebo-controlled PURSUIT trial assessed the efficacy of eptifibatide in 10,948 patients (36 % women) with NSTE-ACS. Fifty-nine percent of the patients underwent coronary angiography, 24 % were treated with PCI, and 14 % with CABG. At 30 days, there was a significant reduction in the primary endpoint of death or MI in men (OR 0.80, 95 % CI 0.70–0.90), but not in women (OR 1.1, 95 % CI 0.9–1.3; *p* values for interaction were not reported). The authors found that the observed treatment effect varied according to geographic regions with the benefit confined to patients from North America. When restricting the analysis to North American patients, there was also a treatment benefit with eptifibatide in women. The lesser benefit in women outside North America has – at least in part – been ascribed to differences in baseline characteristics and the decreased use of invasive procedures. In fact, there was a great variation in the use of cardiac catheterization which was 79 % in North America but only 20 % in Eastern Europe. Furthermore, it could be shown that treatment benefit was confined to patients undergoing PCI with 72 h compared to those treated conservatively [53].

A later meta-analysis (including the PURSUIT trial) on the use of glycoprotein IIb/IIIa inhibitors in 31,402 patients (35 % women) with NSTE-ACS who were not scheduled to undergo routine early revascularization enrolled in 6 trials also noted harm of glycoprotein IIb/IIIa inhibitors in women. There was a significant increase in the composite primary end point of death or MI with glycoprotein IIb/IIIa inhibitors in women (OR 1.15, 95 % CI 1.01–1.30) compared to a benefit in men (OR 0.81, 95 % CI 0.75–0.89, p interaction < 0.0001). However, further analysis revealed that the treatment benefit was limited to patients with a positive troponin. More men in this study presented with elevated baseline troponin. After stratification of patients according to baseline troponin, there was no more evidence of a differential treatment effect. Thus, the gender-specific effects of glycoprotein IIb/IIIa inhibitors in this study were related to differences in baseline troponin between women and men [54].

Another meta-analysis of 6,595 patients (1,771 women) undergoing PCI enrolled in 3 placebo-controlled trials of abciximab did not find a gender-specific difference in clinical outcome. There was a reduction in the composite of death, MI, or urgent revascularization at 30 days in both genders. Regarding bleeding complications, women had a higher risk of major and minor bleeding compared to men. In women, the use of abciximab was associated with a significant increase in minor but not major bleeding [55].

A gender-specific analysis of the ESPRIT trial comparing eptifibatide or placebo in 2,064 patients (562 women) undergoing elective PCI showed that overall women tended to incur more ischemic events. The primary composite endpoint of death, MI, urgent revascularization, or "bail-out" eptifibatide occurred in 10.5 % of women and 7.9 % of men, $p = 0.08$. The relative risk reduction with eptifibatide was greater in women: 30 % in women and 15 % in men, resulting in comparable event rates in women and men at 48 h (6.1 % versus 6.8 %). The p value for interaction did not reach criteria for statistical significance ($p = 0.063$) [56]. Contrasting the results of the PURSUIT trial, the results of the ESPRIT trial have been interpreted as suggestion that glycoprotein IIb/IIIa inhibitors may have the potential to reduce the excess risk in women for inhospital major adverse cardiac events [57].

The routine use of oral $P2Y_{12}$ ADP antagonists has obviated the need for GPIIb/IIIa inhibitors in a broad spectrum of patients undergoing PCI. The ISAR-REACT trial showed that in biomarker-negative patients undergoing PCI after pretreatment with 600 mg clopidogrel, the use of abciximab is of no additional benefit, with consistent results in both genders [58]. The ISAR-REACT 2 trial assessed the value of abciximab after pretreatment with 600 mg clopidogrel in 2,022 patients (498 women) with NSTE-ACS undergoing PCI. In this population, a significant 31 % relative risk reduction in the combined endpoint of death, MI, or urgent revascularization at 30 days with abciximab despite pretreatment with 600 mg clopidogrel was observed [59]. In a subsequent gender-specific analysis, treatment benefit with abciximab was found to be confined to men with no benefit in women (RR women 0.98, 95 % CI 0.56–1.72; RR men 0.69, 95 % CI 0.50–0.94). However, there were several differences in baseline and angiographic factors with a more adverse risk profile in women. After adjustment for these differences, there was no significant interaction between gender and treatment effect of abciximab regarding major adverse cardiac events (MACE; p interaction = 0.71) [60]. Overall, the bleeding risk in women was significantly higher compared to men (RR 5.5, 95 % CI 2.54–11.9). Yet, there was no increase in major or minor bleeding in women treated with abciximab compared to placebo. Finally, the BRAVE-3 trial found no benefit of upstream administration of abciximab in 800 STEMI patients (207 women) pre-treated with 600 mg clopidogrel regarding infarct size [61]. Subgroup analysis did not find a significant interaction for gender and treatment effect ($p=0.14$), although point estimates favored placebo in women and abciximab in men [61].

In summary, no clear evidence for gender-based disparities in the treatment effect of glycoprotein IIb/IIIa inhibitors have been found. Of note, neither subgroup analysis was sufficiently powered to support any definitive conclusion. A nonsignificant p value for a given factor does not prove definitely that there is a lack of a true factor interaction on treatment effect (Table 6.1).

6.6 Anticoagulants

6.6.1 Heparin

Unfractionated heparin (UFH) has been the standard antithrombin agent since the early days of PCI and used as a reference against which new antithrombotic agents have been tested. Unfractionated heparin binds to antithrombin and augments the inactivation of thrombin and to a lesser extent factor Xa and IXa.

Despite its longstanding application, recommendations regarding UFH dose during PCI lack evidence base from large-scale, randomized clinical trials. Current dosing recommendations in Europe are 70–100 U/kg i.v. bolus and 50–70 U/kg i.v. bolus if GP IIb/IIIa inhibitors are co-administered [32]. The ACC/AHA guideline committee recommends the same initial bolus dose but also recommends that subsequent doses be guided according to activated clotting time (ACT), to achieve 250–300 s for HemoTec and 300–350 s for Hemochron device and a target ACT of 200–250 s in case of GPIIb/IIIa co-administration [64]. Yet, the value of ACT guidance has been discussed controversially.

Several studies suggest increased sensitivity of women to heparin. Partial thromboplastin time (PTT) after heparin is longer in women compared to women, even after weight-adjusted dosing [65, 66]. Moreover, women have a nearly fivefold increased risk of heparin-induced thrombocytopenia [67].

6.6.2 Low Molecular Weight Heparin

Compared to UFH, low molecular weight heparin (LMWH) has a higher ratio of anti-factor Xa compared to anti-factor IIa activity and therefore a greater proximal inhibition of the coagulation cascade. Advantages of LMWH over UFH include a more stable and predictable anticoagulant effect, obviating the need for routine monitoring, less platelet activation, and a lower incidence of HIT. Disadvantages in case of bleeding include the lack of complete reversibility with protamine and a long half-life.

Table 6.1 Gender-specific efficacy and safety of antiplatelet medication

Drug	Comparison	Type of study	Indication	No. of individuals	Follow-up	Efficacy endpoint	Relative risk (95 % CI)	Safety endpoint	Relative risk (95 % CI)	Reference
Acetylsalicylic acid										
Acetylsalicylic acid	Placebo	Collaborative meta-analysis	Primary prevention	W = 51,342 M = 44,114	3.6 – 10.1 years	Cardiovascular death, non-fatal MI or non-fatal stroke	W: 0.88 (0.79–0.99) M: 0.86 (0.78–0.94)	Major bleeding	W: 1.68 (1.13–2.52) M: 1.72 (1.35–2.20)	Berger et al., *JAMA* 2006 [26]
	Placebo	Patient-level meta-analysis	Secondary prevention (previous MI, stroke or TIA)	W = 2,908 M = 14,092	NA	Vascular death, MI or stroke	W: 0.81 (0.64–1.02) M: 0.81 (0.73–0.90)	Major bleeding	2.69 (1.25–5.76) *No gender-specific analysis*	ATT Collaborators, *Lancet* 2009 [23]
$P2Y_{12}$ ADP receptor antagonists										
Clopidogrel	Placebo	Randomized, double blind trial	NSTE-ACS undergoing PCI	W = 804 M = 1,854	12 months	Cardiovascular death or MI	W: 0.89 (0.75–1.06) M: 0.77 (0.52–1.15)	Bleeding necessitating transfusion of > 2 blood units or life-threatening	1.12 (0.70–1.78) *No gender-specific analysis*	PCI-CURE trial, Mehta et al. *Lancet* 2001 [62]
	Placebo	Randomized, double blind trial	Planned PCI (14 % recent MI, 53 % unstable angina, 33 % stable angina or other)	W = 606 M = 1,510	12 months	Death, MI or stroke	W: 0.68 (0.41–1.12) M: 0.76 (0.55–1.05)	TIMI major bleeding	1.32 (0.97–1.80) *No gender-related analysis*	CREDO trial, Steinhubl et al., *JAMA* 2002 [36]
	Placebo	Collaborative Meta-analysis	NSTE-ACS, STEMI, planned PCI, established CVD, multiple risk factors for but without CVD	W = 23,533 M = 56,091	8.3 months	Cardiovascular death, MI or stroke	W: 0.93 (0.86–1.01) M: 0.81 (0.70–1.05)	Major bleeding	W: 1.43 (1.15–1.79) M: 1.22 (1.05–1.42)	Berger et al, *JACC* 2009 [38]

(continued)

Table 6.1 (continued)

Drug	Comparison	Type of study	Indication	No. of individuals	Follow-up	Efficacy endpoint	Relative risk (95 % CI)	Safety endpoint	Relative risk (95 % CI)	Reference
Prasugrel	Clopidogrel	Randomized, double blind trial	Acute coronary syndrome patients with scheduled PCI	W = 3,523 M = 10,085	15 months	Cardiovascular death, nonfatal MI or nonfatal stroke	W: 0.88 (0.72–1.05) M: 0.79 (0.71–0.90)	Non-CABG related TIMI major or minor bleeding	W: 1.38 (1.06–1.80) M: 1.31 (1.05–1.64)	TRITON-TIMI 38 trial, Wiviott et al., *NEJM* 2007 [41]
	Clopidogrel	Randomized, double blind trial	NSTE-ACS without revascularization <75 years	W = 2,576 M = 4,604	17 months	Cardiovascular death, nonfatal MI or nonfatal stroke	W:1.02 (0.80.–1.29) M: 0.86 (0.72–1.03)	Non-CABG related TIMI major bleeding	W: 1.13 (0.41–3.11) M: 1.37 (0.80–2.35)	TRILOGY trial, Roe et al., *NEJM* 2012
Prasugrel pretreatment	Deferred Prasugrel loading after angiography	Randomized, double blind trial	NSTE-ACS with positive troponin, scheduled for coronary angiography	W = 1,110 M = 2,923	7 days	Cardiovascular death, MI, stroke, urgent revascularization, or glycoprotein IIb/IIIa inhibitor rescue therapy	W: 1.14 (0.76–1.70) M: 0.99 (0.79–1.24)	TIMI major bleeding	W: 3.61 (1.46–8.95) M: 1.43 (0.82–2.49)	ACCOAST trial, Montalescot et al, *NEJM* 2013 [44]
Ticagrelor	Clopidogrel	Randomized, double blind trial	ACS	W = 5,288 M = 13,336	12 months	Vascular death, nonfatal MI or nonfatal stroke	W: 0.83 (0.71–0.97) M: 0.85 (0.76–0.95)	PLATO major bleeding	W: 1.01 (0.85–1.21) M: 1.05 (0.94–1.16)	PLATO trial, Wallentin et al., *NEJM* 2009 [46]
	In-hospital	Randomized, double blind trial	STEMI within 6 h	W = 369 M = 1,493	Before PCI	Absence of ≥ 70 % ST-segment elevation before PCI Absence of TIMI flow grade at initial angiography	W: 0.87 (0.45–1.68) M: 0.95 (0.68–1.31) W: 1.34 (0.78–2.31) M: 0.88 (0.66–1.17)	Non-CABG related PLATO major bleeding	*No gender-specific analysis*	ATLANTIC trial. Montalescot et al., *NEJM* 2014 [47]

Cangrelor	Placebo/ Clopidogrel	Pooled analysis of 3 randomized, double blind trials	STEMI, NSTE-ACS, stable CAD	W=6,905 M=17,976	48 h	Death, MI, ischemia-driven revascularization, stent thrombosis	W: 0.71 (0.56–0.89) M: 0.85 (0.74–0.99)	GUSTO severe/ moderate bleeding	W: 0.68 (0.47– 0.99) M: 0.41 (0.22–0.74)	Steg et al., *Lancet* 2013 [51]
Glycoprotein IIb/IIIa receptor inhibitors										
Abciximab, Eptifibatide, Lamifiban, Tirofiban	Placebo	Meta-analysis	NSTE-ACS without routine early revascularization	W=10,991 M=20,411	30-day	Death or MI	W: 1.15 (1.01–1.30) M: 0.81 (0.75–0.89)	Major bleeding	W: 2.20 (1.60–2.90) M: 1.60 (1.30–2.00)	Boersma et al., *Lancet* 2002 [63]
Abciximab	Placebo	Meta-analysis	Patients undergoing PCI	W=1,771 M=4,824	6-month	Death, MI or urgent revascularization	W: 0.62 (0.44–0.86) M: 0.59 (0.48–0.73)	TIMI major bleeding	W: 1.02 (0.50–2.16) M: 0.48 (0.28–0.84)	Cho et al., *JACC* 2000 [55]
Eptifibatide	Placebo	Randomized, double blind trial	Elective PCI	W=562 M=1,502	12-month	Death, MIor target vessel revascularization	W: 30 % RRR M: 15 % RRR	TIMI major bleeding	W: 3.07 (0.56–30.9) M: 3.30 (0.63–32.7)	ESPRIT trial, Fernandes et al., *JACC* 2002 [56]
Abciximab	Placebo	Randomized, double blind trial	NSTE-ACS undergoing PCI	W=498 M=1,524	30-day	Death, MIor urgent revascularization	W: 0.98 (0.55–1.74) M: 0.69 (0.50–0.93)	TIMI major bleeding	W: 0.89 (0.31–2.46) M: 1.44 (0.34–6.94)	ISAR-REACT 2 trial. Mehilli et al., *AHJ* 2007 [6]

ACS acute coronary syndrome, *CABG* aortocoronary bypass graft, *M* men, *MI* myocardial infarction, *PCI* percutaneous coronary intervention, *NSTE-ACS* non-ST-segment elevation acute coronary syndrome, *NSTEMI* non-ST-segment elevation myocardial infarction, *STEMI* ST-segment elevation myocardial infarction, *TIMI* thrombolysis in myocardial infarction, *W* women, *OASIS* Organization to Assess Strategies in Acute Ischemic Syndromes

Studies on the pharmacodynamic response according to gender have yielded conflicting results. In a substudy of the open-label TIMI 11A trial, comparing 2 different doses of enoxaparin in 445 NSTE-ACS patients (36 % women), found comparable results for anti Xa activity according to gender [68]. On the other hand, a substudy of the double-blind FRISC trial, comparing dalteparin against placebo in 175 patients with NSTE-ACS (25 % women), found higher anti X activity in women compared with men [69]. Consistent with this finding, there was a large reduction in the primary endpoint of death or MI at 6 days in women enrolled in the main FRISC trial (RR women 0.16, 95 % CI 0.05–0.56, RR men 0.55, 95 % CI 0.28–1.11, *p* values for interactions were not reported) [70].

The value of LMWH in patients undergoing elective PCI was assessed in the open-label STEEPLE trial. In that study, 2 doses of enoxaparin (0.5 and 0.75 mg/kg bodyweight) were compared against UFH. Bleeding according to study definition and GUSTO moderate or severe bleeding (but not TIMI major or minor bleeding) was reduced with the use of the low but not of the high dose of enoxaparin. Yet, enrolment in the low-dose arm was stopped prematurely due to increased mortality. The trial was not sufficiently powered for the assessment of ischemic events. In a multivariate analysis, female gender was an independent predictor for bleeding (HR 1.63, 95 % CI 1.23–2.17). Gender-specific data were not reported [71].

Superiority of LMWH over UFH has been shown in clinical trials of patients with NSTE-ACS receiving conservative treatment [72] and in STEMI patients treated with fibrinolysis [73]. The ExTRACT-TIMI 25 trial compared LMWH with UFH in 20,506 STEMI patients receiving fibrinolysis. In a gender-specific analysis (4,783 women), the relative risk reduction in the primary endpoint of death or nonfatal recurrent MI in women was comparable to that achieved in men (RR women 0.82, 95 % CI 0.74–0.90; RR men 0.84, 95 % CI 0.74–0.95). Due to a higher risk profile, the absolute benefit was higher in women (2.9 % versus 1.9 %). The rate of bleeding was higher with LMWH compared to UFH in the overall population and in women. The rate of bleeding in women and men receiving enoxaparin was comparable [74].

The value of LMWH in the revascularization era with the use of stents and adjunct antithrombotic therapy has diminished. In clinical trials – such as the SYNERGY trial of 10,027 patients with NSTE-ACS (34 % women) – in which prerandomization antithrombotic therapy was not consistent with study treatment and high post-procedural crossover rates, LMWH was not superior to UFH but increased the risk of bleeding [75]. In general, crossover between UFH and LMWH is not recommended and should be avoided [76]. In the SYNERGY trial, no significant interaction for gender and treatment effect regarding the composite of death or MI at 30 days was observed [75].

The value of LMWH compared to UFH in STEMI patients undergoing PCI has been assessed in the open-label ATOLL trial [77]. Among 910 patients, the primary endpoint of death, MI, procedural failure, or major bleeding at 30 days was numerically lower in patients assigned to LMWH, but the benefit was not statistically significant ($p=0.06$). However, there was a significant benefit with LMWH regarding the secondary composite endpoint of death, recurrent ACS, and urgent revascularization and in the primary endpoint when data were analyzed according to per protocol analysis [78]. Subgroup analysis did not find significant heterogeneity for the primary and secondary outcome according to gender. In women, results were directionally the same compared to men [77].

6.6.3 Bivalirudin

Bivalirudin is a synthetic direct thrombin inhibitor with several theoretic advantages over unfractionated heparin: greater thrombin specificity, linear kinetic, shorter half-life, lack of platelet activation, and heparin-induced thrombocytopenia and action on clot bound and circulating thrombin.

Bivalirudin has been suggested as a replacement for heparin as antithrombotic agent during PCI due to reduced bleeding rates (at least compared to a combination of heparin plus glycoprotein IIb/IIIa inhibitors and high heparin doses) while providing similar protection from peri-procedural ischemic complications. Since women are more susceptible to bleeding, the use of bivalirudin seems particularly attractive in this population.

Subgroup analyses of the pivotal bivalirudin trials ACUITY [79], REPLACE-2 [80], and HORIZONS-AMI [81] did not find a significant interaction for gender and treatment effect regarding composite ischemic, bleeding, and net clinical endpoints.

Also in the randomized ISAR-REACT 3 and 4 trials comparing bivalirudin against heparin monotherapy in biomarker-negative patients [82] and bivalirudin against heparin plus abciximab in NSTEMI patients [83], no interaction of gender with treatment effect was observed.

A more refined analysis of the ISAR-REACT 3 trial of biomarker-negative patients aimed to identify subsets of patients at high risk of bleeding or myocardial infarction and to investigate whether such high-risk subsets derive preferential benefit from heparin or bivalirudin. Bivalirudin was found to be most advantageous in reducing the risk of bleeding in patients at low risk, such as younger patients, men, patients with greater body weight, and those with single lesion intervention. Bivalirudin was not helpful in reducing the risk of bleeding in subsets of patients at a higher risk for this event. Moreover, the use of bivalirudin in the subgroup of patients with low bleeding risk was associated with a trend towards an increased risk of myocardial infarction [84].

6.6.4 Fondaparinux

Fondaparinux – a synthetic pentasaccharide – indirectly inhibits factor Xa via binding to antithrombin III.

In the double-blind OASIS 6 trial of 12,092 STEMI patients (3,345 women), the benefit of fondaparinux was limited to patients receiving thrombolysis or no reperfusion therapy. In patients undergoing primary PCI, fondaparinux was associated with potential harm. There was an increased risk of guiding catheter thrombosis and subsequent coronary complications with fondaparinux [85]. The results of death or myocardial infarction were not significantly heterogeneous in women and men.

In the double-blind OASIS 5 trial of 20,078 patients (7,699 women) with NSTE-ACS, the use of fondaparinux over 6 days was noninferior to enoxaparin regarding the composite ischemic endpoint of death, myocardial infarction, or refractory ischemia at 9 days. The rate of major bleeding was significantly lower with fondaparinux, resulting in improved net clinical benefit and decreased mortality at 30 and 180 days. Results for the primary efficacy endpoint and the safety endpoint of major bleeding were consistent in women and men (primary efficacy endpoint: women RR 1.08, 95 % CI 0.89–1.30, men RR 0.97, 95 % CI 0.83–1.12, p interaction = 0.48; major bleeding women RR 0.46, 95 % CI 0.34–0.58, men RR 0.61, 95 % CI 0.49–0.76, p interaction = 0.07) (Table 6.2).

6.7 Duration of Dual Antiplatelet Therapy After Drug-Eluting Stent Implantation

Patients with drug-eluting stenting (DES) implantation require a regimen of dual antiplatelet therapy (DAPT) with ASA plus $P2Y_{12}$ ADP receptor antagonist. While ASA is usually prescribed lifelong, ADP receptor blocker therapy duration has been discussed controversially.

The double-blind DAPT trial of 9,961 DES patients (2,526 women) showed that prolonging DAPT (with clopidogrel or prasugrel) for up to 30 months prevents myocardial infarction and stent thrombosis. However, the DAPT trial also showed that this strategy may cause harm by increasing bleeding and mortality [88]. In the DAPT trial, the effect of prolonged DAPT on the risk of definite or probable stent thrombosis and on MI was not consistent in women and men. There was no difference in the direction of treatment effect but in magnitude: Men showed significant reduction in stent thrombosis and MI, whereas the results was nonsignificant in women (stent thrombosis: HR women 0.73, 95 % CI 0.28–1.91; HR men 0.21, 95 % CI 0.11–0.39, p interaction = 0.04; MI: HR women 0.76, 95 % CI 0.48–1.19, HR men 0.41, 95 % CI 0.31–0.55, p interaction = 0.03). There was no interaction on treatment effect on GUSTO moderate or severe bleeding [88].

In contrast, a number of RCTs have shown that shortening DAPT duration to 6 months is safe, especially after new-generation DES implantation, and that this strategy does not expose the patient to an increased bleeding risk [9–11, 13, 15–17]. The largest and only double blind of these trials, the ISAR-SAFE trial evaluated the value of shortening DAPT duration from 12 to 6 months after DES

Table 6.2 Gender-specific efficacy and safety of anticoagulant drugs

Drug	Comparator	Indication	No. of individuals	Follow-up	Efficacy endpoint	Relative risk (95 % CI)	Safety endpoint	Relative risk (95 % CI)	Reference
Indirect thrombin inhibitors									
Enoxaparin	Unfractionated heparin	STEMI, undergoing thrombolysis	W = 4,783 M = 15,696	30 days	Death or nonfatal MI	W: 0.84 (0.74–0.95) M: 0.82 (0.74–0.90)	TIMI major bleeding	W: 1.64 (1.07–2.51) M: NA	ExTRACT-TIMI 25 trial. Mega et al., *Circulation* 2007 [74]
Enoxaparin	Unfractionated heparin	STEMI	W = 97 M = 353	30 days	Death, recurrent ACS, or urgent revascularization	W: 0.72 (0.32–1.61) M: 0.55 (0.33–0.91)	Major bleeding	0.92 (0.51–1.66) *No gender-specific analysis*	ATOLL trial, Montalescot et al., Lancet 2011 [77]
Dalteparin	Placebo	NSTE-ACS	W = 539 M = 959	6 days	Death or MI	W: 0.16 (0.05–0.56) M: 0.55 (0.28–1.11)	Major bleeding	NA	FRISC trial, Lancet 1996 [70]
Direct thrombin inhibitors									

(continued)

Table 6.2 (continued)

Drug	Comparator	Indication	No. of individuals	Follow-up	Efficacy endpoint	Relative risk (95 % CI)	Safety endpoint	Relative risk (95 % CI)	Reference
Bivalirudin	Heparin + planned GPIIb/IIIa inhibitor	Planned PCI, not for acute MI	W = 1,537 M = 4,465	30 days	Death, MI, or urgent revascularization	W: 0.90 (0.62–1.31) M: 1.16 (0.93–1.44)	Inhospital major bleeding	W: 0.61 (0.38–0.99) M: 0.54 (0.37–0.79)	REPLACE-2 trial, Chacko et al., *Am Heart J* 2006 [80]
	Heparin + planned GPIIb/IIIa inhibitor	NSTE-ACS with early invasive strategy	W = 4,157 M = 9,662	30 days	Death, recurrent MI, or revascularization	W: 1.23 (0.92–1.65) M: NA	Non-CABG TIMI major bleeding	W: 0.31 (0.14–0.65) M: NA	ACUITY trial, Lansky et al., *Am J Cardiol* 2009 [79]
	Heparin + planned GPIIb/IIIa inhibitor	STEMI within 12 h of symptom onset, undergoing PCI	W = 399 M = 1,322	30 days	Death, recurrent MI, target vessel revascularization for ischemia or stroke	W: 0.99 (0.60–1.62) M:1.00 (0.71–1.39)	Major bleeding	W: 0.60 (0.39–0.91) M: 0.56 (0.41–0.77)	HORIZONS-AMI trial, Yu et al., *Catheter Cardiovasc Interv* 2014 [81]
	Unfractionated heparin	Biomarker negative, undergoing PCI	W = 1,075 M = 3,495	1 year	Death, recurrent MI, or target vessel revascularization	W: 0.85 (0.64–1.12) M: 1.03 (0.88–1.21)	Inhospital REPLACE-2 major bleeding	W: 0.69 (0.43–1.13) M: 0.63 (0.42–0.94)	*ISAR*-REACT 3, Kastrati et al., *New Engl J Med*, 2008, Iijima et al., *Eur Heart J* 2009 [84], Schulz et al., Eur Heart J 2010 [86]
	Abciximab plus unfractionated heparin	NSTEMI, undergoing PCI	W = 399 M = 1,322	12 months	Death, recurrent MI, or target vessel revascularization	W: 0.80 (0.55–1.17) M:1.10 (0.86–1.40)	Non-CABG TIMI major bleeding	W: 0.60 (0.26–1.39) M: 0.52 (0.27–1.02)	ISAR-REACT 4 trial, Mehilli et al., *Am Heart J* 2013 [60]

Factor Xa inhibitors									
Fondaparinux	Enoxaparin	NSTE-ACS	W = 7,699 M = 12,379	9 days	Death, MI, or refractory ischemia	W: 1.08 (0.89–1.30) M:0.97 (0.83–1.12)	Major bleeding	W: 0.46 (0.34–0.58) M:0.61 (0.49–0.76)	OASIS-5 Investigators *NEJM* 2006 [87]
	Enoxaparin	STEMI	W = 3,345 M = 8,746	30 days	Death or recurrent MI	W: 0.87 (0.74–1.04) M:0.86 (0.74–1.00)	Modified TIMI major bleeding	0.77 (0.55–1.08) *No gender-specific analysis*	OASIS-6 Investigators, *JAMA* 2006 [85]

NA not available, *CABG* aortocoronary bypass graft, *M* men, *MI* myocardial infarction, *PCI* percutaneous coronary intervention, *NSTEMI* non-ST-segment elevation myocardial infarction, *STEMI* ST-segment elevation myocardial infarction, *TIMI* thrombolysis in myocardial infarction, *W* women, *OASIS* Organization to Assess Strategies in Acute Ischemic Syndromes implantation. At 15 months after DES implantation, there was no difference in the composite net clinical endpoint in patients randomized to either 6 or 12 months of DAPT. However, there was a significant interaction for age and treatment effect regarding net clinical outcome and the combined ischemic endpoint, suggesting a benefit with shorter duration of clopidogrel therapy in older and longer duration in younger patients. There was no significant interaction for gender. Of note, the trial was stopped prematurely after inclusion of 4005 of 6000 patients, and event rates were much lower than expected. Moreover, interpreting subgroup results in an overall negative trial is challenging [89].

Recently, in the double-blind PEGASUS-TIMI 54 trial, 21,162 patients (5,060 women) with myocardial infarction 1–3 years earlier were randomly assigned in a 1:1:1 fashion to either ticagrelor 90 mg twice daily, ticagrelor 60 mg twice daily, or placebo. After a median of 33 months, the primary efficacy end point – the composite of cardiovascular death, myocardial infarction, or stroke – was significantly reduced in both ticagrelor groups. However, increased efficacy occurred at the expense of a doubled risk of major bleeding. Overall mortality was not significantly impacted. Thus, in patients characterized by an excessive risk of ischemic complications and low bleeding risk, the use of ticagrelor beyond 1 year maybe beneficial. There was no heterogeneity of treatment effect according to gender regarding the primary efficacy endpoint and bleeding (Table 6.3) [90].

6.7.1 Triple Therapy

Oral anticoagulation is required in patients with mechanical heart valves, atrial fibrillation and other conditions. A substantial proportion of these patients will have to undergo PCI and are therefore in additional need of dual antiplatelet therapy.

In one open-label trial of 573 patients (115 women), the omission of ASA compared to triple therapy with oral anticoagulation plus clopidogrel and ASA resulted in favorable outcome regarding bleeding complications without increasing ischemic complications. There was no gender-specific treatment effect regarding bleeding events [91].

The other open-label randomized clinical trial regarding triple therapy aimed to assess optimal clopidogrel therapy duration as part of triple therapy. A total of 614 patients (143 women) were randomly assigned to either 6 weeks or 6 months of clopidogrel as part of triple therapy. At 9 months, there was no difference in net clinical outcome between both groups. Overall event rates were higher in women. Again no interaction for gender and treatment effect was observed.

Protein binding of warfarin is influenced by sex hormones. Women and especially old women require a lower warfarin dose compared to men. If hormone replacement therapy is initiated, dose adjustment is required [14].

Table 6.3 Duration of dual antiplatelet therapy

Drug	Duration	Type of study	No. of individuals	Efficacy endpoint	Relative risk (95 % CI)	Safety endpoint	Relative risk (95 % CI)	Reference
Clopidogrel	6 versus 12 months	Randomized, double-blind trial	W = 777 M = 3,223	Composite of death, MI, definite or probable stent thrombosis, or stroke	W: 0.33 (0.07–1.66) M: 1.00 (0.57–1.76)	TIMI major bleeding	W: NA M: 0.66 (0.24–1.87)	ISAR-SAFE trial, Schulz-Schüpke et al., *Eur Heart J*, 2015 [89]
Clopidogrel or prasugrel	12 versus 30 months	Randomized, double-blind trial	W = 2,526 M = 7,435	Stent thrombosis (ARC definite or probable)	W: 0.73 (0.28–1.91 M:0.21 (0.11–0.39)	GUSTO moderate or severe bleeding	W: 1.34 (0.79–2.26) M: 1.76 (1.24,2.50)	DAPT-Trial, Mauri et al., *N Engl J Med*, 2014 [88]
Ticagrelor 60 or 90 mg bid	Placebo	Randomized, double-blind trial	W = 5,060 M = 16,102	Cardiovascular death, MI, or stroke	Ticagrelor 90 mg W: 0.74 (0.57–0.95) M: 0.89 (0.77–1.02)	TIMI major bleeding	W: 2.34 (1.16–4.70) M: 2.78 (1.94–3.97)	Pegasus-Trial, Bonaca et al., *N Engl J Med*, 2015 [90]
					Ticagrelor 60 mg W: 0.98 (0.78–1.24) M: 0.79 (0.69–0.91)		W: 2.51 (1.27–4.98) M: 2.27 (1.57–3.27)	

ARC Academic Research Consortium, *M* men, *MI* myocardial infarction, *TIMI* thrombolysis in myocardial infarction, *W* women

References

1. Califf RM, DeLong ER, Ostbye T, Muhlbaier LH, Chen A, LaPointe NA, Hammill BG, McCants CB, Kramer JM. Underuse of aspirin in a referral population with documented coronary artery disease. Am J Cardiol. 2002;89(6):653–61.
2. Blomkalns AL, Chen AY, Hochman JS, Peterson ED, Trynosky K, Diercks DB, Brogan GX, Jr., Boden WE, Roe MT, Ohman EM, Gibler WB, Newby LK, Investigators C. Gender disparities in the diagnosis and treatment of non-ST-segment elevation acute coronary syndromes: large-scale observations from the CRUSADE (Can Rapid Risk Stratification of Unstable Angina Patients Suppress Adverse Outcomes With Early Implementation of the American College of Cardiology/American Heart Association Guidelines) National Quality Improvement Initiative. J Am Coll Cardiol. 2005;45(6):832–7.
3. Mosca L, Linfante AH, Benjamin EJ, Berra K, Hayes SN, Walsh BW, Fabunmi RP, Kwan J, Mills T, Simpson SL. National study of physician awareness and adherence to cardiovascular disease prevention guidelines. Circulation. 2005;111(4):499–510.
4. Pepine CJ, Kerensky RA, Lambert CR, Smith KM, von Mering GO, Sopko G, Bairey Merz CN. Some thoughts on the vasculopathy of women with ischemic heart disease. J Am Coll Cardiol. 2006;47(3 Suppl):S30–5.
5. Hamm CW, Bassand JP, Agewall S, Bax J, Boersma E, Bueno H, Caso P, Dudek D, Gielen S, Huber K, Ohman M, Petrie MC, Sonntag F, Uva MS, Storey RF, Wijns W, Zahger D, Guidelines ESCCfP. ESC Guidelines for the management of acute coronary syndromes in patients presenting without persistent ST-segment elevation: The Task Force for the management of acute coronary syndromes (ACS) in patients presenting without persistent ST-segment elevation of the European Society of Cardiology (ESC). Eur Heart J. 2011;32(23):2999–3054.
6. Mehilli J, Ndrepepa G, Kastrati A, Neumann FJ, Ten Berg J, Bruskina O, Dotzer F, Seyfarth M, Pache J, Kufner S, Dirschinger J, Berger PB, Schomig A. Sex and effect of abciximab in patients with acute coronary syndromes treated with percutaneous coronary interventions: results from Intracoronary Stenting and Antithrombotic Regimen: Rapid Early Action for Coronary Treatment 2 trial. Am Heart J. 2007;154(1):158.e1–7.
7. Ndrepepa G, Berger PB, Mehilli J, Seyfarth M, Neumann FJ, Schomig A, Kastrati A. Periprocedural bleeding and 1-year outcome after percutaneous coronary interventions: appropriateness of including bleeding as a component of a quadruple end point. J Am Coll Cardiol. 2008;51(7):690–7.
8. Ndrepepa G, Guerra E, Schulz S, Fusaro M, Cassese S, Kastrati A. Weight of the bleeding impact on early and late mortality after percutaneous coronary intervention. J Thromb Thrombolysis. 2015;39(1):35–42.
9. Alexander KP, Chen AY, Newby LK, Schwartz JB, Redberg RF, Hochman JS, Roe MT, Gibler WB, Ohman EM, Peterson ED, Investigators C. Sex differences in major bleeding with glycoprotein IIb/IIIa inhibitors: results from the CRUSADE (Can Rapid risk stratification of Unstable angina patients Suppress ADverse outcomes with Early implementation of the ACC/AHA guidelines) initiative. Circulation. 2006;114(13):1380–7.
10. Ndrepepa G, Schulz S, Neumann FJ, Byrne RA, Hoppmann P, Cassese S, Ott I, Fusaro M, Ibrahim T, Tada T, Richardt G, Laugwitz KL, Schunkert H, Kastrati A. Bleeding after percutaneous coronary intervention in women and men matched for age, body mass index, and type of antithrombotic therapy. Am Heart J. 2013;166(3):534–40.
11. Moukarbel GV, Signorovitch JE, Pfeffer MA, McMurray JJ, White HD, Maggioni AP, Velazquez EJ, Califf RM, Scheiman JM, Solomon SD. Gastrointestinal bleeding in high risk survivors of myocardial infarction: the VALIANT Trial. Eur Heart J. 2009;30(18):2226–32.
12. Sandgren T, Sonesson B, Ahlgren R, Lanne T. The diameter of the common femoral artery in healthy human: influence of sex, age, and body size. J Vasc Surg. 1999;29(3):503–10.
13. Argulian E, Patel AD, Abramson JL, Kulkarni A, Champney K, Palmer S, Weintraub W, Wenger NK, Vaccarino V. Gender differences in short-term cardiovascular outcomes after percutaneous coronary interventions. Am J Cardiol. 2006;98(1):48–53.
14. Rosano GM, Lewis B, Agewall S, Wassmann S, Vitale C, Schmidt H, Drexel H, Patak A, Torp-Pedersen C, Kjeldsen KP, Tamargo J. Gender differences in the effect of cardiovascular drugs:

a position document of the Working Group on Pharmacology and Drug Therapy of the ESC. Eur Heart J. 2015.

15. Oertelt-Prigione S, Regitz-Zagrosek V. Gender aspects in cardiovascular pharmacology. J Cardiovasc Transl Res. 2009;2(3):258–66.
16. Ho PC, Triggs EJ, Bourne DW, Heazlewood VJ. The effects of age and sex on the disposition of acetylsalicylic acid and its metabolites. Br J Clin Pharmacol. 1985;19(5):675–84.
17. Gum PA, Kottke-Marchant K, Welsh PA, White J, Topol EJ. A prospective, blinded determination of the natural history of aspirin resistance among stable patients with cardiovascular disease. J Am Coll Cardiol. 2003;41(6):961–5.
18. Eikelboom JW, Hirsh J, Weitz JI, Johnston M, Yi Q, Yusuf S. Aspirin-resistant thromboxane biosynthesis and the risk of myocardial infarction, stroke, or cardiovascular death in patients at high risk for cardiovascular events. Circulation. 2002;105(14):1650–5.
19. Eikelboom JW, Hankey GJ, Thom J, Bhatt DL, Steg PG, Montalescot G, Johnston SC, Steinhubl SR, Mak KH, Easton JD, Hamm C, Hu T, Fox KA, Topol EJ. Clopidogrel for High Atherothrombotic R, Ischemic Stabilization M, Avoidance I. Incomplete inhibition of thromboxane biosynthesis by acetylsalicylic acid: determinants and effect on cardiovascular risk. Circulation. 2008;118(17):1705–12.
20. Cattaneo M. Letter by cattaneo regarding article, "incomplete inhibition of thromboxane biosynthesis by acetylsalicylic Acid: determinants and effect on cardiovascular risk". Circulation. 2009;119(24):e594; author reply e595–6.
21. Becker DM, Segal J, Vaidya D, Yanek LR, Herrera-Galeano JE, Bray PF, Moy TF, Becker LC, Faraday N. Sex differences in platelet reactivity and response to low-dose aspirin therapy. JAMA. 2006;295(12):1420–7.
22. Mayer K, Bernlochner I, Braun S, Schulz S, Orban M, Morath T, Cala L, Hoppmann P, Schunkert H, Laugwitz KL, Kastrati A, Sibbing D. Aspirin treatment and outcomes after percutaneous coronary intervention: results of the ISAR-ASPI registry. J Am Coll Cardiol. 2014;64(9):863–71.
23. Antithrombotic Trialists C, Baigent C, Blackwell L, Collins R, Emberson J, Godwin J, Peto R, Buring J, Hennekens C, Kearney P, Meade T, Patrono C, Roncaglioni MC, Zanchetti A. Aspirin in the primary and secondary prevention of vascular disease: collaborative meta-analysis of individual participant data from randomised trials. Lancet. 2009;373(9678): 1849–60.
24. Antithrombotic TC. Collaborative meta-analysis of randomised trials of antiplatelet therapy for prevention of death, myocardial infarction, and stroke in high risk patients. BMJ. 2002;324(7329):71–86.
25. Manson JE, Stampfer MJ, Colditz GA, Willett WC, Rosner B, Speizer FE, Hennekens CH. A prospective study of aspirin use and primary prevention of cardiovascular disease in women. JAMA. 1991;266(4):521–7.
26. Berger JS, Roncaglioni MC, Avanzini F, Pangrazzi I, Tognoni G, Brown DL. Aspirin for the primary prevention of cardiovascular events in women and men: a sex-specific meta-analysis of randomized controlled trials. JAMA. 2006;295(3):306–13.
27. Algra A, Greving JP. Aspirin in primary prevention: sex and baseline risk matter. Lancet. 2009;373(9678):1821–2.
28. Ridker PM, Cook NR, Lee IM, Gordon D, Gaziano JM, Manson JE, Hennekens CH, Buring JE. A randomized trial of low-dose aspirin in the primary prevention of cardiovascular disease in women. N Engl J Med. 2005;352(13):1293–304.
29. Rothwell PM, Wilson M, Elwin CE, Norrving B, Algra A, Warlow CP, Meade TW. Long-term effect of aspirin on colorectal cancer incidence and mortality: 20-year follow-up of five randomised trials. Lancet. 2010;376(9754):1741–50.
30. Schomig A, Neumann FJ, Kastrati A, Schuhlen H, Blasini R, Hadamitzky M, Walter H, Zitzmann-Roth EM, Richardt G, Alt E, Schmitt C, Ulm K. A randomized comparison of antiplatelet and anticoagulant therapy after the placement of coronary-artery stents. N Engl J Med. 1996;334(17):1084–9.
31. Bertrand ME, Rupprecht HJ, Urban P, Gershlick AH. Double-blind study of the safety of clopidogrel with and without a loading dose in combination with aspirin compared with

ticlopidine in combination with aspirin after coronary stenting : the clopidogrel aspirin stent international cooperative study (CLASSICS). Circulation. 2000;102(6):624–9.
32. Windecker S, Kolh P, Alfonso F, Collet JP, Cremer J, Falk V, Filippatos G, Hamm C, Head SJ, Juni P, Kappetein AP, Kastrati A, Knuuti J, Landmesser U, Laufer G, Neumann FJ, Richter DJ, Schauerte P, Sousa Uva M, Stefanini GG, Taggart DP, Torracca L, Valgimigli M, Wijns W, Witkowski A, Authors/Task Force m. 2014 ESC/EACTS Guidelines on myocardial revascularization: The Task Force on Myocardial Revascularization of the European Society of Cardiology (ESC) and the European Association for Cardio-Thoracic Surgery (EACTS). Developed with the special contribution of the European Association of Percutaneous Cardiovascular Interventions (EAPCI). Eur Heart J. 2014;35(37):2541–619.
33. Jochmann N, Stangl K, Garbe E, Baumann G, Stangl V. Female-specific aspects in the pharmacotherapy of chronic cardiovascular diseases. Eur Heart J. 2005;26(16):1585–95.
34. Price MJ, Berger PB, Teirstein PS, Tanguay JF, Angiolillo DJ, Spriggs D, Puri S, Robbins M, Garratt KN, Bertrand OF, Stillabower ME, Aragon JR, Kandzari DE, Stinis CT, Lee MS, Manoukian SV, Cannon CP, Schork NJ, Topol EJ, Investigators G. Standard- vs high-dose clopidogrel based on platelet function testing after percutaneous coronary intervention: the GRAVITAS randomized trial. JAMA. 2011;305(11):1097–105.
35. Sibbing D, Braun S, Morath T, Mehilli J, Vogt W, Schomig A, Kastrati A, von Beckerath N. Platelet reactivity after clopidogrel treatment assessed with point-of-care analysis and early drug-eluting stent thrombosis. J Am Coll Cardiol. 2009;53(10):849–56.
36. Steinhubl SR, Berger PB, Mann 3rd JT, Fry ET, DeLago A, Wilmer C, Topol EJ. Observation CICftRoED. Early and sustained dual oral antiplatelet therapy following percutaneous coronary intervention: a randomized controlled trial. JAMA. 2002;288(19):2411–20.
37. Mehta SR, Yusuf S, Peters RJ, Bertrand ME, Lewis BS, Natarajan MK, Malmberg K, Rupprecht H, Zhao F, Chrolavicius S, Copland I, Fox KA. Effects of pretreatment with clopidogrel and aspirin followed by long-term therapy in patients undergoing percutaneous coronary intervention: the PCI-CURE study. Lancet. 2001;358(9281):527–33.
38. Berger JS, Bhatt DL, Cannon CP, Chen Z, Jiang L, Jones JB, Mehta SR, Sabatine MS, Steinhubl SR, Topol EJ, Berger PB. The relative efficacy and safety of clopidogrel in women and men a sex-specific collaborative meta-analysis. J Am Coll Cardiol. 2009;54(21): 1935–45.
39. Zaccardi F, Pitocco D, Willeit P, Laukkanen JA. Efficacy and safety of P2Y12 inhibitors according to diabetes, age, gender, body mass index and body weight: Systematic review and meta-analyses of randomized clinical trials. Atherosclerosis. 2015;240(2):439–45.
40. U.S. Food and Drug Administration Cardiovascular and Renal Drugs Advisory Committee Briefing Document on prasugrel. Available at: http://www.fda.gov/downloads/AdvisoryCommittees/CommitteesMeetingMaterials/Drugs/CardiovascularandRenalDrugsAdvisoryCommittee/ucm129219.pdf.
41. Wiviott SD, Braunwald E, McCabe CH, Montalescot G, Ruzyllo W, Gottlieb S, Neumann FJ, Ardissino D, De Servi S, Murphy SA, Riesmeyer J, Weerakkody G, Gibson CM, Antman EM. Prasugrel versus clopidogrel in patients with acute coronary syndromes. N Engl J Med. 2007;357(20):2001–15.
42. Hochholzer W, Wiviott SD, Antman EM, Contant CF, Guo J, Giugliano RP, Dalby AJ, Montalescot G, Braunwald E. Predictors of bleeding and time dependence of association of bleeding with mortality: insights from the Trial to Assess Improvement in Therapeutic Outcomes by Optimizing Platelet Inhibition With Prasugrel—Thrombolysis in Myocardial Infarction 38 (TRITON-TIMI 38). Circulation. 2011;123(23):2681–9.
43. Wiviott SD, White HD, Ohman EM, Fox KA, Armstrong PW, Prabhakaran D, Hafley G, Lokhnygina Y, Boden WE, Hamm C, Clemmensen P, Nicolau JC, Menozzi A, Ruzyllo W, Widimsky P, Oto A, Leiva-Pons J, Pavlides G, Winters KJ, Roe MT, Bhatt DL. Prasugrel versus clopidogrel for patients with unstable angina or non-ST-segment elevation myocardial infarction with or without angiography: a secondary, prespecified analysis of the TRILOGY ACS trial. Lancet. 2013;382(9892):605–13.

44. Montalescot G, Bolognese L, Dudek D, Goldstein P, Hamm C, Tanguay JF, ten Berg JM, Miller DL, Costigan TM, Goedicke J, Silvain J, Angioli P, Legutko J, Niethammer M, Motovska Z, Jakubowski JA, Cayla G, Visconti LO, Vicaut E, Widimsky P, Investigators A. Pretreatment with prasugrel in non-ST-segment elevation acute coronary syndromes. N Engl J Med. 2013;369(11):999–1010.
45. Teng R, Mitchell P, Butler K. Effect of age and gender on pharmacokinetics and pharmacodynamics of a single ticagrelor dose in healthy individuals. Eur J Clin Pharmacol. 2012;68(8):1175–82.
46. Wallentin L, Becker RC, Budaj A, Cannon CP, Emanuelsson H, Held C, Horrow J, Husted S, James S, Katus H, Mahaffey KW, Scirica BM, Skene A, Steg PG, Storey RF, Harrington RA, Investigators P, Freij A, Thorsen M. Ticagrelor versus clopidogrel in patients with acute coronary syndromes. N Engl J Med. 2009;361(11):1045–57.
47. Montalescot G, van't Hof AW, Lapostolle F, Silvain J, Lassen JF, Bolognese L, Cantor WJ, Cequier A, Chettibi M, Goodman SG, Hammett CJ, Huber K, Janzon M, Merkely B, Storey RF, Zeymer U, Stibbe O, Ecollan P, Heutz WM, Swahn E, Collet JP, Willems FF, Baradat C, Licour M, Tsatsaris A, Vicaut E, Hamm CW, Investigators A. Prehospital ticagrelor in ST-segment elevation myocardial infarction. N Engl J Med. 2014;371(11):1016–27.
48. Bhatt DL, Lincoff AM, Gibson CM, Stone GW, McNulty S, Montalescot G, Kleiman NS, Goodman SG, White HD, Mahaffey KW, Pollack Jr CV, Manoukian SV, Widimsky P, Chew DP, Cura F, Manukov I, Tousek F, Jafar MZ, Arneja J, Skerjanec S, Harrington RA, Investigators CP. Intravenous platelet blockade with cangrelor during PCI. N Engl J Med. 2009;361(24):2330–41.
49. Harrington RA, Stone GW, McNulty S, White HD, Lincoff AM, Gibson CM, Pollack Jr CV, Montalescot G, Mahaffey KW, Kleiman NS, Goodman SG, Amine M, Angiolillo DJ, Becker RC, Chew DP, French WJ, Leisch F, Parikh KH, Skerjanec S, Bhatt DL. Platelet inhibition with cangrelor in patients undergoing PCI. N Engl J Med. 2009;361(24):2318–29.
50. Bhatt DL, Harrington RA, Committee CPE. Investigators. Platelet inhibition with cangrelor during PCI. N Engl J Med. 2013;369(4):393–4.
51. Steg PG, Bhatt DL, Hamm CW, Stone GW, Gibson CM, Mahaffey KW, Leonardi S, Liu T, Skerjanec S, Day JR, Iwaoka RS, Stuckey TD, Gogia HS, Gruberg L, French WJ, White HD, Harrington RA, Investigators C. Effect of cangrelor on peri-procedural outcomes in percutaneous coronary interventions: a pooled analysis of patient-level data. Lancet. 2013;382(9909): 1981–92.
52. Faraday N, Goldschmidt-Clermont PJ, Bray PF. Gender differences in platelet GPIIb-IIIa activation. Thromb Haemost. 1997;77(4):748–54.
53. Inhibition of platelet glycoprotein IIb/IIIa with eptifibatide in patients with acute coronary syndromes. The PURSUIT Trial Investigators. Platelet glycoprotein IIb/IIIa in unstable angina: receptor suppression using integrilin therapy. N Engl J Med. 1998;339(7):436–43.
54. Boersma E, Harrington RA, Moliterno DJ, White H, Simoons ML. Platelet glycoprotein IIb/IIIa inhibitors in acute coronary syndromes. Lancet. 2002;360(9329):342–3.
55. Cho L, Topol EJ, Balog C, Foody JM, Booth JE, Cabot C, Kleiman NS, Tcheng JE, Califf R, Lincoff AM. Clinical benefit of glycoprotein IIb/IIIa blockade with Abciximab is independent of gender: pooled analysis from EPIC, EPILOG and EPISTENT trials. Evaluation of 7E3 for the Prevention of Ischemic Complications. Evaluation in Percutaneous Transluminal Coronary Angioplasty to Improve Long-Term Outcome with Abciximab GP IIb/IIIa blockade. Evaluation of Platelet IIb/IIIa Inhibitor for Stent. J Am Coll Cardiol. 2000;36(2):381–6.
56. Fernandes LS, Tcheng JE, O'Shea JC, Weiner B, Lorenz TJ, Pacchiana C, Berdan LG, Maresh KJ, Joseph D, Madan M, Mann T, Kilaru R, Hochman JS, Kleiman NS, investigators E. Is glycoprotein IIb/IIIa antagonism as effective in women as in men following percutaneous coronary intervention?. Lessons from the ESPRIT study. J Am Coll Cardiol. 2002;40(6):1085–91.
57. Iakovou I, Dangas G, Mehran R, Lansky AJ, Kobayashi Y, Adamian M, Polena S, Collins MB, Roubin GS, Stone GW, Leon MB, Moses JW. Gender differences in clinical outcome after coronary artery stenting with use of glycoprotein IIb/IIIa inhibitors. Am J Cardiol. 2002;89(8): 76–9.

58. Kastrati A, Mehilli J, Schuhlen H, Dirschinger J, Dotzer F, ten Berg JM, Neumann FJ, Bollwein H, Volmer C, Gawaz M, Berger PB, Schomig A. A clinical trial of abciximab in elective percutaneous coronary intervention after pretreatment with clopidogrel. N Engl J Med. 2004;350(3):232–8.
59. Kastrati A, Mehilli J, Neumann FJ, Dotzer F, ten Berg J, Bollwein H, Graf I, Ibrahim M, Pache J, Seyfarth M, Schuhlen H, Dirschinger J, Berger PB, Schomig A. Abciximab in patients with acute coronary syndromes undergoing percutaneous coronary intervention after clopidogrel pretreatment: the ISAR-REACT 2 randomized trial. JAMA. 2006;295(13):1531–8.
60. Mehilli J, Neumann FJ, Ndrepepa G, King L, Schulz S, Maimer Rodrigues da Cunha F, Jochheim D, Byrne RA, Hausleiter J, Ott I, Massberg S, Kastrati A, Pache J. Sex-related effectiveness of bivalirudin versus abciximab and heparin in non-ST-segment elevation myocardial infarction. Am Heart J. 2013;165(4):537–43.
61. Mehilli J, Kastrati A, Schulz S, Frungel S, Nekolla SG, Moshage W, Dotzer F, Huber K, Pache J, Dirschinger J, Seyfarth M, Martinoff S, Schwaiger M, Schomig A. Abciximab in patients with acute ST-segment-elevation myocardial infarction undergoing primary percutaneous coronary intervention after clopidogrel loading: a randomized double-blind trial. Circulation. 2009;119(14):1933–40.
62. Mehta SR, Yusuf S, Peters RJ, Bertrand ME, Lewis BS, Natarajan MK, Malmberg K, Rupprecht H, Zhao F, Chrolavicius S, Copland I, Fox KA. Effects of pretreatment with clopidogrel and aspirin followed by long-term therapy in patients undergoing percutaneous coronary intervention: the PCI-CURE study. Lancet. 2001;358(9281):527–33.
63. Boersma E, Harrington RA, Moliterno DJ, White H, Theroux P, Van de Werf F, de Torbal A, Armstrong PW, Wallentin LC, Wilcox RG, Simes J, Califf RM, Topol EJ, Simoons ML. Platelet glycoprotein IIb/IIIa inhibitors in acute coronary syndromes: a meta-analysis of all major randomised clinical trials. Lancet. 2002;359(9302):189–98.
64. Amsterdam EA, Wenger NK, Brindis RG, Casey DE, Jr., Ganiats TG, Holmes DR, Jr., Jaffe AS, Jneid H, Kelly RF, Kontos MC, Levine GN, Liebson PR, Mukherjee D, Peterson ED, Sabatine MS, Smalling RW, Zieman SJ, American College of C, American Heart Association Task Force on Practice G, Society for Cardiovascular A, Interventions, Society of Thoracic S, American Association for Clinical C. 2014 AHA/ACC Guideline for the Management of Patients with Non-ST-Elevation Acute Coronary Syndromes: a report of the American College of Cardiology/American Heart Association Task Force on Practice Guidelines. J Am Coll Cardiol. 2014;64(24):e139–228.
65. Granger CB, Hirsch J, Califf RM, Col J, White HD, Betriu A, Woodlief LH, Lee KL, Bovill EG, Simes RJ, Topol EJ. Activated partial thromboplastin time and outcome after thrombolytic therapy for acute myocardial infarction: results from the GUSTO-I trial. Circulation. 1996;93(5):870–8.
66. Hirsh J, Warkentin TE, Raschke R, Granger C, Ohman EM, Dalen JE. Heparin and low-molecular-weight heparin: mechanisms of action, pharmacokinetics, dosing considerations, monitoring, efficacy, and safety. Chest. 1998;114(5 Suppl):489S–510.
67. Falvo N, Bonithon-Kopp C, Rivron Guillot K, Todoli JA, Jimenez-Gil M, Di Micco P, Monreal M, Investigators R. Heparin-associated thrombocytopenia in 24,401 patients with venous thromboembolism: findings from the RIETE Registry. J Thromb Haemost. 2011;9(9): 1761–8.
68. Becker RC, Spencer FA, Gibson M, Rush JE, Sanderink G, Murphy SA, Ball SP, Antman EM, Investigators TA. Influence of patient characteristics and renal function on factor Xa inhibition pharmacokinetics and pharmacodynamics after enoxaparin administration in non-ST-segment elevation acute coronary syndromes. Am Heart J. 2002;143(5):753–9.
69. Toss H, Wallentin L, Siegbahn A. Influences of sex and smoking habits on anticoagulant activity in low-molecular-weight heparin treatment of unstable coronary artery disease. Am Heart J. 1999;137(1):72–8.
70. Low-molecular-weight heparin during instability in coronary artery disease, Fragmin during Instability in Coronary Artery Disease (FRISC) study group. Lancet. 1996;347(9001):561–8.

71. Montalescot G, White HD, Gallo R, Cohen M, Steg PG, Aylward PE, Bode C, Chiariello M, King 3rd SB, Harrington RA, Desmet WJ, Macaya C, Steinhubl SR. Enoxaparin versus unfractionated heparin in elective percutaneous coronary intervention. N Engl J Med. 2006;355(10):1006–17.
72. Cohen M, Demers C, Gurfinkel EP, Turpie AG, Fromell GJ, Goodman S, Langer A, Califf RM, Fox KA, Premmereur J, Bigonzi F. A comparison of low-molecular-weight heparin with unfractionated heparin for unstable coronary artery disease. Efficacy and Safety of Subcutaneous Enoxaparin in Non-Q-Wave Coronary Events Study Group. N Engl J Med. 1997;337(7):447–52.
73. Antman EM, Morrow DA, McCabe CH, Murphy SA, Ruda M, Sadowski Z, Budaj A, Lopez-Sendon JL, Guneri S, Jiang F, White HD, Fox KA, Braunwald E, Ex T-TI. Enoxaparin versus unfractionated heparin with fibrinolysis for ST-elevation myocardial infarction. N Engl J Med. 2006;354(14):1477–88.
74. Mega JL, Morrow DA, Ostor E, Dorobantu M, Qin J, Antman EM, Braunwald E. Outcomes and optimal antithrombotic therapy in women undergoing fibrinolysis for ST-elevation myocardial infarction. Circulation. 2007;115(22):2822–8.
75. Ferguson JJ, Califf RM, Antman EM, Cohen M, Grines CL, Goodman S, Kereiakes DJ, Langer A, Mahaffey KW, Nessel CC, Armstrong PW, Avezum A, Aylward P, Becker RC, Biasucci L, Borzak S, Col J, Frey MJ, Fry E, Gulba DC, Guneri S, Gurfinkel E, Harrington R, Hochman JS, Kleiman NS, Leon MB, Lopez-Sendon JL, Pepine CJ, Ruzyllo W, Steinhubl SR, Teirstein PS, Toro-Figueroa L, White H, Investigators ST. Enoxaparin vs unfractionated heparin in high-risk patients with non-ST-segment elevation acute coronary syndromes managed with an intended early invasive strategy: primary results of the SYNERGY randomized trial. JAMA. 2004;292(1):45–54.
76. Task Force on Myocardial Revascularization of the European Society of C, the European Association for Cardio-Thoracic S, European Association for Percutaneous Cardiovascular I, Wijns W, Kolh P, Danchin N, Di Mario C, Falk V, Folliguet T, Garg S, Huber K, James S, Knuuti J, Lopez-Sendon J, Marco J, Menicanti L, Ostojic M, Piepoli MF, Pirlet C, Pomar JL, Reifart N, Ribichini FL, Schalij MJ, Sergeant P, Serruys PW, Silber S, Sousa Uva M, Taggart D. Guidelines on myocardial revascularization. Eur Heart J. 2010;31(20):2501–55.
77. Montalescot G, Zeymer U, Silvain J, Boulanger B, Cohen M, Goldstein P, Ecollan P, Combes X, Huber K, Pollack Jr C, Benezet JF, Stibbe O, Filippi E, Teiger E, Cayla G, Elhadad S, Adnet F, Chouihed T, Gallula S, Greffet A, Aout M, Collet JP, Vicaut E, Investigators A. Intravenous enoxaparin or unfractionated heparin in primary percutaneous coronary intervention for ST-elevation myocardial infarction: the international randomised open-label ATOLL trial. Lancet. 2011;378(9792):693–703.
78. Collet JP, Huber K, Cohen M, Zeymer U, Goldstein P, Pollack Jr C, Silvain J, Henry P, Varenne O, Carrie D, Coste P, Angioi M, Le Breton H, Cayla G, Elhadad S, Teiger E, Filippi E, Aout M, Vicaut E, Montalescot G, Investigators A. A direct comparison of intravenous enoxaparin with unfractionated heparin in primary percutaneous coronary intervention (from the ATOLL trial). Am J Cardiol. 2013;112(9):1367–72.
79. Lansky AJ, Mehran R, Cristea E, Parise H, Feit F, Ohman EM, White HD, Alexander KP, Bertrand ME, Desmet W, Hamon M, Stone GW. Impact of gender and antithrombin strategy on early and late clinical outcomes in patients with non-ST-elevation acute coronary syndromes (from the ACUITY trial). Am J Cardiol. 2009;103(9):1196–203.
80. Chacko M, Lincoff AM, Wolski KE, Cohen DJ, Bittl JA, Lansky AJ, Tsuchiya Y, Betriu A, Yen MH, Chew DP, Cho L, Topol EJ. Ischemic and bleeding outcomes in women treated with bivalirudin during percutaneous coronary intervention: a subgroup analysis of the Randomized Evaluation in PCI Linking Angiomax to Reduced Clinical Events (REPLACE)-2 trial. Am Heart J. 2006;151(5):1032.e1–7.
81. Yu J, Mehran R, Grinfeld L, Xu K, Nikolsky E, Brodie BR, Witzenbichler B, Kornowski R, Dangas GD, Lansky AJ, Stone GW. Sex-based differences in bleeding and long term adverse events after percutaneous coronary intervention for acute myocardial infarction: three year results from the HORIZONS-AMI trial. Catheter Cardiovasc Interv. 2015;85(3):359–68.

82. Kastrati A, Neumann FJ, Mehilli J, Byrne RA, Iijima R, Buttner HJ, Khattab AA, Schulz S, Blankenship JC, Pache J, Minners J, Seyfarth M, Graf I, Skelding KA, Dirschinger J, Richardt G, Berger PB, Schomig A. Bivalirudin versus unfractionated heparin during percutaneous coronary intervention. N Engl J Med. 2008;359(7):688–96.
83. Kastrati A, Neumann FJ, Schulz S, Massberg S, Byrne RA, Ferenc M, Laugwitz KL, Pache J, Ott I, Hausleiter J, Seyfarth M, Gick M, Antoniucci D, Schomig A, Berger PB, Mehilli J. Abciximab and heparin versus bivalirudin for non-ST-elevation myocardial infarction. N Engl J Med. 2011;365(21):1980–9.
84. Iijima R, Ndrepepa G, Mehilli J, Byrne RA, Schulz S, Neumann FJ, Richardt G, Berger PB, Schomig A, Kastrati A. Profile of bleeding and ischaemic complications with bivalirudin and unfractionated heparin after percutaneous coronary intervention. Eur Heart J. 2009;30(3):290–6.
85. Yusuf S, Mehta SR, Chrolavicius S, Afzal R, Pogue J, Granger CB, Budaj A, Peters RJ, Bassand JP, Wallentin L, Joyner C, Fox KA, Group O-T. Effects of fondaparinux on mortality and reinfarction in patients with acute ST-segment elevation myocardial infarction: the OASIS-6 randomized trial. JAMA. 2006;295(13):1519–30.
86. Schulz S, Mehilli J, Ndrepepa G, Neumann FJ, Birkmeier KA, Kufner S, Richardt G, Berger PB, Schomig A, Kastrati A. Bivalirudin vs. unfractionated heparin during percutaneous coronary interventions in patients with stable and unstable angina pectoris: 1-year results of the ISAR-REACT 3 trial. Eur Heart J. 2010;31(5):582–7.
87. Fifth Organization to Assess Strategies in Acute Ischemic Syndromes I, Yusuf S, Mehta SR, Chrolavicius S, Afzal R, Pogue J, Granger CB, Budaj A, Peters RJ, Bassand JP, Wallentin L, Joyner C, Fox KA. Comparison of fondaparinux and enoxaparin in acute coronary syndromes. N Engl J Med. 2006;354(14):1464–76.
88. Mauri L, Kereiakes DJ, Yeh RW, Driscoll-Shempp P, Cutlip DE, Steg PG, Normand SL, Braunwald E, Wiviott SD, Cohen DJ, Holmes Jr DR, Krucoff MW, Hermiller J, Dauerman HL, Simon DI, Kandzari DE, Garratt KN, Lee DP, Pow TK, Ver Lee P, Rinaldi MJ, Massaro JM, Investigators DS. Twelve or 30 months of dual antiplatelet therapy after drug-eluting stents. N Engl J Med. 2014;371(23):2155–66.
89. Schulz-Schupke S, Byrne RA, Ten Berg JM, Neumann FJ, Han Y, Adriaenssens T, Tölg R, Seyfarth M, Maeng M, Zrenner B, Jacobshagen C, Mudra H, von Hodenberg E, Wöhrle J, Angiolillo DJ, von Merzljak B, Rifatov N, Kufner S, Morath T, Feuchtenberger A, Ibrahim T, Janssen PW, Valina C, Li Y, Desmet W, Abdel-Wahab M, Tiroch K, Hengstenberg C, Bernlochner I, Fischer M, Schunkert H, Laugwitz KL, Schömig A, Mehilli J, Kastrati A, Intracoronary Stenting and Antithrombotic Regimen: Safety And EFficacy of 6 Months Dual Antiplatelet Therapy After Drug-Eluting Stenting (ISAR-SAFE) Trial Investigators. ISAR-SAFE: a randomized, double-blind, placebo-controlled trial of 6 versus 12 months of clopidogrel therapy after drug-eluting stenting. Eur Heart J. 2015;36(20):1252–63.
90. Bonaca MP, Bhatt DL, Cohen M, Steg PG, Storey RF, Jensen EC, Magnina G, Bansilal S, Fish PM, Im K, Bengtsson O, Ophuis TO, Budaj A, Theroux P, Ruda M, Hamm C, Goto S, Spinar J, Nicolau JC, Kiss RG, Murphy SA, Wiviott SD, Held C, Braunwald E, Sabatine MS. Long-term use of ticagrelor in patients with prior myocardial infarction. N Engl J Med. 2015. doi:10.1056/NEJMoa1500857.
91. Dewilde WJ, Oirbans T, Verheugt FW, Kelder JC, De Smet BJ, Herrman JP, Adriaenssens T, Vrolix M, Heestermans AA, Vis MM, Tijsen JG, van't Hof AW, ten Berg JM, investigators Ws. Use of clopidogrel with or without aspirin in patients taking oral anticoagulant therapy and undergoing percutaneous coronary intervention: an open-label, randomised, controlled trial. Lancet. 2013;381(9872):1107–15.

Part II

Structural Heart Disease

Aortic Valve Valvuloplasty

7

Cristina Giannini

7.1 Percutaneous Aortic Valvuloplasty in the Transcatheter Aortic Valve Implantation Era

Aortic stenosis (AS) represents the most frequent heart valve disease in developed countries and its prevalence and impact on public health is expected to increase due to aging Western population. A recent meta-analysis described that AS occurs in 12.4 % of the general elderly (≥75 years of age) population and severe AS is present in 3.4 %. Among patients with severe AS, 75.6 % are symptomatic, and 40.5 % of these patients did not undergo surgical aortic valve replacement (SAVR) due to excessive operative risk, advanced age, comorbidities, and patient's preference [1].

Percutaneous balloon aortic valvuloplasty (BAV) was proposed in 1986 by Alain Cribier as a new therapeutic approach in a large number of high-risk candidates mostly elderly, in whom surgical treatment was often referred [2]. However, after initial exciting results surrounding this technique, the interest in BAV waned subsequently because of early recurrence of stenosis. Several studies reported an unacceptable incidence of serious complications around 25 % within the first 24 h and in-hospital mortality between 3.5 and 10 % [3]. Moderate or severe aortic regurgitation was noted in 2 % of the cases. The benefit of the procedure has proved to be of brief duration and 75 % of the patients developed evidence of restenosis within 6 months of valvuloplasty. Furthermore, the long-term outcome was dismal and resembled the natural history of critical AS [4].

The recent introduction of transcatheter aortic valve implantation (TAVI) has renewed interest in the use of BAV, and the number of BAV procedure will continue to increase in the near future. BAV plays an integral role in TAVI, and it is used to

C. Giannini, MD, PhD
Cardio-Thoracic and Vascular Department, Azienda Ospedaliero-Universitaria Pisana, Pisa, Italy
e-mail: crigiannini@hotmail.it

P. Presbitero et al. (eds.), *Percutaneous Treatment of Cardiovascular Diseases in Women*, DOI 10.1007/978-3-319-39611-8_7

allow easier valve delivery, to measure annular size, and to evaluate displacement of the aortic valve leaflets adjacent to the left main coronary artery. In particular, when measurements of the aortic annulus are ambiguous and borderline, supra-aortic angiography during preparatory BAV provides a simple, direct, and effective measure to improve sizing with a reduction of paravalvular leak frequency and severity.

Multiple modifications with technical improvement have been made in the BAV technique over the past years which contributed to a significant reduction of serious adverse events. In particular, the incidence of major vascular complications has been lowered compared with previous series [5]. This improvement may be attributed to the newer balloon catheter that allows the use of a 10-F sheath instead of a 13-F sheath as well as the use of vascular closure devices for arterial hemostasis. Moreover, most of these patients had an assessment of peripheral arteries by multidetector computed tomography as a part of screening for TAVI, thereby allowing to choose the better side for a safer vascular approach [6]. Furthermore, the introduction of rapid ventricular pacing during BAV enables to optimize balloon positioning and stability [5]. These changes and others have led to overall lower complication rates. The study by Eltchaninoff et al., enrolling 323 patients who underwent BAV, showed a lower incidence of major adverse events (6.8 %) as compared with previous studies ranging from 16.2 to 31 % [3, 5, 6].

This marked improvements and the development of TAVI resurged new possible indications in the use of BAV. Currently, the European guidelines recommended BAV with very restrictive indications, as a bridge to SAVR or TAVI in hemodynamically unstable patients who are at high risk for surgery or in patients with symptomatic severe AS who require urgent noncardiac surgery (recommendation class IIb, level of evidence C). Balloon aortic valvuloplasty for acquired AS may be also considered as a palliative measure in selected individual cases when surgery is contraindicated because of severe comorbidities and TAVI is not an option [7]. Data from many studies reported that a considerable proportion of patients referred for TAVI are judged not eligible for the procedure at the time of referral [8]. In these high-risk patients with temporary contraindications to TAVI, BAV can be used as a bridge with the hope that the patient will improve sufficiently to become suitable for intervention. Investigators have widely shown that long-term outcomes in BAV patients' bridge to SAVR or TAVI are superior to outcomes in palliative use alone. Recently, Saia et al. demonstrated that patients successfully bridged to TAVI or SAVR had survival rate equivalent to those who had undergone primary TAVI or SAVR; otherwise, without a definite therapy, the survival rate was equivalent to that of medical therapy alone [9]. Finally, BAV can also help to identify which patients are suitable for a definitive valve intervention (TAVI or SAVR) when other comorbidities such as concomitant chronic obstructive pulmonary disease and severe left ventricular dysfunction raise concerns about symptom reversibility. For those patients who experience symptom relief after BAV, more definitive treatments should be considered.

7.2 Indications of Percutaneous Balloon Aortic Valvuloplasty: Sex-Related Differences

Although gender differences in cardiovascular disease have been explored for a long time, only a limited number of studies have been conducted to show differences between male and female patients with severe AS in terms of clinical presentation and outcome.

It has been reported that women receive medical care later than men, either because they wait longer before visiting a doctor or because it takes longer until they are referred to surgery. In fact, the left ventricle of women adapt differently to AS, developing more pronounced hypertrophy with super normal ejection fraction, which could have influenced the time of the diagnosis with symptoms appearing later and lead to older age at the time of intervention [10]. Bach et al. have showed that women and patients aged >80 years had lower rate referral to a specialist, diagnostic testing, and SAVR compared to men and to patients aged 65–79 years [11]. In particular, SAVR was performed at approximately half the rate in women (1.4 %) compared to men (2.7 %, $p<0.001$), and in patients aged >80 years (1.1 %) compared to those aged 65–79 years (2.5 %, $p<0.001$). Lower rates of SAVR in women may have been due to excessive operative risks that would preclude safe intervention. It has been demonstrated that at presentation, female patients with severe AS tend to be more symptomatic and with more associated advanced diseases and have a higher predicted operative risk related to the presence of more comorbidities, lower body surface area, and older age [12]. A recent meta-analysis including 6.645 patients with symptomatic severe AS reported that at time of referral, women were older, with higher ejection fraction, more severe mean pressure gradients, and smaller valve areas compared to men [13].

The recent introduction of TAVI opened new perspectives for the treatment of female patients with severe AS at a very high surgical risk. In fact, the available TAVI data show that females are more represented than in previous surgical series with the proportion of women similar or even greater than that of men [13]. However, a large proportion of women may be not offered even TAVI because they are judged to be too old and frail at the time of presentation. Despite the higher prevalence of well-known comorbid conditions affecting outcome detected in male patients with AS, other unweighted risk factors are present in women such us advanced age and frailty.

In elderly populations, frailty has emerged as an important risk factor for morbidity and mortality in multiple clinical situations. Recently, several publications reported that frailty is associated with increased mortality and a higher rate of poor outcome in elderly patients undergoing cardiac surgery. In addition, small, single-center studies identified frailty status as independent predictors of adverse short- and long-term outcomes even after TAVI procedures. Plus et al. followed a cohort of 300 high-risk patients undergoing TAVI and showed that frail patients were on average of 2 years older ($p=0.0004$) and more likely to be female ($p=0.01$) [14]. Woman therefore may be more often suited to undergo BAV intervention for palliation of symptoms with the hope to improve sufficiently to become suitable for a definitive therapy compared to men. In line with these findings, recently Ben-Dor et al. reported that women represented more than one half of the total patients screened but not eligible for TAVI and treated with medical therapy plus balloon valvuloplasty [5].

Another possible explanation is that lower body surface area in women, known to be associated with a decreased survival, could influence the therapeutic decision leading to BAV.

However, in the transcatheter valve era, no studies have been conducted to describe gender differences in patients with AS referred for BAV used whether standalone or as a bridge to TAVI.

7.3 Gender Difference During Aortic Balloon Valvuloplasty: Technical Issues

Several studies have emphasized the existence of sex differences in the left ventricular adaptation to AS [10, 13]. In particular, Carroll et al. have observed that women with severe AS are more likely than men to respond to the pressure load with concentric hypertrophy, small-volume, and hyperdynamic ejection performance [10]. All these baseline characteristics are important in understanding the pathophysiology of AS and have practical consequences for the management and choice of BAV. Women patients are highly prone to complication due to stiff wire manipulation and possible LV perforation. Nevertheless, asymmetric LV hypertrophy and small LV outflow tract, frequent among women, should make the procedure more challenging (Fig. 7.1).

Other important issues of BAV procedure in female patients are smaller aortic annulus and smaller vascular access [15]. It has been demonstrated that women with AS have smaller body size and consequently smaller aortic annulus and reduced ileofemoral diameters compared to men [16]. A recent multicenter study, enrolling more than 600 patients with severe AS referred for TAVI, reported that females have smaller aortic annulus and body surface area than men [17]. Smaller aortic annulus has a potential risk of annulus rupture due to the relative balloon oversizing. Annulus rupture or perforation is a rare but catastrophic complication of BAV associated with a high risk of procedural death (Fig. 7.1) [5]. Despite technical improvement, recent reports show similar rates of annulus rupture as compared with previous studies, although this

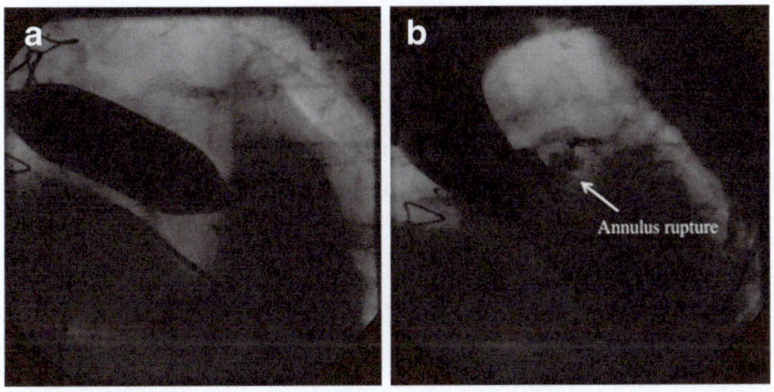

Fig. 7.1 (**a**) BAV performed with a 22 mm balloon catheter in a woman with a mean annuls diameter of 21 mm. (**b**) Annulus rupture through the free LV myocardial occurred after the second aggressive balloon inflation. An evident contrast extravasation (*white arrow*) was identified during angiography. The patient was treated by unplanned TAVI but she died during the procedure

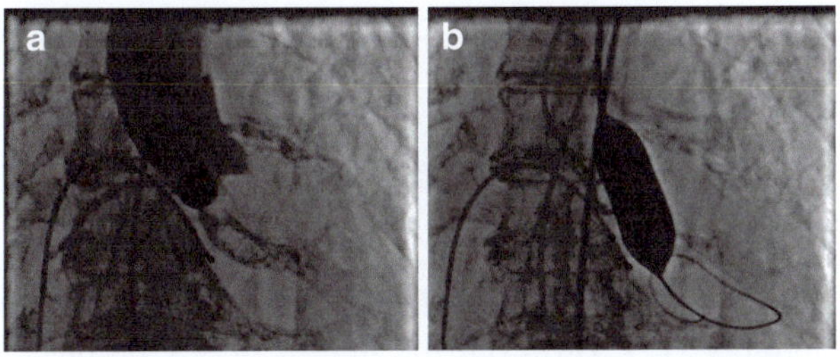

Fig. 7.2 (**a**) Aortic angiography view of a female with a small aortic annulus. At transthoracic echocardiography mean annulus diameter was 19 mm. (**b**) Moderately aggressive BAV was performed successfully with the utilization of undersized balloon (18 mm balloon catheter) to reduce the risk of annulus damage

complication remains infrequent [6]. Accurate measurement of the aortic root using multidetector CT or transesophageal echocardiography is crucial for appropriate device sizing allowing to avoid this drawback. Furthermore, a moderately aggressive BAV technique, meaning utilization of balloons often undersized without the pursuit of achieving excellent hemodynamic results, allows to reduce the chances of annulus damage (Fig. 7.2).

Vascular access is also an important issue in female patients undergoing BAV. Reduced ileofemoral diameters increase the sheath to femoral artery ratio, resulting in a higher risk of vascular complications which have been shown to be associated with significant increase in mortality [18]. Recently the introduction of newer balloon catheters that allow the use of a 10-F sheath instead of a 13-F sheath may contribute to reduce the incidence of vascular complications even in patients of small body size. Moreover, the precise assessment of ileofemoral diameter and calcification with the use multidetector computer tomography, in patients screened but not eligible for TAVI and treated with BAV, let to choose the better side for a safer vascular approach.

In the TAVI setting, the limited availability of device plays a crucial role, representing a major limitation for transarterial approach, especially for women with small femoral arteries. In such selected case, when alternative TAVI approaches are not available, BAV may also be considered a palliative measure.

Acute coronary occlusion from embolic calcium is another rare potential problem during BAV. In fact, Ben-Dor et al. reported an incidence of coronary occlusion/dissection after BAV about 0.6 % [5]. The shorter distance between coronary ostia and aortic annulus in female patients with small body size could increase the risk of coronary occlusion by calcium embolization [16]. Furthermore, the more advanced aortic disease in women associated with higher trans-aortic gradients and higher degree of leaflet calcifications may contribute to a higher incidence of coronary occlusion compared with men [13].

7.4 Impact of Female Gender on BAV Outcome

Predictors of mortality in patients undergoing BAV have been previously reported (Otto 1994).

Otto et al. analyzed the largest series of nonsurgical patients treated with BAV in 24 centers in North America and identified the female gender as an independent predictor of mortality [19]. However, the impact of sex on outcome after BAV remains unclear and to be defined. Recently, Ben-Dor et al. analyzed a large cohort of patients screened but not eligible for TAVI and treated with balloon valvuloplasty and reported that women had a higher survival rates compared to men [5]. Several reports confirmed this result, demonstrating that the female sex is associated with a better outcome even among patients undergoing TAVI [13]. Furthermore, in the retrospective subanalysis of the PARTNER trial, female subjects had a lower late mortality with TAVI versus SAVR [20].

Nevertheless, female gender is actually considered a risk factor for surgical procedure, even in isolated valve operation, both in the Society of Thoracic Surgeon (STS) predicted risk of mortality score and in the EuroSCORE II. Others studies, however, questioned this finding, reporting a significant better long-term survival in women compared with men after SAVR with a bioprosthesis [21]. A randomized controlled trial conducted in female high-risk patients with AS is necessary to study differences in mortality between treatment modalities.

Conclusion

With the recent introduction of TAVI, there has been resurgence in the use of BAV, either as a bridge to TAVI in patients at high risk of periprocedural complications or as an additional selection tool whenever there are doubts about the indications to TAVI.

In this setting, the effect of gender may be relevant to understand timing and opportunity of percutaneous intervention, but none of the studies have investigated gender-specific differences in outcomes after BAV. In the future, it seems mandatory to collect more prospective data to accurately evaluate risk and strategy for patients with severe AS with regard to sex.

References

1. Osnabrugge RL, Mylotte D, Head SJ, et al. Aortic stenosis in the elderly: disease prevalence and number of candidates for transcatheter aortic valve replacement: a meta-analysis and modeling study. J Am Coll Cardiol. 2013;62:1002–12.
2. Cribier A, Savin T, Saoudi N, Rocha P, Berland J, Letac B. Percutaneous transluminal valvuloplasty of acquired aortic stenosis in elderly patients: an alternative to valve replacement? Lancet. 1986;1:63–7.
3. Safian RD, Berman AD, Diver DJ, et al. Balloon aortic valvuloplasty in 170 consecutive patients. N Engl J Med. 1988;319:125–30.
4. Lieberman EB, Bashore TM, Hermiller JB, et al. Balloon aortic valvuloplasty in adults: failure of procedure to improve long-term survival. J Am Coll Cardiol. 1995;26:1522–8.
5. Ben-Dor I, Pichard AD, Satler LF, et al. Complications and outcome of balloon aortic valvuloplasty in high-risk or inoperable patients. JACC Cardiovasc Interv. 2010;3:1150–6.
6. Eltchaninoff H, Durand E, Borz B, et al. Balloon aortic valvuloplasty in the era of transcatheter aortic valve replacement: acute and long-term outcomes. Am Heart J. 2014;167:235–40.
7. Vahanian A, Alfieri O, Andreotti F, et al. Guidelines on the management of valvular heart disease (version 2012): the Joint Task Force on the Management of Valvular Heart Disease of the European Society of Cardiology (ESC) and the European Association for Cardio-Thoracic Surgery (EACTS). Eur J Cardiothorac Surg. 2012;42:S1–44.
8. De Carlo M, Giannini C, Ettori F, et al. Impact of treatment choice on the outcome of patients proposed for transcatheter aortic valve implantation. EuroIntervention. 2010;6:568–74.
9. Saia F, Marrozzini C, Moretti C, et al. The role of percutaneous balloon aortic valvuloplasty as a bridge for transcatheter aortic valve implantation. EuroIntervention. 2011;7:723–9.
10. Carroll JD, Carroll EP, Feldman T, et al. Sex-associated differences in left ventricular function in aortic stenosis of the elderly. Circulation. 1992;86:1099–107.
11. Bach DS, Radeva JI, Birnbaum HG, Fournier AA, Tuttle EG. Prevalence, referral patterns, testing, and surgery in aortic valve disease: leaving women and elderly patients behind? J Heart Valve Dis. 2007;16:362–9.
12. Fuchs C, Mascherbauer J, Rosenhek R, et al. Gender differences in clinical presentation and surgical outcome of aortic stenosis. Heart. 2010;96:539–45.
13. Conrotto F, D'Ascenzo F, Presbitero P, et al. Effect of gender after transcatheter aortic valve implantation: a meta-analysis. Ann Thorac Surg. 2015;99:809–16.
14. Puls M, Sobisiak B, Bleckmann A, et al. Impact of frailty on short- and long-term morbidity and mortality after transcatheter aortic valve implantation: risk assessment by Katz Index of activities of daily living. EuroIntervention. 2014;10:609–19.
15. Buja P, Napodano M, Tamburino C, et al. Comparison of variables in men versus women undergoing transcatheter aortic valve implantation for severe aortic stenosis (from Italian Multicenter CoreValve Registry). Am J Cardiol. 2013;111:88–93.
16. Watanabe Y, Hayashida K, Lefèvre T, et al. Transcatheter aortic valve implantation in patients of small body size. Catheter Cardiovasc Interv. 2014;84:272–80.

17. Ferrante G, Pagnotta P, Petronio AS, et al. Sex differences in postprocedural aortic regurgitation and mid-term mortality after transcatheter aortic valve implantation. Catheter Cardiovasc Interv. 2014;84(2):264–71.
18. Hayashida K, Lefèvre T, Chevalier B, et al. True percutaneous approach for transfemoral aortic valve implantation using the Prostar XL device: impact of learning curve on vascular complications. JACC Cardiovasc Interv. 2012;5:207–14.
19. Otto CM, Mickel MC, Kennedy JW, et al. Three-year outcome after balloon aortic valvuloplasty. Insights into prognosis of valvular aortic stenosis. Circulation. 1994;89:642–50.
20. Williams M, Kodali SK, Hahn RT, et al. Sex-related differences in outcomes after transcatheter or surgical aortic valve replacement in patients with severe aortic stenosis: insights from the PARTNER trial (Placement of Aortic Transcatheter Valve). J Am Coll Cardiol. 2014;63:1522–8.
21. Kulik A, Burwash IG, Kapila V, Mesana TG, Ruel M. Long-term outcomes after valve replacement for low-gradient aortic stenosis: impact of prosthesis-patient mismatch. Circulation. 2006;114:I553–8.

8 Transcatheter Aortic Valve Implantation

Martine Gilard and Jacques Boschat

Transcatheter aortic valve replacement (TAVI) is becoming a widespread therapeutic alternative to surgery for patients with symptomatic aortic stenosis (AS) who are deemed to be at high or prohibitive surgical risk, with more than 80,000 procedures performed to date in over 40 countries worldwide [1]. A lower risk profile and lower mortality have been reported in women than men after TAVI at medium-term follow-up [2], while other studies found similar or worse survival compared with males [3]. In this setting, the effect of gender may be relevant to understanding the timing and appropriateness of percutaneous coronary intervention (PCI).

At present, a small number of registries have investigated gender-specific differences in outcome after TAVI, reporting variable results [4–9]. Some data are available from the randomized PARTNER trial [10], and four meta-analyses have so far been published [1, 11–13]. The available TAVI data show a greater proportion of women than in previous coronary clinical trials, in which the inclusion rate of female patients has historically been low. In the FRANCE 2 registry, 49 % of participants were female [4]. In the PARTNER trial, in the subgroup of patients at high surgical risk who were assigned to undergo TAVI, 42.2 % were female; 39.3 % of patients treated via a femoral approach were female, compared with 49 % in the apical arm [10].

M. Gilard (✉)
Department of Cardiology, CHRU Brest, Brest, France
e-mail: martine.gilard@chu-brest.fr

J. Boschat
Department of Cardiology, University of Brest, Brest, France

P. Presbitero et al. (eds.), *Percutaneous Treatment of Cardiovascular Diseases in Women*,
DOI 10.1007/978-3-319-39611-8_8

8.1 Indications for TAVI in Women

Although gender differences in cardiovascular disease have long been studied, only a small number of studies investigated differences between male and female AS patients, in terms of clinical presentation and outcome after surgical aortic valve replacement (SAVR). Female patients with symptomatic AS tend to be older, more symptomatic, and with greater associated advanced disease burden [5]. Despite this, it has been shown that women who underwent SAVR had outcomes similar to those for men [14].

8.1.1 Comorbidities

The management of female AS patients at high surgical risk should take account of clinical presentation and associated comorbidity factors. The greater number of women included in TAVI series compared with coronary artery disease (CAD) series may depend on several factors. The lower body surface area (BSA) in female patients, which is known to be associated with poorer post-SAVR survival, may have influenced therapeutic decision-making in favor of TAVI.

Available registry data show fundamental differences in comorbidity factors (Table 8.1):

Table 8.1 Patient characteristics in FRANCE 2

	Female ($n=1967$)	Male ($n=2005$)	p value
Age, years	84.0 ± 6.6	81.6 ± 7.5	<0.001
Body mass index, kg/m^2	25.7 ± 5.4	26.3 ± 4.5	<0.001
Logistic EuroSCORE, %	21.4 ± 13	22.2 ± 15	0.97
Clinical history			
Coronary artery disease	918 (47.9 %)	1341 (69.0 %)	<0.001
Chronic obstructive pulmonary disease	397 (20.3 %)	503 (25.1 %)	0.003
Peripheral vascular disease	278 (14.2 %)	521 (26.1 %)	<0.001
Creatinine before procedure >200 mmol/l	120 (6.1 %)	220 (11.0 %)	<0.001
Cerebrovascular disease	191 (9.8 %)	198 (9.9 %)	0.91
Echocardiographic findings			
Mean gradient, mm Hg	51.0 ± 17.7	45.4 ± 14.8	<0.001
Effective orifice area indexed, cm^2/m^2	0.4 ± 0.2	0.4 ± 0.2	0.041
Ejection fraction, %	56.6 ± 13.3	50.1 ± 14.3	<0.001
Transfemoral TAVI approach	1536 (78.7 %)	1365 (68.4 %)	<0.001
Edwards SAPIEN/Medtronic CoreValve	73.2 %, 26.8 %	60.4 %, 39.6 %	<0.001
Echocardiographic findings, postprocedural			
Effective orifice area indexed, cm^2/m^2	1.1 ± 0.3	1.0 ± 0.3	0.13
Ejection fraction, %	58.2 ± 11.6	52.9 ± 12.9	<0.001
Pulmonary artery pressure, mm Hg	40.5 ± 12.1	41.2 ± 13.2	0.31
Moderate to severe aortic regurgitation	196 (11.8 %)	294 (17.1 %)	<0.001

- In the FRANCE 2 registry, female patients were older (84 vs. 81.6 years; $p<0.001$), with less frequent history of CAD (47.9 % vs. 69 %; $p<0.001$), chronic obstructive pulmonary disease (COPD), peripheral vascular disease (PVD), or renal failure (creatinine >200 μmol/l: 6.1 % vs. 11.0 %; $p<0.001$) [4].
- In contrast, the UK registry found higher female rates of COPD (25.1 % vs. 20.8 %; $p=0.04$) and chronic renal disease (6.8 % vs. 3.7 %; $p=0.006$) [7].
- In the Italian Observational Multicenter Registry (OBSERVANT Research Group), female TAVI patients had a different risk profile from males, with greater age (82.4 vs. 81.1 years; $p=0.005$), lower body weight (67.6 vs. 74.5 kg; $p<0.001$), and lower preoperative hemoglobin level (11.4 vs. 11.8 g/dL; $p<0.001$) but with similar New York Heart Association (NYHA) class (class III, 45 % vs. 43.4 %; class IV, 15.5 % vs. 13.8 %), frailty score (2 (partially self-sufficient), 24.8 % vs. 16.2 %) and European system for cardiac operative risk evaluation (EuroSCORE) (14.6 vs. 15.9; NS), and less frequent renal dysfunction, COPD, arteriopathy, or history of cardiovascular surgery or PCI ($p<0.01$) [6].
- Canadian and German registry data were similar to those of FRANCE 2 [8, 9].

The major findings of recent meta-analyses were significant sex differences in terms of age, CAD, COPD, and PVD [13, 15] (Table 8.2). In O'Connor's meta-analysis, 48.6 % ($n=5502$) of the 11,310 patients included in the final cohort were women. Men had higher rates of risk factors than women, with higher prevalences of diabetes and of history of myocardial infarction, PCI, coronary artery bypass graft, PVD, poor left ventricular systolic function (left ventricular ejection fraction <30 %) and three-vessel coronary artery disease, higher logistic EuroSCORE, and greater prevalence of pulmonary disease [1].

The difference in clinical presentation between men and women may partly be due to women having lower rates of specialist referral and thus receiving medical care later than men. They wait longer before consulting a doctor [16].

8.1.2 Left Ventricle Evolution

Several studies have emphasized the existence of sex differences in the left ventricle adaptation to AS. On average, women with AS develop thicker ventricles with better conservation of ejection fraction and less fibrosis than male counterparts [15]. Hence, despite being uniformly labeled as "severe AS patients" when presenting for aortic valve replacement (AVR), women and men may show markedly different phenotypes when the complete physiological picture of ventricular performance and valvulo-arterial impedance is considered.

Pressure overload leading to cardiac remodeling is largely influenced by gender; for example, hypertrophy is more frequently associated with the left ventricular dilation and systolic dysfunction in males, whereas geometry is more favorable to conserving systolic pump performance in women. Initial studies suggested that the

Table 8.2 Clinical baseline characteristics of patients enrolled in registries [3, 5, 9, 11], trial [12], and meta-analysis [13, 15]

	Age (year)		EuroSCORE (%)		COPD (%)		Previous MI (%)		Previous PCI (%)		Previous cardiac surgery (%)		NYHA III/IV	
	F	M	F	M	F	M	F	M	F	M	F	M	F	M
Hayashida [3]	83.8	82.4	22.3	26.2	38.2	36.4	7.6	21.7	25.2	35.6	13.7	26.4	86.3	82.9
Buja [5]	82	80	23	23	17	26	13	32	22	36	6.3	28	74	66
Al-Lamee [9]	82.6	80.8	21	21.8	21.8	25.1	13	29.5	17	18	12.7	40.9	20.1	19
Sherif [11]	82.8	80.3	21	20	20.8	28.3	11.5	21.9	30.2	40.5	13.9	33.6	90.7	85
Williams [12]	84.5	82.9	27.5	30.7	22.5	15	18.4	32.5	27.2	38.2	19	59.7	93.9	94.5
Zhao [13]	82.1	80.6	22.7	24	24.2	38.6	19.5	34.3	27.3	44.1	n.r	n.r	79.9	75.3
O'Connor [15]	83.3	81.6	22.2	23.9	28.2	31.4	14.6	28.6	17.6	23.4	14.1	41.1	n.r	n.r

All values are means

COPD chronic obstructive pulmonary disease, *MI* myocardial infarction, *PCI* percutaneous coronary intervention, *NYHA* New York Heart Association, *n.r.* not reported loss of the left ventricular mass after AVR is more frequent and rapid in women, allowing better normalization of ventricle biomechanics than in men. Taken together, these translational data point to the intriguing possibility that women with AS may exhibit a positive differential treatment response to TAVI.

8.2 Specific Female Anatomical Features for TAVI

The literature is unanimous in finding fundamental sex differences in ultrasound data and the size of arterial approaches.

8.2.1 Mean Aortic Valve Gradient

In the FRANCE 2 registry, mean aortic valve gradient was greater in women than in men (51 vs. 45 mmHg; $p<0.001$), as was mean ejection fraction (56 % vs. 50 %; $p<0.001$). Findings were similar in the other registry reports and in O'Connor's meta-analysis (61 % vs 55 %; $p<0.001$) [1]. Overall, mean aortic orifice diameter is 21 mm in women and 23 mm in men, which probably explains the observed difference in choice of valve for AVR. Thus, percentage use of CoreValve and SAPIEN implants was, respectively, 35.2 % and 64.8 % in women and 31.4 % and 67.9 % in men ($p<0.001$) in the 11,310 patients analyzed by O'Connor. Small (23 mm) valves are more often used in female patients (31.2 % vs. 10.8 %; $p<0.001$) [15]. The FRANCE 2 results are in agreement with the above: women, 26.8 % CoreValve and 73.2 % SAPIEN; men, 39.6 % and 60.4 %, respectively; $p<0.001$ [4].

8.2.2 Access

The most frequently used approach is femoral, but its safety greatly depends on iliofemoral axis assessment. Vascular axis diameters should be measured and tortuosity and calcification assessed. For this, CT angiography provides precious precise information. Minimum femoral dimensions are defined by the manufacturer's specifications based on introducer sheath size, which, in published studies, was 6 mm for 18Fr sheaths for the Medtronic CoreValve and 6–7 mm for Edwards SAPIEN XT. However, these sheath diameters are based on the devices' internal diameters. Moreover, excessive calcification at the femoral access site constitutes a risk factor independently of any major vascular complication.

The approach was more often femoral in women in the FRANCE 2 study (78.7 % vs. 68.4 % in men; $p<0.001$), probably due to a higher rate of peripheral vascular disease in males (14.2 % in women vs. 26.1 % in men; $p<0.001$) [4]. However, femoral approaches were globally smaller in women: 7.2 vs. 7.9 mm on the left and 7.5 vs. 7.7 mm on the right ($p<0.001$) [1].

The presence and degree of femoral and aortoiliac atheroma are an important factor to be taken into account in selecting the approach. Framingham's data are useful here: prevalence of abdominal aortic plaque, and of any aortic plaque, was higher in women than in men ($p<0.02$). Total plaque volume, both absolute and normalized to BSA, was larger in women than in men on thoracoabdominal aortic cardiac MRI ($p<0.05$) [17].

8.2.3 Coronary and Aortic Valve Calcifications

There are differences in the aortic valve itself, not only in terms of orifice size but also of degree of calcification. Because calcium is detectable noninvasively with CT imaging, it is possible to use the extent and distribution of calcification in cardiac valves, coronary arteries, and aorta as a diagnostic tool in risk stratification.

A significant gender difference in total coronary and aortic valve calcification in patients with severe AS was recently reported [18]. Men had more severe aortic and coronary calcification than women. Valvular calcification in AS patients has been linked to systemic calcified atherosclerosis. The identification of oxidized lipoproteins, inflammatory cells, and proteins activated by macrophages in aortic valve calcification suggests a similarity to the pathogenesis of coronary artery calcification. Furthermore, highly calcified stenotic aortic valves show greater oxidized low-density lipoprotein concentrations as well as increased expression of metalloproteinases [18].

The persistence of gender difference in coronary calcification in severe AS suggests that this cardioprotection against calcification continues beyond the menopause, and perhaps calcification itself may be either a delayed process or a process that continues once initiated.

8.3 Technical Issues and Complications

8.3.1 Procedural Device Success

Procedural device success rates are reportedly similar in women and men, with 97 % success [1]. The majority of registries and trials performed TAVI via the transfemoral approach [3–10], and this was more common in women than in men in the FRANCE 2 series (78.7 % vs. 68.4 %; $p<0.001$) and in O'Connor's meta-analysis (70.4 % vs. 67.9 %; $p=0.004$). In the majority of studies, implanted valves included the SAPIEN and SAPIEN XT devices in 23-, 26-, and 29-mm sizes (Edwards Lifesciences) and the CoreValve device in 23-, 26-, 29-, and 31-mm sizes (Medtronic).

8.3.2 Type of Device

Balloon-expandable devices were used more frequently than self-expandable valves [1, 4, 8], and a higher proportion of women than men received balloon-expandable valves [1].

8.3.3 Post-procedural Aortic Regurgitation

It remains unclear whether factors related to aortic valve implantation could contribute to differential mortality between men and women. Postprocedural aortic regurgitation (AR ≥ 2) has emerged as a predictor of increased mortality after TAVI in several studies [2, 5, 19] and was less frequent in women than men in a CoreValve registry (20.9 % vs. 29.6 %; $p=0.01$) [20]; AR grade 3/4 was also less frequent in women than men in a balloon-expandable device study (1.6 % vs. 3.1 %) [8]. The same finding was reported in O'Connor's meta-analysis: AR > 2 in 2.7 % of females vs. 4.6 % of males ($p<0.001$) [1].

8.3.4 Contrast-Induced Nephropathy

Contrast-induced nephropathy (CIN) is the third most common cause of acute renal failure and is associated with increased morbidity and in-hospital mortality. Some recent studies identified female gender as a risk factor for CIN. In O'Connor's meta-analysis, renal insufficiency (CrCL < 60 ml/mn/1.73 m^2) was more frequent in women than in men (66.1 % vs. 64.3 %; $p=0.04$) [1].

The impact of female gender on onset and clinical outcome of CIN after TAVI in patients with preexisting renal impairment was recently reported [21]. The women had significantly smaller BSA (1.8 vs. 1.95 m^2; $p=0.002$), lower hemoglobin levels (11.5 vs. 12.7 g/dL; $p<0.001$), and lower estimated glomerular filtration rate (34.2 vs. 49.4 mL/min/1.73 m^2; $p=0.002$). The frequency of CIN within 72 h after exposure to contrast medium was significantly greater in women (62.1 % vs. 26.9 %; $p=0.009$) [21].

8.3.5 Valve Migration

There was no difference in the incidence of valve migration or embolization, conversion to conventional surgery, or procedure-related death [1]. However, there was a higher rate of major vascular complications and major bleeding in women (Table 8.3).

8.3.6 Vascular Complications

There was an almost twofold higher rate of vascular complications in women in the FRANCE 2 registry (4.3 % vs. 1.9 %; $p<0.001$) [4]. In Stangl's meta-analysis, vascular complications were defined on Valve academic research consortium (VARC) criteria in eight studies and also used the following definitions: vascular rupture with fatal bleeding or need for surgical or percutaneous repair [3] and severe peripheral vascular complications (e.g., iliac artery rupture) [9]; there was a 1.72-fold greater vascular complications rate in women (odds ration (OR), 1.72 [95 % confidence interval (CI),

Table 8.3 Outcomes in France 2

	Female (n=1967)	Male (n=2005)	p value
Adverse events <24 h			
Major and life-threatening bleeding	85 (4.3 %)	38 (1.9 %)	0.001
Major vascular event	90 (4.6 %)	39 (1.9 %)	<0.001
Postprocedural pacemaker implantation (before 1 month)			
PPI total	184 (9.3 %)	257 (12.8 %)	<0.001
PPI in Medtronic CoreValve prosthesis	83 (15.8 %)	145 (18.2 %)	0.30
PPI in Edwards SAPIEN prosthesis	101 (17.0 %)	112 (9.3 %)	0.040
Combined safety end point at 1 month	448 (22.8 %)	407 (20.3 %)	0.058
Death			
At 1 month			
From any cause	187 (9.5 %)	184 (9.2 %)	0.27
From cardiovascular cause	125 (6.4 %)	133 (6.6 %)	0.35
From 1 month to 1 year			
From any cause	193(9.8 %)	291 (14.5 %)	<0.001
From cardiovascular cause	95 (4.8 %)	152 (7.6 %)	0.004
At 1 year (cumulative)			
From any cause	380 (19.3 %)	475 (23.7 %)	0.021
From cardiovascular cause	220 (11.2 %)	285 (14.2 %)	0.036

1.41, 2.09]) [12]. Vascular complications are related to smaller vessel size in women [2], introducer sheath to femoral artery ratio, and femoral artery calcium score [22].

8.3.7 Bleeding Complications

Women experienced higher rates of major and life-threatening bleeding in three meta-analyses [1, 11, 13]. Major bleeding at 30 days was significantly more frequent in female patients (10.5 % vs. 8.5 %; p=0.003) [1]. A significantly higher risk of major bleeding was also reported in meta-analyses by Conrotto (OR, 1.55 [95 % CI, 1.03, 2.34]) and Zhao (RR 0.82 [95 % CI, 0.68, 0.98]) [11, 13]. The mechanism for this is probably comparable to peri-PCI bleeding, in which female gender is a significant risk factor (smaller BSA and older age in female patients) [1].

Cardiac tamponade is more frequent in female than in male patients (1.3 % vs. 0.7 %; p=0.002) [1]. There are many predisposing factors for the development of tamponade in TAVI: calcified aortic annulus and fragile and scarred myocardium due to likely coexistence of ischemic heart disease with previous infarcts. Some cases of cardiac tamponade implicate temporary pacemakers.

8.3.8 Stroke

Stroke is a major complication of TAVI, associated with poor prognosis. However, recent reports have shown that stroke rates are decreasing, with reported in-hospital incidence of 1 % with a femoral approach [23]. This progressive drop can be attributed to multiple factors, such as technological progress, increased operator experience, better patient selection, standardized postprocedural neurological evaluation, antithrombotic treatment, and protection devices.

The vast majority of cases of stroke seem to be ischemic, occurring within the first 30 days; later excess stroke is attributable to hemorrhagic events [24]. O'Connor's study was the first meta-analysis to demonstrate a significantly higher rate of stroke in women undergoing TAVI [1]. This increased stroke risk seems to be associated with self-expandable but not balloon-expandable valves, without a clear explanation. There are no data for gender differences according to type of stroke.

8.3.9 Permanent Pacemaker

The FRANCE 2 registry reported more frequent postprocedural pacemaker implantation in men (12.8 % vs. 9.3 %; $p<0.001$) [4]; for women, rates of pacemaker implantation were higher in case of balloon-expandable valves (SAPIEN, Edwards Lifesciences, Irvine, CA), which may illustrate the impact of balloon expansion on smaller aortic roots (Table 8.3).

However, in contrast, in O'Connor's meta-analysis, in a sub-analysis of procedural and 30-day outcome according to valve type, pacemaker implantation was significantly more common in men in the self-expandable valve group (26.4 % vs. 19.4 %; $p<0.001$), while there was no significant sex difference in the balloon-expandable valve group (9.3 % vs. 8.4 %; $p=0.15$) [1].

These results are consistent with Zhao's meta-analysis including 1719 men and 2145 women. In studies that predominantly used the CoreValve, heart block requiring permanent pacemaker implantation was a common complication after TAVI, with an incidence of 31.3 % for men and 24.7 % for women. However, the rate of postprocedural pacemaker implantation was much lower in studies mainly using the Edwards valve: 8.0 % in men and 7.4 % in women [11].

8.4 Outcome in Women

Most follow-up studies according to gender concern short- (30 days) or medium-term (1–2 years) results; there are no long-term (5 years) data [3–10].

8.4.1 30-Day Outcome

Hayashida provided the first precise description of sex-related differences, in 260 patients with severe AS undergoing TAVI using both the Edwards valve and the CoreValve. Female gender was associated with lower comorbidity and lower EuroSCORE (22.3 ± 9.0 % vs. 26.2 ± 13.0 %; $p<0.005$), although no significant relationship with 30-day mortality was seen (12.2 % vs. 17.8 %; $p=0.207$) [2].

In the OBSERVANT registry (725 patients), EuroSCOREs did not differ according to gender (15.9 ± 16.1 vs. 14.6 ± 12.0; $p=0.23$), and female gender did not impact risk-adjusted 30-day mortality [6].

Humphries' study, with balloon-expandable valves in a majority of patients and more apical approaches in women than men (52 % vs. 38 %), showed significantly greater 30-day mortality in men (11.2 % vs. 6.5 %; $p=0.05$). After adjusting for grade 3/4 AR, mitral regurgitation grade 3/4, access route, estimated glomerular filtration rate, heart failure, chronic obstructive pulmonary disease, prior myocardial infarction, coronary artery disease, STS-PROM score, AVA index, mean aortic gradient, prior revascularization, porcelain aorta, ejection fraction, and site, the female odds ratio (OR) for 30-day mortality was 0.39 (95 % CI, 0.19, 0.80). In a parsimonious model, with only the first five covariates, the female OR was 0.37 (95 % CI, 0.19, 0.72) [8].

In the FRANCE 2 registry (3972 patients), we sought to clarify the independent impact of gender on cardiovascular outcome. Absolute 1-month mortality was similar in men and women (Table 8.3). A significant interaction between gender and EuroSCORE clearly emerged, with higher EuroSCORE proving predictive of excess mortality solely in male patients (hazard ratio [HR], 3.44 [95 % CI, 1.77, 6.69]; $p<0.001$). In this model, female gender was associated with an HR of 2.59 [95 % CI, 1.30, 5.17] ($p=0.013$). The other independent predictors for 1-month mortality were apical approach (HR, 1.78 [95 % CI, 1.10–2.87]; $p=0.020$) and moderate to severe postprocedural AR (HR, 2.46 [95 % CI, 1.57–3.85]; $p<0.001$) [4].

In a retrospective sub-analysis of high-risk symptomatic AS in the PARTNER trial, male and female subjects had similar 30-day and periprocedural mortality (6 % vs. 6.8 %) [10].

In O'Connor's meta-analysis there was no impact of gender on short-term mortality despite the fact that female patients had significantly higher rates of periprocedural adverse events (men, 6.5 % vs. women, 6.5 %; $p=0.93$). In an analysis of the associations of these periprocedural events with 30-day mortality, no significant differences were observed between women and men with respect to the impact of major vascular complications (OR, 2.57; 95 % CI, 1.87, 3.57; $p<0.001$ vs. OR, 2.78; 95 % CI, 1.85, 4.12; $p<0.001$) or major bleeding (OR, 9.64; 95 % CI, 7.27, 12.79; $p<0.001$ vs. OR, 10.20; 95 % CI, 7.64, 13.65; $p<0.001$). However, stroke appeared to have a more significant impact on short-term mortality in men than in women (OR, 15.4; 95 % CI, 11.59, 20.48; $p<0.001$ vs. OR, 20.65; 95 % CI, 15.30, 27.87; $p<0.001$). This may in some part explain the lack of sex difference at 30 days despite more periprocedural events [1].

8.4.2 Medium-Term Outcome

The effect of gender may be relevant to understanding the timing and appropriateness of PCI, but only a small number of studies, reporting variable results, have investigated gender-specific differences in medium-term outcome after TAVI [2–4, 6–10].

A recent meta-analysis on the topic reported better medium-term survival for women [13]. One of the most intriguing questions that it left unsolved, however, is the effect of female gender itself on outcome after TAVI; some of the included studies were adjusted for confounding variables [1, 4, 13, 20].

In the UK National Institute for Cardiovascular Outcomes Research, survival status was obtained in 1625 patients (99.9 %). For survivors, median follow-up was 475 days (interquartile range, 377–820 days). For the 433 patients who died, median time to death was 140 days (interquartile range, 28–382 days); of these, 237 (55.0 %) were men and 196 (45.0 %) women. There was no difference in survival between the sexes ($p=0.331$). One-year mortality in men and women, respectively, was 22.4 % (range, 19.4–25.4 %) and 21.9 % (range, 18.7–25.1 %). On Cox proportional hazards analysis, female gender gave a hazard ratio of 0.911 (range, 0.754–1.100) [7].

In the FRANCE 2 registry, women showed lower 1-year mortality (19.3 % vs. 23.7 %; $p=0.021$). Independent predictors of 1-month to 1-year mortality were female gender (HR, 0.71 [95 % CI, 0.57, 0.88]; $p<0.002$), age >85 years (HR, 1.29 [95 % CI, 1.04, 1.59]; $p=0.020$), EuroSCORE (HR, 1.36 [95 % CI, 1.09, 1.68]; $p=0.006$), hostile thorax (HR, 1.42 [95 % CI, 1.10, 1.83]; $p=0.007$), New York Heart Association functional class III or IV (HR, 1.43 [95 % CI, 1.10, 1.86]; $p=0.008$), renal failure (HR, 1.86 [95 % CI, 1.38, 2.52]; $p<0.001$), and moderate to severe postprocedural AR (HR, 1.68 [95 % CI, 1.32, 2.16]; $p<0.001$). No significant interactions were detected [4].

Twelve studies, totaling 7091 patients, reported on late mortality in Stangl's meta-analysis. Although the lengths of the observation periods differed between studies, a survival advantage for women was apparent: 737 out of 3733 women and 870 out of 3358 men died during follow-up, which corresponds to a 30 % lower risk in women (OR, 0.70 [95 % CI, 0.59, 0.82]). There was a moderate level of heterogeneity ($Q=19.31$, DF = 11 ($P=0.06$); I2 = 43.04 %, 95 % CI, 0.00, 71.03), therefore an M–H random model was used. Several factors may explain better outcome in women: differences in baseline characteristics and major bleeding complications (less frequent in women).

In a recent collaborative patient-level meta-analysis of 11,310 patients, median follow-up was 387 days (interquartile range, 192–730 days). The Kaplan–Meier survival curve showed a significant survival advantage for women (log-rank $p<0.001$) (Fig. 8.1). The 1- and 2-year survival estimates were 82.7 % (95 % CI, 81.6 %, 84.0 %) and 74.0 % (95 % CI, 72.5 %, 75.4 %), respectively, for women and 78.2 % (95 % CI, 77.0 %, 79.3 %) and 67.8 % (95 % CI, 66.3, 69.3 %), respectively, for men. In the Cox model for all-cause mortality, adjusted HR for female gander was 0.79 (95 % CI, 0.73, 0.86; $p<0.001$).

Independent predictors of late mortality are listed in Table 8.4. Female gander was consistently associated with improved survival, regardless of valve type or access route. The most important finding of this study was that female gender was associated with survival advantage even after adjustment for baseline demographic and clinical factors and valve type [1]. For the authors, female patients continued to show better late survival despite significantly higher rates of periprocedural adverse events (which had less impact than for men). Women also had longer life expectancy and significantly lower incidence of postprocedural moderate to severe paravalvular aortic incompetence, probably because of more frequent under-sizing in men due to larger annular diameters, which appeared specifically associated with balloon-expandable valves, as reported by Ferrante [20]. Postprocedural AR ≥ 2 has been shown to be associated with poor outcome [1, 4, 5].

Whether sex differences in postprocedural AR ≥ 2 could contribute to a mortality difference between women and men was recently investigated [20]. Six hundred

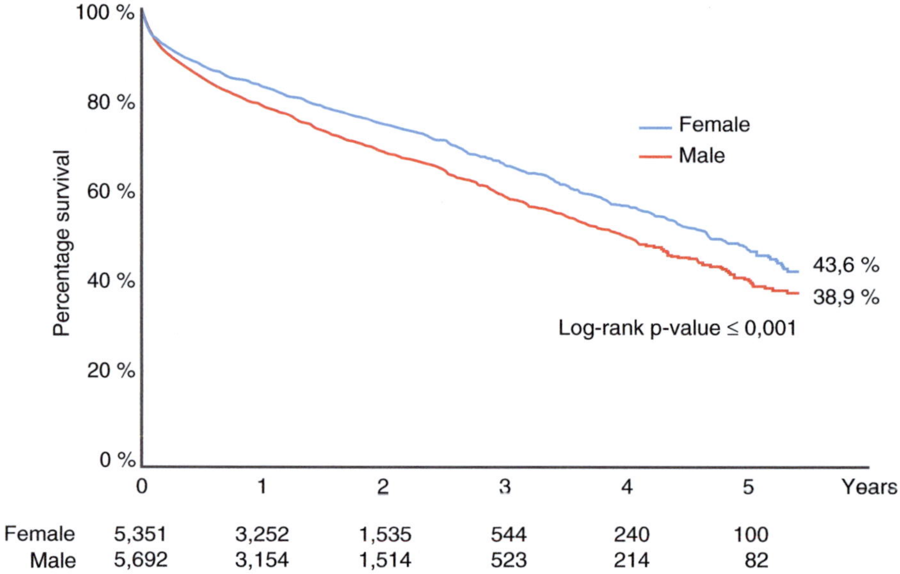

Fig. 8.1 Kaplan–Meier plot of all-cause mortality (Modified and reproduced from O'Connor [1], with permission)

Table 8.4 Predictors of long-term all-cause mortality

	Death (*n*=3072)	No death (*n*=8417)	*p* value	HR (95 % CI) multivariate model (Cox)	*p* value
Age, years	82.2±8.2	83.1±7.2	<0.001	1.00 (1.00–1.02)	0.002
Women	1359 (44.2)	4037 (50.1)	<0.001	0.79 (0.72–0.87)	<0.001
BMI, kg/m²	26.7±5.4	25.9±5.5	<0.001	0.98 (0.98–0.99)	<0.001
Peripheral vascular disease	1069 (34.9)	2287 (28.5)	<0.001	1.11 (1.01–1.21)	0.026
Previous PCI	658 (23.4)	1526 (19.4)	<0.001	0.93 (0.84–1.03)	0.17
Pulmonary disease	1070 (34.8)	2258 (28.0)	<0.001	1.32 (1.22–1.44)	<0.001
Renal insufficiency (CrCl <60 ml/min/1.73 m²)	2138 (70.8)	4952 (63)	<0.001	1.22 (1.11–1.35)	<0.001
Transfemoral access	1911 (62.2)	5745 (71.3)	<0.001	0.77 (0.71–0.85)	<0.001
Aortic incompetence (grade ≥2)	658 (26.1)	1486 (20.9)	<0.001	1.74 (1.46–2.07)	<0.001

Modified and reproduced from O'Connor [1], with permission
Values are mean ± SD or *n* (%)
CI confidence interval, *HR* hazard ratio

fifty-six AS patients (53.1 % female, 46.9 % male) underwent TAVI with the CoreValve (92.8 %) or Edwards SAPIEN system (7.2 %). Postprocedural AR $\geq$ 2 was less frequent in women than in men (20.9 % vs. 29.6 %; $p=0.01$). After a median follow-up of 434 days, all-cause mortality tended to be lower in women than in men (20.7 % vs. 26.6 %; log-rank $p=0.10$) and was significantly higher in patients with AR $\geq$ 2 than in those without (34.8 % vs. 19.7 %; log-rank $p<0.001$). AR $\geq$ 2 [HR, 1.73; 95 % CI, 1.22, 2.43; $p=0.002$] but not female gender ($p=0.17$) was an independent predictor of all-cause mortality on multivariate Cox regression. The predictive value of AR $\geq$ 2 was restricted to men (HR, 2.96, $p<0.001$ in men; HR, 0.86, $p=0.60$ in women; p for interaction $=0.002$).

Women, as compared to men, present a trend toward lower mortality following TAVI. A significantly lower incidence of postprocedural AR $\geq$ 2 in women may contribute to this finding.

Take-Home Messages

There are significant sex differences in complications and prognosis after TAVI. Although men have lower risks for major/life-threatening bleeding and major vascular complication after TAVI, they have less favorable short- and medium-term survival.

Comorbidities differ between the sexes. Female patients have less coronary artery disease, peripheral vascular disease, cerebrovascular disease, and elevated creatinine

Complications are not the same. Females have higher risk for major/life-threatening bleeding, major vascular complications, and permanent pacemaker.

Women have significantly better late survival. Lower 1-year mortality in women remains significant after adjustment for confounders.

The logistic EuroSCORE is not a good predictor of mortality and appears unsuitable for 1-month prognosis estimation in female patients. The best way to determine gender impact on TAVI outcome will be to develop a TAVI-specific long-term mortality risk model utilizing a truly unselected patient population. It would be interesting to see whether female gender emerges as a "protective" factor in such a model.

It is tempting to speculate that technical improvements in the TAVI procedure, reduction in sheath and valve sizes, and consequent decrease in vascular complications may further enhance the female advantage in outcome.

Additional investigations into treatment disparities and long-term outcome in women with severe AS treated by TAVI are warranted, because the cost-effectiveness of TAVI procedures in women could be further increased by women's longer life expectancy.

Ongoing trials comparing conventional surgery with TAVI in medium-risk patients may be a way to demonstrate that women can benefit from earlier TAVI than men.

References

1. O'Connor S, Morice MC, Gilard M, et al. Revisiting sex equality with transcatheter aortic valve replacement outcomes: a collaborative, patient-level meta-analysis of 11310 patients. J Am Coll Cardiol. 2015;66:221–8.
2. Hayashida K, Morice MC, Chevalier B, et al. Sex-related differences in clinical presentation and outcome of transcatheter aortic valve implantation for severe aortic stenosis. J Am Coll Cardiol. 2012;59:566–71.
3. Buja P, Napodano M, Tamburino C, et al. Italian Multicenter CoreValve Registry Investigators. Comparison of variables in men versus women undergoing trans-catheter aortic valve implantation for severe aortic stenosis (from Italian Multicenter CoreValve registry). Am J Cardiol. 2013;111:88–93.
4. Bière L, Launay M, Pinaud F, et al. Influence of sex on mortality and perioperative outcomes in patients undergoing TAVR : insights from the France 2 registry. J Am Coll Cardiol. 2015;65:755–7.
5. Gilard M, Eltchaninoff H, Iung B, et al. Registry of transcatheter aortic-valve implantation in high-risk patients. N Engl J Med. 2012;366:1705–15.
6. Onorati F, D'Errigo P, Barbanti M, et al. Different impact of sex on baseline characteristics and major periprocedural outcomes of transcatheter and surgical aortic valve interventions: results of the multicenter Italian OBSERVANT registry. J Thorac Cardiovasc Surg. 2014;147:1529–39.
7. Al-Lamee R, Broyd C, Parker J, et al. Influence of gender on clinical outcomes following transcatheter aortic valve implantation from the UK transcatheter aortic valve implantation registry and the National Institute for Cardiovascular Outcomes Research. Am J Cardiol. 2014;113:522–8.
8. Humphries KH, Toggweiler S, Rodés-Cabau J, et al. Sex differences in mortality after transcatheter aortic valve replacement for severe aortic stenosis. J Am Coll Cardiol. 2012;60:882–6.
9. Sherif MA, Zahn R, Gerckens U, et al. Effect of gender differences on 1-year mortality after transcatheter aortic valve implantation for severe aortic stenosis: results from a multi center real-world registry. Clin Res Cardiol. 2014;103:613–20.
10. Williams M, Kodali SK, Hahn RT, et al. Sex-related differences in outcomes after transcatheter or surgical aortic valve replacement in patients with severe aortic stenosis: insights from the PARTNER trial (Placement of Aortic Transcatheter Valve). J Am Coll Cardiol. 2014;63:1522–8.
11. Zhao ZG, Liao YB, Peng Y, et al. Sex-related differences in outcomes after transcatheter aortic valve implantation: a systematic review and meta-analysis. Circ Cardiovasc Interv. 2013;6:543–51.
12. Stangl V, Baldenhofer G, Laule M, et al. Influence of sex on outcome following transcatheter aortic valve implantation (TAVI): systematic review and meta-analysis. J Interv Cardiol. 2014;27:531–9.
13. Conrotto F, D'Ascento F, Presbitero P, et al. Effect of gender after transcatheter aortic valve implantation: a meta-analysis. Ann Thorac Surg. 2015;99:809–16.
14. Hartzell M, Malhotra R, Yared K, et al. Effect of gender on treatment and outcomes in severe aortic stenosis. Am J Cardiol. 2011;107:1681–6.
15. Carroll JD, Carroll EP, Feldman T, et al. Sex-associated differences in left ventricular function in aortic stenosis of the elderly. Circulation. 1992;86:1099–107.
16. Bach DS, Radeva JI, Birnbaum HG, et al. Prevalence, referral patterns, testing, and surgery in aortic valve disease: leaving women and elderly patients behind? J Heart Valve Dis. 2007;16:362–9.
17. Oyama N, Gona P, Salton CJ, et al. Differential impact of age, sex and hypertension on aortic atherosclerosis :the Framingham heart study. Arterioscler Thromb Vasc Biol. 2008;28:155–9.

18. Liyanage L, Lee NJ, Cook T. The impact of gender on cardiovascular system calcification in very elderly patients with severe aortic stenosis. Int J Cardiovasc Imaging. 2016;32(1):173–9.
19. Kodali SK, Williams MR, Smith CR, et al. Two-year outcomes after transcatheter or surgical aortic-valve replacement. N Engl J Med. 2012;366:1686–95.
20. Ferrante G, Pagnotta P, Petronio A. Sex differences in postprocedural aortic regurgitation and mid-term mortality after transcatheter aortic valve implantation. Catheter Cardiovasc Interv. 2014;84:264–71.
21. Madershahian N, Scherner M, Rudolph T. Impact of sex on the risk to develop contrast-induced nephropathy after transcatheter aortic valve implantation. Innovations. 2014;9:87.
22. Hayashida K, Lefevre T, Chevalier B, et al. Transfemoral aortic valve implantation new criteria to predict vascular complications. J Am Coll Cardiol Intv. 2011;4:851–8.
23. Webb J, Gerosa G, Lefèvre T, et al. Multicenter evaluation of a next-generation balloon-expandable transcatheter aortic valve. J Am Coll Cardiol. 2014;64:2235–43.
24. Makkar RR, Fontana GP, Jalaihawi H, et al. Transcatheter aortic-valve replacement for inoperable severe aortic stenosis. N Engl J Med. 2012;366:1696–704.

Mitral Valvuloplasty for Mitral Stenosis

9

Benjamin Beska, Christopher Eggett, and Vijay Kunadian

9.1 Introduction

Mitral valve stenosis (MS) is a progressive condition associated with significant cardiovascular complications. It is rare in developed countries with a prevalence of around 0.02–0.2 % [1]. However, it remains a very common disease in the developing world, mostly due to the high prevalence of rheumatic fever and is therefore still responsible for a large burden of disease worldwide [1]. The established gold standard management of MS is percutaneous balloon mitral valvuloplasty (PBMV), and this chapter will discuss its use in women.

9.2 Mitral Stenosis

Rheumatic heart disease is still by far the most common cause of MS with an estimated 12 million people affected and 1.4 million deaths per year worldwide. The high incidence of rheumatic fever in developing countries, in addition to socioeconomic factors such as household overcrowding and poor hygiene, may go some way to explaining the large differences in prevalence across the world [1, 2]. Even in developed countries, rheumatic heart disease accounts for 85.4 % of all cases of MS [3]. Degenerative causes, the second most common cause, account for only 12.5 % [3]. Despite the ease of diagnosis and the effectiveness of the current

B. Beska
Faculty of Medical Sciences, Newcastle University, Newcastle upon Tyne, UK

C. Eggett • V. Kunadian, MBBS, MD, FRCP, FACC, FESC (✉)
Faculty of Medical Sciences, Institute of Cellular Medicine, Newcastle University, 3rd Floor William Leech Building, Newcastle upon Tyne NE2 4HH, UK

Cardiothoracic Centre, Freeman Hospital, Newcastle upon Tyne Hospitals NHS Foundation Trust, Newcastle upon Tyne, UK
e-mail: vijay.kunadian@ncl.ac.uk

P. Presbitero et al. (eds.), *Percutaneous Treatment of Cardiovascular Diseases in Women*,
DOI 10.1007/978-3-319-39611-8_9

approach to management, it remains an important cause of morbidity [1]. The female predominance of rheumatic heart disease is well established, particularly in those of childbearing age, which may explain the higher proportion of MS in this group, occurring two to three times more commonly than in men [4].

The pathophysiology is well described and is characterised by continued inflammation and injury, predominately affecting the mitral valve, which progresses over decades to cause leaflet thickening, chordal shortening and commissural fusion [1]. The clinical syndrome associated with MS results from the gradual reduction of the normal mitral valve area (MVA) from 4–6 cm^2 to 1.5 cm^2, when symptoms are usually present due to the increasing pressure gradient across the valve and the overall reduction in effective diastolic flow [1].

9.3 Mitral Valvuloplasty: An Overview

9.3.1 Inoue Technique

Since it was first described by Inoue in 1984, PBMV has proved itself to be a safe, effective therapy associated with good short- and long-term outcomes [5]. The technique uses a transvenous approach and an atrial trans-septal puncture with the advancement and dilatation of a single Inoue balloon across the mitral valve [2]. The balloon is formed from a rubber and polyester mesh with a thicker band at its centre, a unique design that constricts the inflation and forces the balloon into an hourglass shape which helps balloon positioning during intervention.

9.3.2 Double-Balloon Technique and Variations

The double-balloon technique is an alternative and involves the passage of two smaller balloons via two catheters which are inflated simultaneously. It carries the risk of left ventricular perforation by the guide wire, which is thicker than the one required by the Inoue technique, or the tips of the balloons. Although few formal comparisons between the two approaches exist, both techniques have been shown to be effective with the double-balloon technique shown to provide slightly better haemodynamic results at the expense of ease of use. The better results are likely due to the mismatch between the round Inoue balloon and the oval shape of the mitral valve, with the double-balloon technique allowing for more effective dilatation [6].

9.3.3 Metallic Commissurotomy

The cost of Inoue and double-balloon techniques, and their single-use nature, remains a problem in the developing world where the largest proportion of cases exists. Metallic, reusable devices that can be autoclaved have similar properties after multiple uses [7], may help address this problem and improve the cost efficiency of mitral valvuloplasty. The short-term results of these devices are good and achieve a post-procedural MVA comparable with Inoue and multi-balloon techniques. Although studies of long-term results are sparse, metallic devices have low complication rates with good long-term symptom improvement [7].

9.4 Indication for Mitral Valvuloplasty

9.4.1 Non-rheumatic Mitral Stenosis

In non-rheumatic MS, which is mostly age related, there is calcification predominately of the annulus extending into the leaflets, causing rigidity and narrowing without commissural fusion. PBMV is not recommended and is usually avoided in these cases. However, although some case reports have suggested its use in the palliative management of poor surgical candidates with severe non-rheumatic MS, surgical intervention is still seen as first line.

9.4.2 Rheumatic Mitral Stenosis

The investigation, indications and management of rheumatic MS are detailed comprehensively in joint guidelines from the American Heart Association (AHA) and American College of Cardiology (ACC) as well as guidelines from the European Society of Cardiology (ESC) [8, 9]. Patient selection for PBMV is very important in achieving the best outcomes, with echocardiographic assessment playing a key role.

9.4.2.1 2D Transthoracic Echocardiography (TTE)

TTE is the technique of choice in evaluating symptomatic patients for PBMV and allows for a quantitative calculation of the severity and consequences of MS and semi-qualitative assessment of valve anatomy. PBMV is indicated in symptomatic patients with severe MS (MVA $\leq$1.5 cm^2 or a pressure half-time of $\geq$150 ms), favourable valve anatomy and without a left atrial thrombus in situ [8, 9]. The AHA/ACC guidelines suggest with a weight of evidence that intervention should be considered in very severe disease (MVA $\leq$1.0 cm^2 or a pressure half-time of $\geq$220 ms) in asymptomatic patients with favourable anatomy and no left atrial clot [9]. In comparison, the ESC guidelines recommend that truly asymptomatic patients should not be considered unless there is a risk of thromboembolism or haemodynamic decompensation [8]. PBMV can be offered to those with high surgical risk or in those that, despite unfavourable anatomy, have favourable clinical characteristics defined by the ESC as absence of old age, New York Heart Association (NYHA) class IV, severe pulmonary hypertension, atrial fibrillation (AF) or history of commissurotomy [8, 9].

9.4.2.2 Exercise Echocardiography

Exercise echocardiography should be used in those who complain of exertional symptoms out of proportion with the degree of stenosis to uncover any hidden haemodynamically significant MS that may then require intervention. Even in patients with an MVA above 1.5 cm^2 on TTE, the AHA/ACC guidelines suggest that a mitral valve gradient >15 mmHg during exercise echocardiography or a pulmonary artery wedge pressure >25 mmHg may be an indication for PBMV, as intervention can lead to a clinical improvement.

9.4.2.3 Assessment of Haemodynamic Severity

The assessment of haemodynamic severity should be carried out with echocardiography by preferably calculation of MVA with planimetry or alternatively by determination of the pressure half-time, assessed with the Bernoulli equation [8, 9]. Both are well established and effective methods in determining disease severity [8, 9].

9.4.2.4 Transoesophageal Echocardiography (TOE)

TOE should be performed to exclude a left atrial or left atrial appendage thrombus prior to PBMV [8, 9]. This is due to the high risk of embolisation of the clot caused by the guide wires or balloon catheters. If a clot is identified, the patient should be warfarinised, the prothrombin time international normalised ratio (INR) controlled at a higher-than-normal level for 3–6 months; after which TOE is repeated to confirm dissipation of the thrombus; only then can the procedure can go ahead.

9.4.2.5 Changing Signs and Symptoms

Worsening features of MS may be an indication for a previously stable patient with an established diagnosis to require intervention. Concurrent or new-onset mitral regurgitation or other valve lesion, atrial fibrillation (AF), fever, anaemia, hyperthyroidism or post-operative state may worsen severity, and in these cases, the use of TTE assessment with a view for intervention with PBMV is needed [9].

9.4.2.6 Contraindications

It is important to be aware of contraindications when considering a patient for PBMV. Contraindications include [8] persistent left atrial thrombus, more than moderate mitral regurgitation, severe calcification, absence of commissural fusion, severe aortic valve disease, combined tricuspid stenosis and regurgitation and concomitant coronary artery disease requiring coronary artery bypass grafting.

9.5 Anatomical Considerations During Mitral Valvuloplasty

Mitral valve morphology and the presence of mitral valve calcification are two important predictors of procedural success, and favourable anatomical characteristics play an important role in the decision to intervene.

9.5.1 Mitral Valve Morphology

A number of scoring systems have been developed to aid clinical decision-making, the most well used being the Wilkins score (Table 9.1). The assessment of valve anatomy with this scoring system takes into account leaflet calcification, leaflet thickening, leaflet mobility and subvalvular deformity with each graded qualitatively on a 1–4 scale. An inverse relationship exists between the Wilkins score and the success of PBMV with a cut-off of ≤8 reflecting good short- and long-term outcomes [10]. However, the score's predictive ability is not absolute, with some of those both around the cut-off score (in the so-called Wilkins score grey zone) and above it achieving good outcomes. AHA/ACC guidelines therefore recommend that severely symptomatic patients that are poor surgical candidates may benefit from PBMV even with suboptimal anatomy [8]. In a study of 1050 consecutive patients undergoing PBMV in a tertiary centre, the baseline Wilkins score was found to be significantly lower (7.47 vs. 8.02, $P = 0.002$) in women than in men [11], suggesting that in this cohort females with MS requiring intervention had more favourable valve anatomy.

9.5.2 Mitral Valve Area

The MVA, as previously discussed, is important in determining the haemodynamic severity of MS. Women have been shown, in limited studies, to have a larger pre-procedural MVA than men [11, 12].

Table 9.1 Assessment of mitral valve anatomy by the Wilkins score

Grade	Mobility	Subvalvular thickening	Thickening	Calcification
1	Highly mobile valve with only leaflet tips restricted	Minimal thickening just below the mitral leaflets	Leaflets near normal in thickness (4–5 mm)	A single area of increased echo brightness
2	Leaflet mid and base portions have normal mobility	Thickening of chordal structures extending up to one-third of the chordal length	Mid leaflets normal, considerable thickening of margins (5–8 mm)	Scattered areas of brightness confined to leaflet margins
3	Valve continues to move forward in diastole, mainly from the base	Thickening extending to the distal third of the chords	Thickening extending through the entire leaflet (5–8 mm)	Brightness extending into the mid portion of the leaflets
4	No or minimal forward movement of the leaflets in diastole	Extensive thickening and shortening of all chordal structures extending down to the papillary muscles	Considerable thickening of all leaflet tissue (>8–10 mm)	Extensive brightness through much of the leaflet tissue

Reproduced with permission from Wilkins et al. [25]
The Wilkins score is the sum of the four items and ranges between 4 and 16

9.5.3 Mitral Valve Calcification

In a previous study, Cruz-Gonzalez et al. found that in a series of 1015 patients that underwent Wilkins scoring prior to the procedure, women scored lower on the calcium component than men [11]. Later, Dreyfus et al. stratified 464 patients undergoing echocardiographic assessment into three groups depending on the extent of valve calcification [13]. The group with no mitral valve calcification had the highest proportion of females (81 %) compared with the group with the most significant calcium burden which had the lowest (66 %). Females with valve calcification were not found by Bouleti et al. to be a predictive factor for poor late functional results after PBMV ($p=0.18$) [14].

9.5.4 Annular Calcification

Annular calcification, a feature increasingly associated with non-rheumatic, senile MS, causes narrowing without fusion of thc commissurcs. It usually causes mitral regurgitation, and little is known about its natural history, but it has been found to be more frequent in patients diagnosed with MS than previously thought [15]. It is associated with coronary artery disease, stroke and chronic kidney disease rather than rheumatic fever [15]. The use of PBMV is avoided in these cases [9].

9.5.5 Commissural Calcification

Commissural calcification has been associated with poorer outcomes after PBMV, and the indication for the procedure in these circumstances is ambiguous [16]. Significant commissural calcification is often considered a relative contraindication [16]. Commissural splitting is the usual mechanism by which the procedure increases MVA and PBMV is unlikely to be able to split commissures able to resist deformation due to significant calcium deposits. However, it should be noted that no current well-used echocardiographic scoring system includes an assessment of commissural calcium, but some scoring systems have been proposed to be used alongside Wilkins scoring. The initial studies investigating the impact of commissural calcification found that calcification of the commissures was associated with a lower procedural success, a higher occurrence of mitral regurgitation and a lower midterm survival [13, 17]. Current guidance from the ESC states that PBMV should still be considered in those with unfavourable anatomy (such as mitral commissural calcification) but with favourable clinical characteristics [8].

9.6 Technical Issues Associated with Mitral Valvuloplasty

9.6.1 Pregnancy

MS is one of the most common lesions found during pregnancy [1]. Pregnancy is a state that increases a woman's intravascular volume by 30–50 % and cardiac output by 70 % [2, 18]. This haemodynamic disturbance exacerbates the pathophysiology of MS causing a gradual increase in the mitral valve pressure gradient and left atrial pressure, which may cause a relatively mild, asymptomatic MS to become decompensated and present during pregnancy [2, 18]. Without intervention, women with MS and mild heart failure (NYHA class I or II) have a maternal mortality of 0.4 %, rising to 6.8 % to those with severe heart failure (NYHA class III or IV).

This usually results from progressive heart failure, particularly during the second and third trimesters, and acute pulmonary oedema [19]. Obstetric risk mostly results from the risk of acute heart failure during delivery or immediately afterwards, with the risk to the fetus increasing with NYHA class but usually resulting from prematurity, intrauterine growth retardation and stillbirth [19]. For mild MS in pregnancy, symptoms can be managed with medical therapy alone and are unlikely to cause serious problems [18]. ESC guidelines recommend that pregnant women with severe symptomatic disease should be considered for active intervention with PBMV if the procedure can be carried out by a skilled operator using minimum radiation and with abdominal and pelvic shielding [19]. In terms of timing, the procedure should be delayed until after between 12 and 14 weeks to prevent radiation exposure during organogenesis and preferably performed after 20 weeks [8].

PBMV for symptom relief during pregnancy has been shown to have high procedural success rates and excellent short- and long-term maternal and fetal outcomes, with results comparable between pregnant and non-pregnant women [1]. Incidence of major complications is low with immediate symptomatic improvement and almost no adverse effect on the outcome of pregnancy [20]. A 17-year follow-up study of children born from mothers who received PBMV agreed with the previous literature and found that development was normal in all cases with no long-term radiation-induced or haematological disease [20]. As pre-pregnancy symptoms predict the likelihood of serious adverse outcomes, it is advisable to counsel women with an established diagnosis of MS, even if asymptomatic, against pregnancy and consider routine, pre-pregnancy intervention [18].

9.6.2 Atrial Fibrillation

Atrial fibrillation (AF) is commonly associated with MS, occurring in between 40 and 75 % of patients with symptoms [1]. Its pathophysiology in rheumatic MS is unique and likely stems from persistent rheumatic inflammation, left atrial fibrosis and remodelling in addition to an increased left atrial size and left atrial hypertension resulting from the MS itself [1, 18]. A large left atrial size is an independent predictor of systemic embolism, death and development of AF regardless of MVA or the mitral valve pressure gradient.

The issue with AF in MS is twofold. One, it predisposes to thrombus formation in the left atria due to blood stasis and hypercoagulability resulting in thromboembolic complications [18]. Two, it reduces cardiac output and precipitates symptoms, reducing exercise capacity and increasing morbidity [1]. It indicates the beginnings of a more severe, symptomatic phase of disease, and the AHA/ACC guidance recommends that in asymptomatic patients with new-onset AF, the need for PBMV should be considered as expectant management [8]. Those with AF have worse immediate and long-term outcomes after PBMV, likely due to AF being a marker for unfavourable clinical and morphological features [21]. The presence of AF is an independent predictor for long-term major adverse cardiovascular outcomes after PBMV.

9.6.3 Balloon Size

Selection of an appropriate balloon size is important in ensuring adequate splitting of the commissures without extensive damage, which may lead to iatrogenic mitral regurgitation and thus poorer outcomes [2]. With the final MVA associated with long-term outcomes, a delicate balance is required. It has been previously suggested that an echocardiographic measurement of mitral valve diameter may provide a more accurate way of selecting balloon size [2]. Indeed, the MVA is routinely assessed in the workup for PBMV anyway. In a randomised control trial comparing current methods with novel, echocardiographic methods, the authors concluded that echocardiographic balloon sizing is a reasonable method that results in good PBMV outcomes and a good post-procedural MVA and may decrease the risk of iatrogenic mitral regurgitation [22]. It is important to mention, however, that the literature on balloon sizing is limited, and the study was not adequately powered to make a definitive conclusion due to its small sample size ($n = 86$). In addition, women may have a larger pre-procedural MVA than men [11, 12], and this may not be taken account of in the current balloon reference size method.

9.6.4 3D Echocardiography

Echocardiography is the main diagnostic imaging method used in MS and to evaluate patients' need for PBMV. 2D imaging is currently the main method used, but 3D echocardiography is increasingly being utilised and may allow greater accuracy [9], achieving excellent images of mitral valve anatomy (Fig. 9.1). 3D echocardiography in comparison allows for a more accurate and reproducible calculation of MVA by planimetry than 2D imaging with excellent interobserver and intraobserver agreement. Recently introduced real-time 3D TOE improves image quality further and provides very detailed anatomical images for the operator [4]. Schlosshan et al. found that 3D TOE allows for excellent assessment of commissural fusion and a more accurate calculation of MVA than 2D imaging which tended to overestimate [23]. Post-procedure 3D echocardiography allows for an accurate assessment of the success of PBMV by unique visualisation of the extent of commissural splitting.

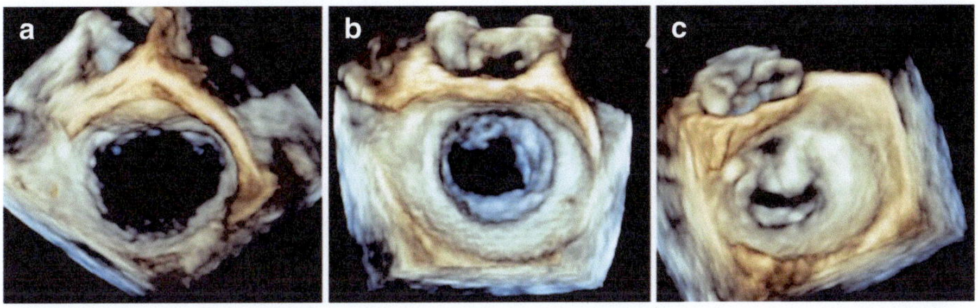

Fig. 9.1 3D echocardiography visualising the mitral valve orifice showing increasing stenosis and deformity of the valve. Image A shows a normal mitral valve appearance; image B shows mild calcification of the mitral valve leaflets; and image C shows severe stenosis affecting the haemodynamics of the mitral valve

9.7 Outcomes

PBMV results in a very high rate of procedural success, defined as a post-procedural MVA of >1.5 cm^2, in nearly 90 % of patients. Very good short- and long-term outcomes have been consistently described in a large body of literature, and it is established that it is a safe, effective technique in the management of MS. It should be noted that given the higher incidence of MS in females, the patient samples studied in these series are gender-biased with the significant majority of participants being female.

Tomai et al. recently set out to report the very long-term results in 482 patients, 83.3 % female, up to 20 years after PBMV, the longest follow-up reported so far [24]. The study found a 20-year rate of cardiovascular survival without re-intervention of 36 % and that a large proportion of patients still had a good outcome two decades after intervention, agreeing with previous studies that were limited by a shorter follow-up. Although the number of procedures is decreasing over time because of the decreasing incidence of rheumatic MS, in those that require intervention, the procedure is still valuable and effective.

The literature evaluating the relationship between sex and PBMV is limited and inconsistent. Tomai et al. found that male gender was an independent predictor for poorer long-term outcomes ($p = 0.004$). A previous study by Bouleti et al. ($n = 2014$, 83 % female) also found this association, which may be due to a link between valve calcification and sex, with the impact of valve anatomy being more significant in men [14]. In contrast, Cruz-Gonzalez et al. directly compared male and female outcomes in 1015 patients (83 % female), and although they also found that women had less mitral calcification, they were also less likely to achieve procedural success and had poorer long-term outcomes and were more likely to need to undergo surgical valve replacement, probably due to a lower post-procedural MVA [11].

Take-Home Messages

MS is a common worldwide cause of morbidity, even though it is now rare in the West and is most often caused by rheumatic heart disease in women. It is associated with significant morbidity and mortality but can be successfully managed with PBMV with very good short- and long-term outcomes in symptomatic patients with severe MS (MVA <1.5 cm^2) and favourable anatomy.

Echocardiography is the key when investigating disease and considering patients for PBMV, particularly for the assessment of mitral valve morphology and commissural calcification, which are important predictors of long-term outcome, as well as Wilkins scoring. 3D echocardiography is increasingly used for pre-procedural imaging, and its popularity can only increase given the high-quality images it can possibly obtain.

PBMV can be successfully carried out during pregnancy, but AF, which is common in MS, may affect the procedural outcomes and careful consideration of balloon size needs to be made in women.

Although gender-specific outcomes are not well characterised due to conflicting studies, short- and long-term outcomes are excellent with a large body of literature confirming the safety and effectiveness of the procedure, with cohorts made up mainly of female participants.

Conclusion

Despite the falling incidence of MS, particularly of rheumatic origin, in the Western world, PBMV remains a safe procedure with good outcomes in the management of rheumatic MS in women.

References

1. Chandrashekhar Y, Westaby S, Narula J. Mitral stenosis. Lancet. 2009;374(9697):1271–83.
2. Nobuyoshi M, Arita T, Shirai S, Hamasaki N, Yokoi H, Iwabuchi M, et al. Percutaneous balloon mitral valvuloplasty: a review. Circulation. 2009;119(8):e211–9.
3. Iung B, Baron G, Butchart EG, Delahaye F, Gohlke-Barwolf C, Levang OW, et al. A prospective survey of patients with valvular heart disease in Europe: The Euro Heart Survey on Valvular Heart Disease. Eur Heart J. 2003;24(13):1231–43.
4. Shiota T. Role of modern 3D echocardiography in valvular heart disease. Korean J Intern Med. 2014;29(6):685–702.
5. Reyes VP, Raju BS, Wynne J, Stephenson LW, Raju R, Fromm BS, et al. Percutaneous balloon valvuloplasty compared with open surgical commissurotomy for mitral stenosis. N Engl J Med. 1994;331(15):961–7.
6. Sakr SA, Ramadan MM, Osama M. A novel technique for multi-track percutaneous balloon mitral valvoplasty. Int Heart J. 2013;54(4):196–201.
7. Harikrishnan S, Bhat A, Tharakan J, Titus T, Kumar A, Sivasankaran S, et al. Percutaneous transvenous mitral commissurotomy using metallic commissurotome: long-term follow-up results. J Invasive Cardiol. 2006;18(2):54–8.

8. Joint Task Force on the Management of Valvular Heart Disease of the European Society of C, European Association for Cardio-Thoracic S, Vahanian A, Alfieri O, Andreotti F, Antunes MJ, et al. Guidelines on the management of valvular heart disease (version 2012). Eur Heart J. 2012;33(19):2451–96.
9. Nishimura RA, Otto CM, Bonow RO, Carabello BA, Erwin 3rd JP, Guyton RA, et al. 2014 AHA/ACC Guideline for the Management of Patients With Valvular Heart Disease: a report of the American College of Cardiology/American Heart Association Task Force on Practice Guidelines. Circulation. 2014;129(23):e521–643.
10. Cavalcante JL, Rodriguez LL, Kapadia S, Tuzcu EM, Stewart WJ. Role of echocardiography in percutaneous mitral valve interventions. JACC Cardiovasc Imaging. 2012;5(7):733–46.
11. Cruz-Gonzalez I, Jneid H, Sanchez-Ledesma M, Cubeddu RJ, Martin-Moreiras J, Rengifo-Moreno P, et al. Difference in outcome among women and men after percutaneous mitral valvuloplasty. Catheter Cardiovasc Interv. 2011;77(1):115–20.
12. Yetkin E, Qehreli S, Ileri M, Senen K, Enen, Atak R, et al. Comparison of clinical echocardiographic and hemodynamic characteristics of male and female patients who underwent mitral balloon valvuloplasty. Angiology. 2001;52(12):835–9.
13. Dreyfus J, Cimadevilla C, Nguyen V, Brochet E, Lepage L, Himbert D, et al. Feasibility of percutaneous mitral commissurotomy in patients with commissural mitral valve calcification. Eur Heart J. 2014;35(24):1617–23.
14. Bouleti C, Iung B, Laouenan C, Himbert D, Brochet E, Messika-Zeitoun D, et al. Late results of percutaneous mitral commissurotomy up to 20 years: development and validation of a risk score predicting late functional results from a series of 912 patients. Circulation. 2012;125(17):2119–27.
15. Akram MR, Chan T, McAuliffe S, Chenzbraun A. Non-rheumatic annular mitral stenosis: prevalence and characteristics. Eur J Echocardiogr. 2009;10(1):103–5.
16. Maisano F. Expanding the indications for percutaneous mitral commmissurotomy in rheumatic mitral stenosis: look carefully at the commissures, and proceed cautiously and skilfully. Eur Heart J. 2014;35(24):1575–7.
17. Sarath Babu D, Ranganayakulu KP, Rajasekhar D, Vanajakshamma V, Pramod Kumar T. Assessment of mitral valve commissural morphology by transoesophageal echocardiography predicts outcome after balloon mitral valvotomy. Indian Heart J. 2013;65(3):269–75.
18. Carabello BA. Modern management of mitral stenosis. Circulation. 2005;112(3):432–7.
19. European Society of G, Association for European Paediatric C, German Society for Gender M, Regitz-Zagrosek V, Blomstrom Lundqvist C, Borghi C, et al. ESC guidelines on the management of cardiovascular diseases during pregnancy: the Task Force on the Management of Cardiovascular Diseases during Pregnancy of the European Society of Cardiology (ESC). Eur Heart J. 2011;32(24):3147–97.
20. A G, W K, Fa N, Me F. Mitral balloon valvuloplasty during pregnancy: the long term up to 17 years obstetric outcome and childhood development. Pak J Med Sci. 2014;30(1):86–90.
21. Leon MN, Harrell LC, Simosa HF, Mahdi NA, Pathan A, Lopez-Cuellar J, et al. Mitral balloon valvotomy for patients with mitral stenosis in atrial fibrillation: immediate and long-term results. J Am Coll Cardiol. 1999;34(4):1145–52.
22. Sanati HR, Zahedmehr A, Shakerian F, Bakhshandeh H, Firoozi A, Kiani R, et al. Percutaneous mitral valvuloplasty using echocardiographic intercommissural diameter as reference for balloon sizing: a randomized controlled trial. Clin Cardiol. 2012;35(12):749–54.
23. Schlosshan D, Aggarwal G, Mathur G, Allan R, Cranney G. Real-time 3D transesophageal echocardiography for the evaluation of rheumatic mitral stenosis. JACC Cardiovasc Imaging. 2011;4(6):580–8.
24. Tomai F, Gaspardone A, Versaci F, Ghini AS, Altamura L, De Luca L, et al. Twenty year follow-up after successful percutaneous balloon mitral valvuloplasty in a large contemporary series of patients with mitral stenosis. Int J Cardiol. 2014;177(3):881–5.
25. Wilkins GT, et al. Percutaneous balloon dilatation of the mitral valve: an analysis of echocardiographic variables related to outcome and the mechanism of dilatation. Br Heart J. 1988;60(4):299–308.

Treatment of Mitral Regurgitation 10

Anna Sonia Petronio

10.1 Introduction

Mitral regurgitation (MR) is caused by primary valve abnormalities (degenerative mitral regurgitation, DMR) or is secondary to left ventricular failure and enlargement (functional mitral regurgitation, FMR).

Degenerative MR involves primary abnormalities of the leaflets, most commonly from myxomatous degeneration, whereas in FMR, the valve apparatus is normal, and insufficiency occurs as a consequence of adverse left ventricular (LV) remodelling, with papillary muscle displacement, leaflet tethering and annular dilatation.

Regardless of its aetiology, severe MR is associated with deterioration of LV function and congestive heart failure, leading to high rates of morbidity and mortality [1, 2].

Nevertheless, different aetiologies of MR influence indication and treatment, for European and American guidelines indicate surgery as the best treatment (class Ia), while in functional MR it is considered less effective (class IIb) [3]. As a matter of fact, the long-term success of the surgical treatment in ischemic or non-ischemic FMR is not significantly better than medical therapy, and this is one of the reasons why approximately the 40 % of patients are not treated [1]. These patients more frequently are older, with a poor ejection fraction and comorbidities.

Moreover though mitral valve surgery has been proven to be effective also in octogenarians, it is important to remind that in these cohorts of patients, the mortality is considerable, and age is one of the mortality predictors [4].

Recently mitral percutaneous valve repair (PMVR) has been taken into account as a possible safer procedure for these elderly, high-risk patients [5]. Though there

A.S. Petronio, MD, FESC
Cardiac Catheterization Laboratory, Cardiothoracic and Vascular Department, University of Pisa, Pisa 56100, Italy
e-mail: as.petronio@gmail.com

P. Presbitero et al. (eds.), *Percutaneous Treatment of Cardiovascular Diseases in Women*, DOI 10.1007/978-3-319-39611-8_10

are few more new devices that currently recently arrived on the market, until now the more widely used procedure is the leaflet repair by MitraClip.

The safety and efficacy of the percutaneous correction with MitraClip has been proven by many studies, and the randomised EVEREST II trial demonstrated higher safety but less efficacy versus the surgery defined as lower reduction of the regurgitation [6, 7]. The follow-up at 4 years has confirmed the success of the percutaneous approach and its durability [8]. Though it is important to underline that this randomised trial includes a wider population of DMR (72 % versus 28 %), while in real world practice, the percutaneous approach is more frequently used in FMR [4, 9].

In a recent review of nearly 3000 patients evaluated in 16 studies, this procedure showed a low 30-day mortality although the 90 % of the population was at high risk and the majority were FMR. Nevertheless at follow-up, the patient had a worse prognosis than patient with lower risk, mostly due to their comorbidities [10].

10.2 Gender Differences

While gender difference was described in mitral valve surgery, little is known on PMVR. The surgical experience revealed some gender-specific differences regarding valve pathology, surgical technique and outcome at follow-up. Recently in an experience with a cohort of more than 3500 patients treated with minimal invasive MV surgery, women were 5 years older, with a higher EuroSCORE, higher amount of calcified leaflet and apparatus and more frequent valve stenosis, while men showed a larger annulus dilatation. These differences turned out to a higher number of mitral valve replacements (MVRs) than repair and a long-term worse survival when compared to men ($p<0.0001$) [11]. The difference can be observed early after the operation, with survival curves diverging already a few months later. This can be explained by greater preoperative risk and a higher incidence of MV replacement in females [12].

Very little has been analysed on gender differences in high-risk patients treated with MitraClip both during the procedure and at follow-up. At the moment, there is no prospective study evaluating likelihood differences in females.

Nevertheless recently few papers about gender differences have been published on retrospective analysis from registries and multicenter experience [13–15].

	Female	Male	P	Female	Male	P	Female	Male	P
	Hofman [15]			Estévez [14]			Attizani [13]		
Female patients, n	205	362	<0.0001	64	109	<0.0001	65	106	<0.0001
Age, %	76	72	<0.0001	79	74	0.001	74	71	0.01
EuroSCORE, %	I 24	I 23	0.6	I 19	I 18	0.6	II 8	II 8	0.8
MR aetiology, FMR, %	68	83	0.004	48	58	0.2	75	82	0.3
COPD, %	–	–	–	27	14	0.03	22	22	0.4
Previous MI, %	21	38	<0.0001	20	46	0.001	20	42	0.003
Renal failure, %	34	46	0.007	39	48	0.04	55	43	0.2
Ejection fraction (<40 %), %	37	62	0.007	48	42	0.06	38	34	0.05

	Female	Male	P	Female	Male	P	Female	Male	P
Procedural success, %	99	99	0.9	97	98	0.6	98	99	0.6
>1 clip implanted, %	28	46	<0.0001	30	40	0.2	37	48	0.15
1 year overall survival, %	81	82	0.6	79	82	0.8	86	87	0.7

On the other hand, unlike percutaneous aortic stenosis, PMVR includes a wide, various range of patients with MR with different aetiologies in which gender characteristics are differently represented and should not be evaluated as a hole.

10.3 Procedural Results and Outcome

10.3.1 Procedural Details

In all cohort of patients where a gender analysis was carried out, there is a wider representative of FMR for in real-world experience, this is the most commonly treated MR. The 60 % of this pathology is ischemic, and in all studies on FMR, the population is mainly represented by males with previous myocardial infarction, wider ventricle and annulus dimensions and poor EF percentage. Conversely women are older and have small BSA and smaller annulus dimensions and are affected more by DMR. As DMR is usually well treated by surgery, this cohort has less comorbidities, but is significantly older.

These differences in aetiology and basal characteristics mainly determine some procedural differences. In the gender analysis from the ACCESS data in 2013, on 567 patients (205 female, 362 male), while the procedural success was similar, >2 clips were used more in male than in female (42 % versus 27 %) with a shorter fluoroscopy time (<0.0364) in the latter [15] (Fig. 10.1). Moreover in another study, a negative correlation between BSA and post-procedural gradient was found, and the correlation was highly significant when authors divided the population in quartiles; most patients in the first quartile were women (54.5 % versus 9 %, $p<0.0001$), and a trend towards a higher gradient and deployment of fewer clips was found. Nevertheless the procedural results and success were similar [14]. It seems important then to balance in women with small BSA and especially DMR the degree of MR reduction with the increase of gradient.

10.3.2 Outcome and Follow-Up

Differently from surgery, all studies on gender behaviour after PMVR experienced that both genders respond similarly irrespective to the older age of women cohort [13, 15]. In all studies, 1-month or 1-year follow-up shows similar if not superimposable curves. Nor combined endpoints or rehospitalisation seems to be different

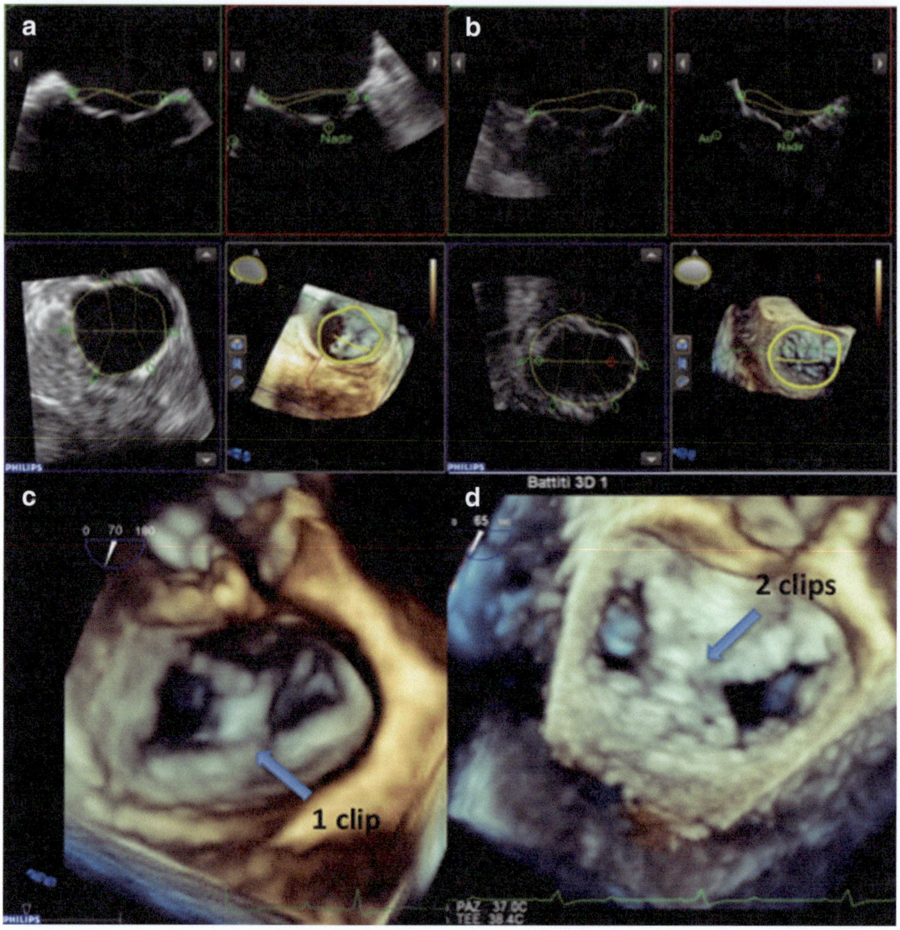

Fig. 10.1 Transoesophageal three-dimensional echocardiographic reconstruction of the mitral valve annulus in a woman (**a**) and in a man (**b**) affected by functional mitral regurgitation. The mitral valve quantification showed smaller annulus dimensions in the woman compared to man. Due to a smaller annulus, the woman was treated with *1 clip* (**c**), while the man with *2 clips* (**d**)

between the two. The only trend to a less clinical improvement was identified in women with very little BSA though death and readmission did not differ [14]. This last observation could be related to higher frailty in this group of old women that can explain the more difficult recovery after treatment. Probably due to a smaller annulus dimension, though women were treated with <2 clips at midterm follow-up, no differences were found in the degree of the reduction of MR and NYHA class improvement. This last observation could be, if widely proven, of great importance for this particular population is the someone that in the surgical experience generally is treated with MVR and worse prognosis [11].

Conclusion

These preliminary results reassure the potential of MitraClip therapy as an alternative to surgery in high-risk patients regardless of the gender. Conversely to surgery and despite to higher-risk patients, this new therapy relatively novel and considerably less invasive can attenuate differences observed in old women who undergo conventional MV surgery.

By the way as previously mentioned, more studies are essential as there is still a lack of information on gender differences especially according to the different aetiologies in MR.

References

1. Mirabel M, Iung B, Baron G, Messika-Zeitoun D, Détaint D, Vanoverschelde JL, Butchart EG, Ravaud P, Vahanian A. What are the characteristics of patients with severe, symptomatic, mitral regurgitation who are denied surgery? Eur Heart J. 2007;28:1358–65.
2. Grigioni F, Enriquez-Sarano M, Zehr KJ, Bailey KR, Tajik AJ. Ischemic mitral regurgitation: long-term outcome and prognostic implications with quantitative Doppler assessment. Circulation. 2001;103:1759–64.
3. Vahanian A, Alfieri O, Andreotti F, Antunes MJ, Barón-Esquivias G, Baumgartner H, Borger MA, Carrel TP, De Bonis M, Evangelista A, Falk V, Lung B, Lancellotti P, Pierard L, Price S, Schäfers HJ, Schuler G, Stepinska J, Swedberg K, Takkenberg J, Von Oppell UO, Windecker S, Zamorano JL, Zembala M, ECfPG, JTFotMoVHDotESoC, EAfC-TS. Guidelines on the management of valvular heart disease (version 2012): the Joint Task Force on the Management of Valvular Heart Disease of the European Society of Cardiology (ESC) and the European Association for Cardio-Thoracic Surgery (EACTS). Eur J Cardiothorac Surg. 2012;42:S1–44.
4. Schillinger W, Hünlich M, Baldus S, Ouarrak T, Boekstegers P, Hink U, Butter C, Bekeredjian R, Plicht B, Sievert H, Schofer J, Senges J, Meinertz T, Hasenfuß G. Acute outcomes after MitraClip therapy in highly aged patients: results from the German TRAnscatheter Mitral valve Interventions (TRAMI) Registry. EuroIntervention. 2013;9:84–90.
5. Feldman T, Wasserman HS, Herrmann HC, Gray W, Block PC, Whitlow P, St Goar F, Rodriguez L, Silvestry F, Schwartz A, Sanborn TA, Condado JA, Foster E. Percutaneous mitral valve repair using the edge-to-edge technique: six-month results of the EVEREST Phase I Clinical Trial. J Am Coll Cardiol. 2005;46:2134–40.
6. Feldman T, Foster E, Glower DD, Glower DG, Kar S, Rinaldi MJ, Fail PS, Smalling RW, Siegel R, Rose GA, Engeron E, Loghin C, Trento A, Skipper ER, Fudge T, Letsou GV, Massaro JM, Mauri L, Investigators EI. Percutaneous repair or surgery for mitral regurgitation. N Engl J Med. 2011;364:1395–406.
7. Glower DD, Kar S, Trento A, Lim DS, Bajwa T, Quesada R, Whitlow PL, Rinaldi MJ, Grayburn P, Mack MJ, Mauri L, McCarthy PM, Feldman T. Percutaneous mitral valve repair for mitral regurgitation in high-risk patients: results of the EVEREST II study. J Am Coll Cardiol. 2014;64:172–81.
8. Mauri L, Foster E, Glower DD, Apruzzese P, Massaro JM, Herrmann HC, Hermiller J, Gray W, Wang A, Pedersen WR, Bajwa T, Lasala J, Low R, Grayburn P, Feldman T, Investigators EI. 4-year results of a randomized controlled trial of percutaneous repair versus surgery for mitral regurgitation. J Am Coll Cardiol. 2013;62:317–28.
9. Maisano F, Franzen O, Baldus S, Schäfer U, Hausleiter J, Butter C, Ussia GP, Sievert H, Richardt G, Widder JD, Moccetti T, Schillinger W. Percutaneous mitral valve interventions in the real

world: early and 1-year results from the ACCESS-EU, a prospective, multicenter, nonrandomized post-approval study of the MitraClip therapy in Europe. J Am Coll Cardiol. 2013;62:1052–61.

10. Vakil K, Roukoz H, Sarraf M, Krishnan B, Reisman M, Levy WC, Adabag S. Safety and efficacy of the MitraClip® system for severe mitral regurgitation: a systematic review. Catheter Cardiovasc Interv. 2014;84:129–36.
11. Seeburger J, Raschpichler M, Garbade J, Davierwala P, Pfannmueller B, Borger MA, Mohr FW, Misfeld M. Minimally invasive mitral valve surgery in octogenarians-a brief report. Ann Cardiothorac Surg. 2013;2:765–7.
12. Vassileva CM, Stelle LM, Markwell S, Boley T, Hazelrigg S. Sex differences in procedure selection and outcomes of patients undergoing mitral valve surgery. Heart Surg Forum. 2011;14:E276–82.
13. Attizzani GF, Ohno Y, Capodanno D, Cannata S, Dipasqua F, Immé S, Mangiafico S, Barbanti M, Ministeri M, Cageggi A, Pistritto AM, Giaquinta S, Farruggio S, Chiarandà M, Ronsivalle G, Scandura S, Tamburino C, Capranzano P, Grasso C. Gender-related clinical and echocardiographic outcomes at 30-day and 12-month follow up after MitraClip implantation in the GRASP registry. Catheter Cardiovasc Interv. 2015;85:889–97.
14. Estévez-Loureiro R, Settergren M, Winter R, Jacobsen P, Dall'Ara G, Sondergaard L, Cheung G, Pighi M, Ghione M, Ihlemann N, Moat NE, Price S, Streit Rosenberg T, Di Mario C, Franzen O. Effect of gender on results of percutaneous edge-to-edge mitral valve repair with MitraClip system. Am J Cardiol. 2015;116:275–9.
15. Ilona H. Analysis of outcomes at 12 months by gender in the ACCESS-EUROPE Phase I Study. PCR London Valves; 2013.

Surgical and Percutaneous Treatment of Tricuspid Valve Insufficiency

11

Alessandra Sala and Francesco Maisano

The prevalence of tricuspid regurgitation (TR) in the general population is 24 % with gender-specific incidence of 28 % in women and 19 % in men [1].

Functional tricuspid regurgitation (FTR) is the most common etiology of tricuspid valve pathology. FTR has been disregarded for a very long time, due to firm belief that treatment of left-sided pathologies would lead to the resolution of tricuspid insufficiency. A more aggressive surgical approach has been proposed, but surgical treatment is still strongly avoided in response to reports underlining poor outcomes. Interest has been growing in the field of tricuspid valve pathology and treatment, with increased attention over surgical indications and possibly exploiting new percutaneous procedures.

11.1 Anatomy

The tricuspid valve orifice is roughly triangular, largest among the four cardiac valves, and delimited by three leaflets: the anterior is the largest one, has a quadrangular shape, and is interposed between the atrioventricular orifice and the conus arteriosus; the posterior leaflet is the smallest one, triangular in shape, and characterized by multiple scallops; the septal leaflet is the least mobile, has a semicircular shape, and is parallel to the membranous interventricular septum. The subvalvular apparatus is made up of chordae tendineae, which directly attach to the leaflets, preventing their prolapse into the right atrium, and papillary muscles that originate within the right ventricle and vary in number (from two to nine). There are three

A. Sala
Department of Cardiovascular and Thoracic Surgery, San Raffaele University Hospital, Milan, Italy

F. Maisano (✉)
Cardiovascular Surgery Clinic, UniversitätsSpital Zürich, Zurich, Switzerland
e-mail: francesco.maisano@usz.ch

P. Presbitero et al. (eds.), *Percutaneous Treatment of Cardiovascular Diseases in Women*, DOI 10.1007/978-3-319-39611-8_11

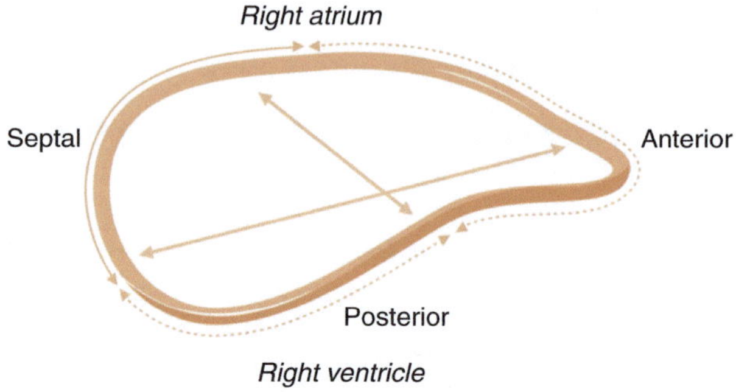

Fig. 11.1 Tricuspid annulus

groups of papillary muscles: anterior, posterior (frequently bifid or trifid), and septal ones. The septal leaflet also receives chordae tendineae from the interventricular septum. The tricuspid valve annulus is a complex 3D structure, elliptical in shape, the highest point being anterolateral, and the lowest aspect being the posteroseptal one (Fig. 11.1). This specific non-planar configuration should be taken into account when analyzing pathologically dilated annuli, which tend to lose their physiologic 3D shape and acquire a more oval and bidimensional shape.

When dealing specifically with women, not many anatomical differences are noted, with the exception of smaller body size (smaller body mass index (BMI)), hence smaller hearts, impacting on the dimensions of the tricuspid apparatus. However, females are subjected to complex cyclical sex hormone status, which plays an important protective role until menopause onset; estrogen has inhibitory effects on smooth muscle cell proliferation and vasodilator effects, exerting protection against deterioration of RV relaxation and function [2].

11.2 Epidemiology

Worldwide incidence of tricuspid regurgitation is 1 %. Prevalence of moderate to severe FTR is 0.8 %, affecting approximately 1.6 million individuals in the United States, and increases with advancing age. Tricuspid regurgitation is frequently present in patients with a clinical history of mitral valve disease, and more than 30 % of patients with mitral stenosis have at least moderate TR. Severe TR has been reported in 23–37 % of patients after mitral valve replacement for rheumatic valve disease, in most cases being diagnosed as late as 10 years, on average, following the procedure. Furthermore, up to 14 % of patients undergoing surgery for functional mitral regurgitation secondary to dilated cardiomyopathy reported grade 3 or higher TR.

Prevalence of significant TR is reported to be 4.3 times greater in women than in men, especially in redo cardiac surgery series [3]. Further assessing possible clinical characteristics, gender, together with age and BMI, plays an important role as determinant of TR; more than a moderate degree of TR correlates with increasing age and with female sex, while an inverse association is generally seen between TR severity and BMI. All such associations require further investigations [4].

11.3 Etiology

Tricuspid insufficiency is the most common pathology affecting the tricuspid valve. Secondary TR or FTR is the major etiology of tricuspid insufficiency in Western countries, accounting for 75 % of cases.

FTR is not related to primary leaflet pathology but secondary to other disease processes causing RV dilation, distortion of the subvalvular apparatus, tricuspid annular dilation, or a combination of these factors. Among the most relevant secondary causes are left-sided heart diseases (left ventricular dysfunction or mitral valve disease), any primary cause of pulmonary hypertension (chronic lung disease or pulmonary thromboembolism), and any cause of right ventricular (RV) dysfunction (myocardial disease or RV ischemia).

On the contrary, less common causes of tricuspid valve pathology (8–10 % of cases), affecting the valvular complex directly, include rheumatic disease, myxomatous degeneration, congenital anomalies (Ebstein's anomaly, ASD), endocarditis, carcinoid disease, and iatrogenic causes (pacemaker leads, defibrillators, drugs) [5].

11.4 Pathophysiology

In order for the three leaflets to correctly coapt during ventricular systole, all of the valvular complex components need to be functioning correctly.

The main mechanisms underlining FTR and preventing normal leaflet coaptation are two: annular dilation and leaflet tethering. The tricuspid annulus (TA) is a component of both the valvular complex and the right ventricle; therefore, upon ventricular or annular dilation, there will be leakage of the tricuspid valve. Assessing pathologically dilated annuli shows a dilation occurring mainly in the septal-lateral direction, involving the free wall of the right ventricle, at the anterior and posterior annular portion (Fig. 11.2). This results in a more circular shape, as compared to a more elliptical shape of healthy subjects. Patients with FTR have a peculiar asymmetric reduction in TA contraction, possibly related to a circular dilated TA, contributing to the extent of TR [6]. Flattening of the valvular annulus and progressive RV dilation cause consequent stretching and displacement of the papillary muscles, leading to an increased tethering effect on the valvular leaflets.

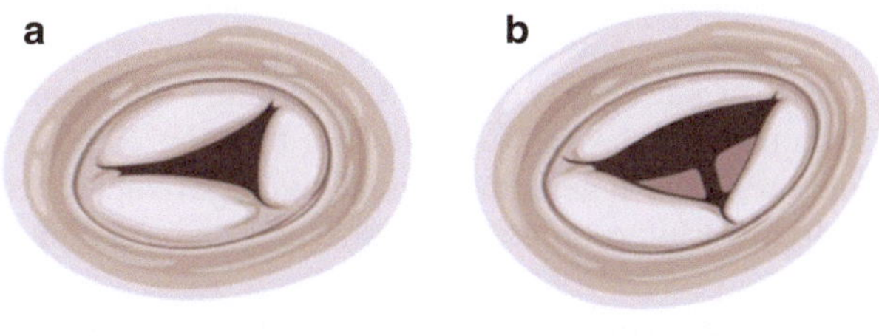

Fig. 11.2 Tricuspid valve. (**a**) Normal tricuspid valve. (**b**) Dilated tricuspid valve annulus

Table 11.1 Guidelines for treatment of tricuspid regurgitation

2012 ESC/EACTS guidelines
Class I: Severe primary or secondary TR undergoing left-sided valve surgery *Class I:* Symptomatic patients with severe isolated primary TR without severe RV dysfunction *Class IIa:* Moderate primary TR undergoing left-sided valve surgery
Class IIa: Mild or moderate secondary TR with dilated annulus (>40 mm or >21 mm/m^2) undergoing left-sided valve surgery
Class IIa: Severe TR, symptomatic or with progressive right ventricular dilation/dysfunction, after left-sided valve surgery
2014 AHA/ACC guidelines
Class I: Severe TR undergoing left-sided valve surgery
Class IIa: Mild, moderate, or greater functional TR at the time of left-sided valve surgery with either tricuspid annular dilation or prior evidence of right heart failure (HF) *Class IIa:* Severe primary TR unresponsive to medical treatment
Class IIb: Moderate functional TR and pulmonary artery hypertension at the time of left-sided valve surgery
Class IIb: Asymptomatic/minimally symptomatic severe primary TR and moderate or greater RV dilation and/or systolic dysfunction
Class IIb: Reoperation for isolated tricuspid valve repair or replacement for persistent symptoms due to severe TR in patients with previous left-sided valve surgery and without severe pulmonary hypertension or significant RV systolic dysfunction

ESC/EACTS European Society Cardiology/European Association Cardio-Thoracic Surgery, *AHA/ACC* American Heart Association/American College Cardiology, *TR* tricuspid regurgitation, *RV* right ventricle, *HF* heart failure

11.5 Surgical Indications

The European guidelines (2012 ESC/EACTS) define the most recent indications for surgical therapy of TR.

Current European and US guidelines (AHA/ACC) are reported in Table 11.1 [7].

Both guidelines pose surgical indication in patients with severe TR undergoing concomitant left-sided valve surgery. European guidelines are more aggressive in posing sufficient level of evidence for surgical treatments of patients with moderate TR and annular dilation (always in a setting of left-sided valve surgery) or cases of reoperations. Elseways, the AHA/ACC guidelines do not consider there is enough evidence to recommend correction of isolated FTR. Intervention is considered feasible in patients with less than severe TR with concomitant left heart surgery and initial signs of RV dysfunction or annular dilation, or in severe cases of primary TR nonresponsive to medical therapy. An even lower recommendation (IIb) is for cases of moderate TR or of reinterventions. The main underlining reason for this conservative approach and for late intervention is the certainty that simply treating left-heart valves is sufficient to improve tricuspid valve function. Reported evidence that TR does not simply regress suggests that a more aggressive approach on the tricuspid valve may help in early postoperative course and may prevent residual or progressive TR.

All studies conducted analyzing the proper timing for FTR surgical treatment took into consideration the importance of assessing preoperatively the annulus dimension (dilation) rather than simply the entity of the regurgitant jet, based on the dependence of the latter on many variables (preload, afterload, and ventricular function) which may interfere with adequate TR severity grading. Dilation of the tricuspid annulus >40 mm or, more importantly in women with small BMI, indexed tricuspid annular dimension (>21 mm/m^2), is used as a marker for the choice of surgical treatment, with good clinical efficacy and late functional results.

11.6 Natural History

Patients suffering from TR can result completely asymptomatic for the disease or can present with varying degrees of heart failure. Presenting symptoms of fatigue and weakness are related to a decreased cardiac output, while right-sided heart failure leads to ascites, congestive hepatosplenomegaly, pleural effusions, and peripheral edema. Further findings are atrial fibrillation and jugular venous distension.

Even if severe, tricuspid insufficiency can be tolerated functionally for many years. The importance of tricuspid regurgitation, regardless of the etiology, as a pathology that impacts on long-term survival is reported: more than moderate TR is to be considered a predictor of mortality, with a relevant difference in survival between severe TR (63.9 %) and no TR (91.7 %) [8].

Conservative treatment has always been considered the gold standard for TR, with pharmacological therapy being the first available choice, based on diuretics with fluid and sodium restriction. Although this approach improves peripheral edema and heart failure symptomatology, the decrease in cardiac output may further exacerbate fatigue and dyspnea. Another category of drugs useful in reducing right ventricular overload and ventricular remodeling are angiotensin converting enzyme (ACE-I) inhibitors but an excessive reduction in central venous pressure may result in worsening of TR severity. These findings suggest surgery as the most effective treatment for symptomatic TR.

11.7 Surgical Treatment

Timing of surgical intervention remains controversial, as the tricuspid valve can be approached with an isolated surgical technique, concomitantly to left heart procedures or late after mitral valve surgery.

Isolated significant TR, in the absence of left heart disease, should be surgically addressed early in the course of the disease before the occurrence of irreversible right ventricular dysfunction and prominent pulmonary hypertension. Survival rate in treated patients is higher than in those with severe TR medically managed. Higher mortality in the untreated population is related to the main consequences of long-standing severe TR, including hepatic failure, protein-losing enteropathy, and renal dysfunction [9].

Surgical treatment of secondary TR remains an object of debate. Surgical abstention continues in many centers to the present day. This is the case of mitral valve repair (MVR) or replacement, in which up to 43 % of patients also suffer from TR, contributing to poor postoperative hemodynamic results (even after successful mitral valve repair), and increasing severity of TV insufficiency. Many studies, assessing both moderate and severe TR, have demonstrated how concomitant TV repair is reasonable and provides an opportunity to prevent progression and development of right ventricular dysfunction (progression of 2 TR grades in 48 % of untreated patients) and significantly improves New York Heart Association (NYHA) functional class and survival in patients with right ventricle remodeling [10].

New onset TR is significant (incidence of 27 %) more than 5 years following left-sided valve surgery. The main preoperative factors increasing the risk of developing late FTR are atrial fibrillation, previous MV surgery, bigger LA dimensions, enlarged right ventricle, and dilated tricuspid annulus. All patients that develop FTR have lower event-free survival and poorer prognosis. Tricuspid regurgitation is an independent factor for persistent or recurrent congestive heart failure and all-cause death [11]. Many retrospective studies have demonstrated very poor outcomes for reoperation in this category of patients, with an average in-hospital mortality rate of 25 % and a 45 % 5-year survival. This is especially true in the female population, in which poorer outcomes following heart valve surgery have been described. Women more commonly undergo redo cardiac surgeries in this context, and those subjected to TV replacement have a trend toward higher in-hospital mortality. On the other hand, long-term mortality rate has not been associated to gender [12].

Poor outcome of tricuspid valve repair long after left-sided valve surgery is mainly related to delayed surgical approach, long-standing pharmacological management, refractivity to medical therapy, and development of hepatorenal dysfunction. Right ventricular dilation and dysfunction tend to be prominent at this stage, resulting in a poor postoperative response. The vicious circle should be interrupted early on in disease progression, especially considering the low risk of tricuspid valve repair, the high prevalence of late secondary TR, and the inability of reliably predicting which patients will develop secondary TR. Tricuspid valve surgical repair requires no more than 30 min, with limited impact on the time of cardiopulmonary bypass and can be performed on a beating heart without the need of prolonged clamp time. All these factors render increased mortality for concomitant mitral and tricuspid valve repair negligible, but more importantly offer a survival benefit by preventing late secondary TR, a condition characterized by high mortality and morbidity, especially in women.

11.8 Surgical Options

Current surgical therapy for functional TR mainly focuses on correction of annular dilatation, by TV annuloplasty, reducing the anteroseptal diameter, valve cross-sectional area, and restoring the three-dimensional valve anatomy. Annuloplasty can either be performed with suturing techniques or with ring implantation.

Surgical exposure of the tricuspid valve is accomplished through a full sternotomy approach or less invasive right minithoracotomy. Cannulation for conventional

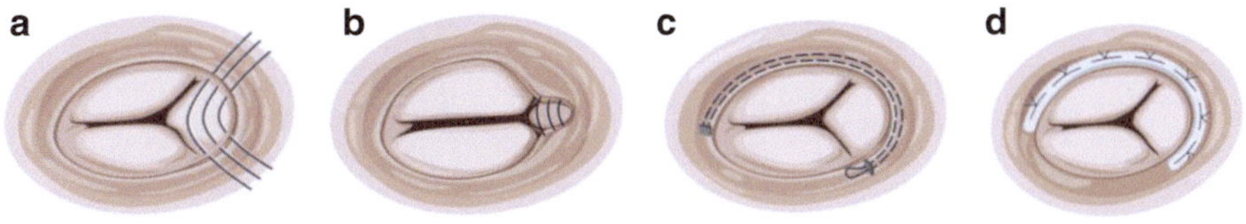

Fig. 11.3 Annuloplasty techniques. (**a**) Kay bicuspidalization suture placement. (**b**) Kay bicuspidalization suture tying. (**c**) De Vega repair. (**d**) Prosthetic ring annuloplasty

sternotomy is performed as a bicaval one to isolate the right atrium; femoral vein and artery cannulation are generally used in case of minithoracotomy. Whenever left-sided valve repair or replacement is performed, cold cardioplegic arrest should be gained. Adequate tricuspid valve exposure allows correct assessment of the regurgitation mechanism and avoids suture misplacement. Particular attention is used in preventing damage to the right coronary artery that lies adjacent to the anterior valve leaflet hinge, to the bundle of His, and to the atrioventricular node, which is found in the atrial septum bordering the septal leaflet. Right minithoracotomy approach is generally preferred in the reoperative setting, avoiding adhesions and the possibility of injuring the right ventricle during sternotomy.

11.8.1 Suturing Techniques

The two most used suture techniques are the modified Kay bicuspidalization surgery and De Vega annuloplasty (Fig. 11.3). The former is accomplished by passing pledgeted mattress sutures from the anterior-posterior to the posteroseptal commissure; when the suture is pulled, the posterior leaflet will be obliterated. The latter is characterized by two parallel running sutures, placed at the junction of the annulus and RV free wall, going from the anteroseptal to the posteroseptal commissure, both in the same clockwise direction; when tightened, it produces a pursed-string effect, reducing the length of the anterior and posterior annulus. Both these techniques are preferably performed in mild to moderate TR, since their durability is variable.

11.8.2 Ring Annuloplasty

Prosthetic ring annuloplasty permanently fixes the annulus in systolic position by suturing a flexible or rigid ring and reducing the overall annulus diameter (Fig. 11.3d). The length of the base of the septal leaflet (the intertrigonal distance) determines the size of the ring or band. The prosthetic ring is sutured with multiple interrupted pledgeted sutures, all inserted prior to seating the ring. Different prosthetic rings are currently available: flexible, rigid, or 3D rings. 3D rings (Edwards MC3 and Contour 3D) are the latest ideated following close analysis of the alteration of the three-dimensional shape in pathologic tricuspid annuli. Normal 2D rings would lead to fixation of the valve in the pathological horizontal plane, with reported

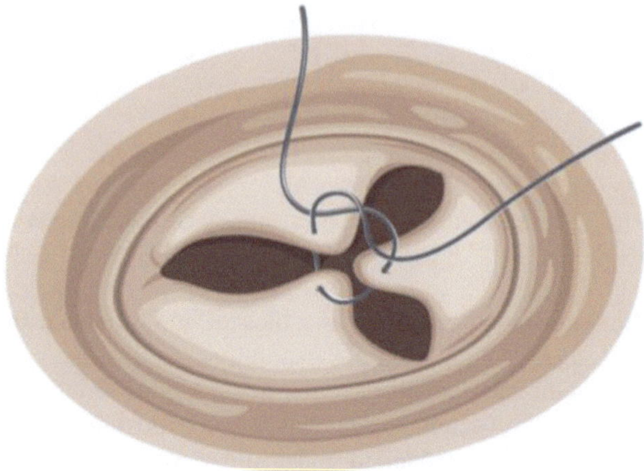

Fig. 11.4 Clover technique

recurrent TR in 20–30 % of patients. These remodeling annuloplasty rings have shown superiority, with freedom from recurrent TR at 3 years in 87.8 % of cases. Moreover, ring annuloplasty in general is associated with improved long-term survival and event-free survival and correlates with a trend toward fewer TV reoperations.

Another available surgery is the Clover technique, gained by stitching the free edges of the leaflets together, leading to a valve with three orifices (Fig. 11.4). A tricuspid ring should always be implanted in order to correct annular dilation and deformation and stabilize the repair, preventing further dilation.

None of the current surgical options have demonstrated to reach optimal repair results, with residual TR being reported in 14 % of patients early after surgery [13]. All currently available surgical options fail to address RV dilatation and leaflet tethering, which seems to be the major determinant of recurrent or residual TR. Dreyfus et al. analyzed this aspect proposing tricuspid anterior leaflet augmentation with an autologous pericardial patch, to increase the surface area of the anterior cusp. As a consequence, there is increased surface area of coaptation with the septal and posterior leaflets and concomitant reduced tension within the right ventricle.

11.8.3 Valve Replacement

Even though TV repair is preferred to replacement, whenever feasible, tricuspid valve replacement represents another surgical option. Hesitance with this approach is related to the high immediate perioperative morbidity and mortality rate and an increased risk of death (up to 3 % per year) in medium- to long-term outcomes. Valves are fixed with pledgeted mattress sutures, using an everting suture technique for mechanical valves and an intra-annular technique for bioprostheses. Tricuspid leaflets are generally left in place, preserving the subvalvular apparatus; however, if there is concern of the billowing of the anterior leaflet, possibly causing obstruction of the right ventricular outflow tract, then a portion of the leaflet can be excised.

Valve replacement can be performed with either biologic or mechanical valves. Mechanical valves have not been proven to be inferior with respect to biologic ones; however, due to lower flow rates in the right heart, there is an increased risk of thromboembolic events, posing indication to anticoagulation therapy with higher international normalized ratio (INR) ranges [14]. On the other hand, biologic valves undergo degeneration in time, with the formation of a pannus on the ventricular side of the prosthesis. Nowadays, various case reports have been published describing transvenous transcatheter valve-in-valve implantation following bioprosthetic valve failure, showing feasibility and effective outcomes. Such promising results require further evaluation but contribute to tipping the scale in favor of biologic prostheses and propose a new percutaneous approach for high-risk candidates.

11.9 Percutaneous Options

Notwithstanding the importance of early intervention, patients currently referred for tricuspid valve surgery are high-risk individuals, frequently elderly, with a high percentage of reoperations, high pulmonary artery pressure, end-stage functional class, and concomitant pathologies. Such patients are commonly considered too high risk for open surgery, regardless of the mortality rate of tricuspid surgery. In this context, the need for percutaneous solutions is increasingly evident, and different approaches are being investigated and proposed, in order to at least provide symptom alleviation and improvement of the quality of life in such population.

Transcatheter devices that have been successfully implanted are the Mitralign device and the TriCinch system. The former has been implanted in two patients for severe TR and works by plicating the posterior annulus, replicating the Kay bicuspidalization procedure. In-hospital results presented showed the ability in reducing right atrial pressure and annular area. The TriCinch system is designed to cinch the anteroposterior dimension of the annulus in order to improve leaflet coaptation [15]. The delivery system allows transfemoral fixation of a stainless steel corkscrew into the anteroposterior TV annulus, connected to a self-expanding nitinol stent that, once tension and remodeling are applied to the TV, is deployed in the inferior vena cava via a Dacron band. Results of three patients, which reached the 6-months follow-up within the CE Mark study, showed sustained improvement in symptomatology and quality of life. Furthermore, bicaval stents, in the superior and inferior vena cavae, have been implanted in three patients up to date, aimed at reducing venous hypertension in the hepatorenal system. Results report 30 days improvement of NYHA functional class, RV function, RV and right atrial volumes, and diameter of the hepatic veins.

Few data are currently available regarding the feasibility and efficacy of percutaneous tricuspid valve treatment, together with many challenging aspects that still need to be addressed: very large annulus diameter with an uncomfortable TA angulation and low flow within the right ventricle with very prominent trabeculation.

Hence, new percutaneous TV technologies and procedures are needed to provide alternative options to patients currently neglected to surgery, to offer a valuable option in order to ameliorate their clinical condition and life expectancy.

Take Home Message

Treatment for tricuspid regurgitation is a relevant topic for both cardiac surgeons and cardiologists. Current surgical indications tend to be conservative, while based on more available evidences, an early and aggressive approach improves functional outcome and overall survival. This being even more true in the female population, which more commonly develops moderate to severe TR, at an advanced age, with prominent RV dilation and dysfunction, possibility related to hormonal changes in menopause. Furthermore, women are also frequently delayed for surgery, with detrimental effects on early outcome and survival. The availability of updated surgical indications and of proven transcatheter therapies will improve the management of patients with significant tricuspid regurgitation, with approaches tailored to the stage of the disease.

References

1. Tei C, Kisanuki A, Minagoe S, Shibata K, Yutsudou T, Otsuji Y, et al. Incidence of tricuspid regurgitation in normal subjects according to a new Doppler echographic criterion. J Cardiol. 1987;17(3):551–8.
2. Hayashi S, Yamada H, Nishio S, Hotchi J, Bando M, Takagawa Y, et al. Age- and gender-specific changes of tricuspid annular motion velocities in normal hearts. Journal of Cardiology. 2015;65:397–402.
3. Pfannmueller B, Eifert S, Seeburger J, Misfeld M, Borger M, Mende M, et al. Gender-dependent differences in patients undergoing tricuspid valve surgery. Thorac Cardiovasc Surg. 2013;61(1):37–41.
4. Singh JP, Evans JC, Levy D, Larson MG, Freed LA, Fuller DL, et al. Prevalence and clinical determinants of mitral, tricuspid, and aortic regurgitation (the Framingham Heart Study). Am J Cardiol. 1999;83(6):897–902.
5. Rogers JH, Bolling SF. The tricuspid valve. Current perspective and evolving management of tricuspid regurgitation. Circulation. 2009;119:2718–25.
6. Fukuda S, Saracino G, Matsumura Y, Daimon M, Tran H, Greenberg NL, et al. Three-dimensional geometry of the tricuspid annulus in healthy subjects and in patients with functional tricuspid regurgitation. Circulation. 2006;114:I-492–8.
7. Vahanian A, Alfieri O, Andreooti F, Antunes M, Barón-Esquivias G, Baumgartner H, et al. Guidelines on the Management of Valvular Heart Disease (Version 2012). Eur Heart J. 2012;33:2451–96.
8. Nath J, Foster E, Heindenreich PA. Impact of tricuspid regurgitation on long-term survival. J Am Coll Cardiol. 2004;43:405–9.
9. Lee JW, Song JM, Park JP, Lee JW, Kang DH, Song JK. Long-term prognosis of isolated significant tricuspid regurgitation. Circ J. 2010;74:375–80.

10. Dreyfus GD, Corbi PJ, Chan KMJ, Bahrami T. Secondary tricuspid regurgitation or dilation: which should be the criteria for surgical repair? Ann Thorac Surg. 2005;79:127–32.
11. Kwak JJ, Kim YJ, Kim MK, Kim HK, Park JS, Kim KH, et al. Development of tricuspid regurgitation late after left-sided valve surgery: a single-center experience with long-term echocardiographic examinations. Am Heart J. 2008;155(4):732–7.
12. Leviner D, Medalion B, Baruch I, Glik I, Biderman P, Fukes A, et al. Tricuspid valve replacement: the effect of gender on operative results. J Heart Valve Dis. 2014;23(2):209–15.
13. McCarthy PM, Bhudia SK, Rajeswaran J, Hoercher KJ, Lytle BW, Cosgrove DM, et al. Tricuspid valve repair: durability and risk factors for failure. J Thorac Cardiovasc Surg. 2004;127:674–85.
14. Hwang HY, Kim KH, Kim KB, Ahn H. Propensity score matching analysis of mechanical versus bioprosthetic tricuspid valve replacement. Ann Thorac Surg. 2014;97:1294–9.
15. Latib A, Agricola E, Pozzoli A, Denti P, Taramasso M, Spagnolo P, et al. First-in-man implantation of a tricuspid annular remodeling device for functional tricuspid regurgitation. JACC Cardiovasc Interv. 2015;8(13):e211–4.

Left Atrial Appendage Closure

12

W. Hamm and A. Bauer

12.1 Introduction

Atrial fibrillation (AF) is the most common arrhythmia worldwide affecting about 2–3 % of the population in Europe and North America [19]. Due to the relative stasis in the left atrial appendage during AF, there is a tendency of clot formation. These clots might dislodge and cause embolic strokes. Atrial fibrillation is associated with a fivefold increased risk of cerebral ischaemia and a twofold increased mortality rate [18]. Also, strokes related to AF are more severe with patients having a 50 % greater likelihood of becoming disabled or handicapped [8].

Oral anticoagulation is an established and highly effective treatment for prevention of stroke. Until recently, coumarin derivatives, such as warfarin, were predominantly used as anticoagulants. However, the use of warfarin is limited by its substantial bleeding risk, the need of strict coagulation monitoring as well as several food and medication interactions. In the last years, novel oral anticoagulants (NOACs) have emerged as an alternative for vitamin K antagonists. Although having an improved efficacy/safety ratio, less food and drug interactions as well as no need for monitoring, there is still a substantial bleeding risk. Especially patients with a history of severe gastrointestinal bleeding or other contraindications against long-term oral anticoagulation represent a challenge.

Since echocardiographic and autopsy studies suggested that the left atrial appendage (LAA) is the main source of thromboembolism in patients with (nonvalvular) AF [10], mechanical approaches have been developed to close the LAA. As surgical strategies to exclude the LAA from systemic circulation are limited by their invasiveness and significant rates of incomplete exclusion, minimally invasive techniques have been developed over the past two decades.

W. Hamm (✉) • A. Bauer
Cardiology, LMU Munich, Klinikum Grosshadern, Munich, Germany
e-mail: wolfgang.hamm@med.uni-muenchen.de

P. Presbitero et al. (eds.), *Percutaneous Treatment of Cardiovascular Diseases in Women*,
DOI 10.1007/978-3-319-39611-8_12

12.2 Procedure of Percutaneous LAA Occlusion

The principle of percutaneous left atrial appendage occlusion is the insertion of a plug in the LAA orifice via a percutaneous trans-septal access. The procedure is usually performed under general anaesthesia or conscious sedation with fluoroscopic and transoesophageal echocardiography (TEE) guidance. Venous access is mostly obtained via the right femoral vein, allowing a more direct trans-septal approach compared to the left femoral vein. Trans-septal puncture is performed via the fossa ovalis guided by bicaval and short-axis TEE views. Before or immediately after trans-septal puncture, intravenous heparin is administered with a target-activated clotting time >250 s. Then, a marker pigtail catheter is advanced into the LAA, and angiograms are performed in various projections to allow for determination of LAA anatomy and measurements. A J-tipped stiff wire is advanced into the left upper pulmonary vein serving as rail for sheath access. After sizing has been completed based on the diameter of the LAA ostium, the occluder is delivered. Final release of the device is performed after position, anchoring and sealing of the occluder has been controlled by TEE and angiography.

After 3–6 months, TEE control or cardiac computed tomography angiography is usually performed to assess for residual leak as well as potential thrombus formation on the device.

12.3 LAA Occlusion Devices

12.3.1 The PLAATO Device

The PLAATO device (Percutaneous *LAA T*ranscatheter *O*cclusion device (Appriva Medical Inc.)) was the first percutaneous device designed to be placed in the LAA orifice. An expandable nitinol-covered cage serves as scaffold, which is overgrown by tissue over time and thereby isolates the LAA from the rest of the atrium. The first human implant was performed in 2001. However, although feasibility of the device was positively evaluated in a non-randomised study [11], it was withdrawn from the market for unspecified commercial reasons.

12.3.2 The Amplatzer Cardiac Plug

The Amplatzer Cardiac Plug (ACP, St. Jude Medical) was modelled after an atrial septal occluder and consists of a lobe and disc connected by a central waist. The matrix is made of a nitinol mesh; polyester patches are sewn on the lobe and disc. The second generation of the Amplatzer Cardiac Plug (ACP 2 or Amulet™, see Fig. 12.1, Panel b1) has a greater diameter of the distal lobe and waist, an increased number of stabilising wires and an inversed disc end-screw to lower the profile protruding into the left atrium [2].

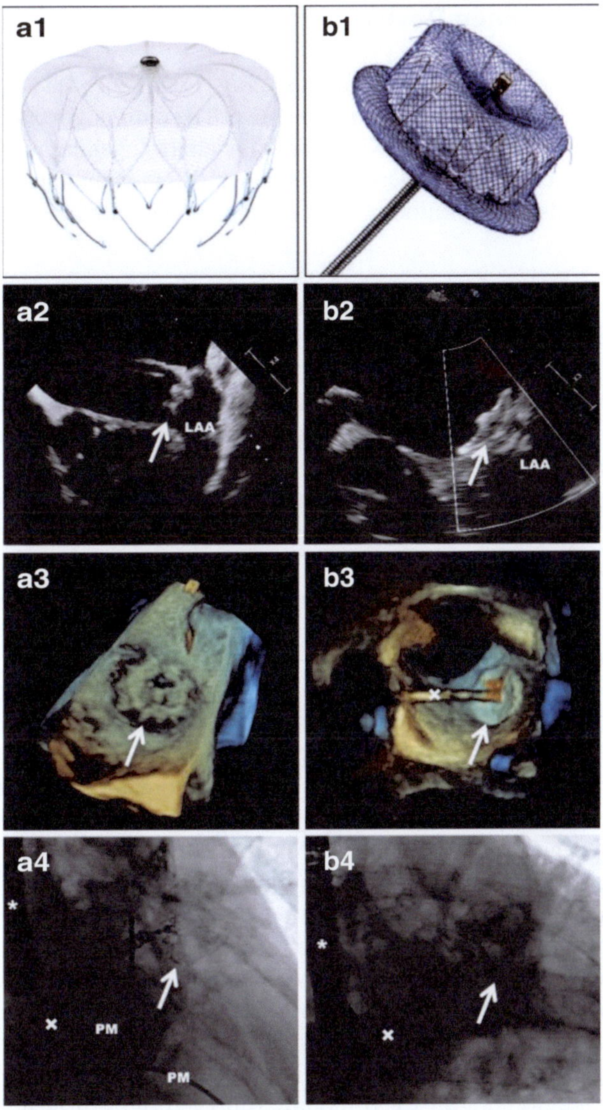

Fig. 12.1 Panel (**a1**) shows the Watchman device (Boston Scientific), and Panel (**b1**) shows the Amplatzer Cardiac Plug 2 (ACP 2 or Amulet™, St. Jude Medical). Below are images of two patients who received the respective LAA occluder because of contraindications for long-term oral anticoagulation: 2D transoesophageal echocardiography (Panels **a2** and **b2**), 3D transoesophageal echocardiography (Panels **a3** and **b3**) and fluoroscopy (Panels **a4** and **b4**). The occluder is marked by an *arrow*. * TEE probe; × delivery system; *LAA* left atrial appendage; *PM* pacemaker leads

12.3.3 The Watchman Device

The Watchman device (Boston Scientific; see Fig. 12.1, Panel a1) is a further development of the PLAATO device described above. The current generation consists of a self-expanding nitinol scaffold with fixation anchors engaging the LAA tissue to stabilise the device. A polyethylene terephthalate (PET) membrane covers the nitinol frame, prevents embolisation of thrombi and allows endothelialisation.

12.3.4 The Lariat System: A Hybrid Procedure (Surgical/Interventional)

The Lariat suture delivery device (SentreHEART) uses a combination of an epicardial and trans-septal access. A magnet-tipped wire is passed to the epicardial side of the LAA via a pericardial access. It meets a second magnet-tipped wire introduced via a trans-septal access. In a next step, a sling is advanced over the epicardial guide wire and tightened around the ostium of the LAA. A non-absorbable polyester suture finally ligates the appendage from the rest of the atrium.

12.4 Clinical Evidence

12.4.1 Watchman Device

In a pilot study, successful implantation of the Watchman device was observed in 66 of 75 patients. Due to device migration after placement, the original device and delivery system have been modified [15]. The PROTECT AF trial was the first randomised controlled trial testing LAA closure by the Watchman device versus long-term warfarin therapy [14]. 707 patients with non-valvular AF from 59 centres worldwide were randomised (2:1) to receive the Watchman device or control treatment (warfarin). Patients in the device group took warfarin for 45 days to allow endothelialisation of the device. Warfarin was discontinued in case of complete closure or significantly decreased flow around the device as assessed by transoesophageal echocardiography. Patients in the device group were then treated with aspirin and clopidogrel for 6 months followed by aspirin indefinitely. The main results of the study were published in 2009. During a median follow-up of 18 months, the device group proved to be non-inferior with respect to occurrence of stroke, systemic thromboembolism and cardiovascular mortality [5]. Later on the 4-year results were published which even showed superiority of the device group with respect to the composite primary endpoint as well as all-cause mortality [14].

A major concern of the PROTECT AF trial was the substantial number of safety events. Serious pericardial effusions occurred in 22 of the 463 patients randomised to LAA occlusion. Of these 7 underwent surgical intervention. Consequently, the

PREVAIL trial (Prospective Randomized Evaluation of the Watchman LAA Closure Device in Patients With Atrial Fibrillation versus long-Term Warfarin Therapy) was designed to address efficacy and safety of the Watchman device compared with long-term warfarin therapy [6]. Early safety events (defined as 7-day occurrence of death, ischaemic stroke, systemic embolism, procedure- or device-related complications requiring major cardiovascular or endovascular intervention) occurred in 2.2 % of patients in the Watchman arm, significantly lower than in early results of the PROTECT AF trial.

The majority of data about LAA occlusion have compared devices versus warfarin therapy. However, the patient population which would benefit the most of an LAA occluder has not been studied extensively: patients with contraindications to long-term oral anticoagulation. The ASA Plavix Feasibility Study (ASAP) focused on patients considered ineligible for warfarin to determine whether implantation of a Watchman device could be safely performed without a transition period with warfarin [13]. After device implantation, patients were treated with clopidogrel for 6 months and ASA indefinitely. Of the 150 enrolled patients which were followed up for a mean of 14.4 months, three of four strokes that occurred were ischaemic (1.7 % per year) reflecting a 77 % reduction from the expected rate of 7.3 % based on the respective $CHADS_2$ scores of the patient cohort.

A recent meta-analysis included 2406 patients (5931 patient years of follow-up) from the PROTECT AF and PREVAIL trials and their respective registries (Continued Access to PROTECT AF registry and Continued Access to PREVAIL registry) [4]. In patients with non-valvular AF at increased risk for stroke and bleeding, LAA closure with the Watchman device resulted in improved rates of haemorrhagic stroke (hazard ratio [HR]: 0.22; $p=0.004$), cardiovascular/unexplained death (HR: 0.48; $p=0.006$) and non-procedural bleeding (HR: 0.51; $p=0.006$). While rates of all-cause stroke or systemic embolism (SE) were similar between the device and control group, more ischaemic strokes or SE could be observed in the device group (HR: 1.95; $p=0.05$).

12.4.2 Amplatzer Cardiac Plug

The procedural feasibility and safety of ACP implantation was initially evaluated in a retrospective pre-registry data collection [12]. Despite a 96 % closure rate (137 of 143 patients), serious complications were observed in ten patients (three ischemic strokes, two device embolisms, five pericardial effusions). Urena and colleagues reported a 98.1 % successful implantation rate in 52 patients who did not tolerate or desire long-term anticoagulation. There was one stroke (1.9 %), one transient ischaemic attack (1.9 %) and one major bleeding event (1.9 %) [16]. A comparison of safety and efficacy of first- versus second-generation Amplatzer occluders showed similarly high success rates. However, Amulet (second generation) was not superior regarding the combined endpoint death, stroke, cardiac tamponade and bail out by surgery [3]. A clinical trial comparing the ACP with optimal medical treatment is presently on hold.

12.5 Indication of the Procedure in Women

Indications for LAA occlusion do not differ between men and women. Generally, any prophylactic treatment for stroke prophylaxis in AF patients that has potential side effects is only reasonable if the risk for thromboembolic events exceeds a certain threshold. This also applies to catheter-based LAA occlusion. Current ESC guidelines recommend a CHA_2DS_2-VASc >2 as threshold value, while the more recent EHRA/EAPCI expert consensus document on catheter-based LAA occlusion found a threshold value of >1 reasonable [9]. Considering the fact that simply female gender increases the CHA_2DS_2-VASc score by one point, women are more likely to fulfil the criteria for stroke prophylaxis including LAA occlusion than men. Generally, LAA occlusion is a treatment option in two types of patients: patients in whom LAA occlusion is an alternative to oral anticoagulation and in patients in whom it is not.

1. In the first type of patients, data from randomised trials comparing catheter-based LAA occlusion with warfarin therapy are available, generally demonstrating non-inferiority of device therapy. Studies comparing LAA occlusion with novel oral anticoagulants are lacking. Accordingly, oral anticoagulation currently remains the standard of therapy. Nevertheless, it is consensus that advantages and disadvantages of LAA occlusion should be discussed with a patient on an individual basis [9]. LAA occlusion might be the preferable treatment option in patients with high bleeding risk (e.g. HAS-BLED score ≥3) or renal failure. However, randomised studies are lacking.
2. Patients with high thromboembolic risk but contraindications to oral anticoagulation (e.g. history of significant bleeding event) currently represent the most accepted clinical indication. However, it needs to be emphasised that these patients have been excluded from randomised trials on LAA occlusion. Observational studies suggest that LAA occlusion in these patients is effective (ASAP registry).

In summary, oral anticoagulation remains the standard therapy for stroke prevention in AF patients. Nevertheless, LAA occlusion is a valid treatment alternative that should be evaluated on an individual basis.

12.6 Anatomical Special Features of Women for the Procedure

There is controversial data whether different LAA morphology is associated with an increased stroke risk and whether morphologic parameters might serve for preoperative selection of the LAA closure device. In many studies, classification of LAA morphology included LAA with an obvious band (Chicken Wing) and LAA without an obvious band (Wind Sock, Cauliflower, Cactus) [17]. However, conflicting data regarding associations of different LAA morphologies with increased stroke risk might, at least in part, be explained by non-standardised classification criteria as well as variation in and overlap of morphological categories [7]. There is no substantial data supporting a clinical relevant difference of LAA anatomy in men and women. However, women are on average smaller and might therefore have a more complex anatomy. There is also data that women are exposed to a higher risk for complications during invasive procedures [1].

Current recommendations regarding the assessment of LAA anatomy include pre-procedural transoesophageal echocardiographic imaging to assess suitability for occluder implantation as well as to exclude pre-existing LAA thrombi. Due to its superior spatial resolution, cardiac computed tomography angiography (CCTA) also helps to examine LAA anatomy and dimension.

12.7 Outcomes in Women

Most recent evidence comes from a patient-level meta-analysis including 2406 patients with 5931 patient years of follow-up from the PROTECT AF and PREVAIL studies and their respective registries [4]. During a mean follow-up of 2.69 years, patients undergoing LAA occlusion with the Watchman device had significantly fewer haemorrhagic strokes (0.15 vs. 0.96 events/100 patient years) and cardiovascular/unexplained deaths (1.1 vs. 2.3 events/100 patient years) compared to warfarin therapy. However, all-cause stroke or systemic thromboembolism was similar between both treatment arms (1.75 vs. 1.87 events/100 patient years) [4]. Although women are more likely to fulfil the criteria for stroke prophylaxis in AF than men, women are underrepresented. Only 33 % of patients studied in randomised trials on LAA occlusion were female. However, subgroup analyses revealed that efficacy of LAA occlusion was not affected by gender ($p = 0.679$). There are also no data that female gender is associated with increased complication rate.

Take-Home Messages

- Catheter-based LAA occlusion is an effective interventional treatment option for prophylaxis of thromboembolic events in AF patients.
- Randomised trials only exist for one device and in patients who are eligible for oral anticoagulation. LAA occlusion has been exclusively compared to oral anticoagulation with warfarin. In a meta-analysis of these studies, LAA occlusion proved to be non-inferior to warfarin with respect to the reduction of all-cause stroke.
- Randomised studies comparing LAA occlusion with novel oral anticoagulants are lacking. The same is true for patients with contraindications to oral anticoagulation, in whom only observational data exist.
- Treatment decision for or against LAA occlusion should be based on an individual risk benefit evaluation, taking into account the individual risks for thromboembolic and bleeding events. A high risk for thromboembolic

events (CHA_2DS_2-VASc score >2) and a high bleeding risk (HAS-BLED >3) or contraindication to oral anticoagulation represent the most accepted indication for LAA occlusion.

- Women are underrepresented in clinical trials of LAA occlusion. However, existing data supports the view that LAA occlusion is equally safe and effective in men and women.

References

1. Applegate RJ, et al. Vascular complications in women after catheterization and percutaneous coronary intervention 1998–2005. J Invasive Cardiol. 2007;19(9):369–74.
2. Freixa X, et al. The Amplatzer™ Cardiac Plug 2 for left atrial appendage occlusion: novel features and first-in-man experience. EuroIntervention : J EuroPCR Collab Work Group Interv Cardiol Eur Soc Cardiol. 2013;8(9):1094–8.
3. Gloekler S, et al. Early results of first versus second generation Amplatzer occluders for left atrial appendage closure in patients with atrial fibrillation. Clin Res Cardiol. 2015;104(8): 656–65.
4. Holmes DR, et al. Left Atrial Appendage Closure as an alternative to warfarin for stroke prevention in atrial fibrillation: a patient-level meta-analysis. J Am Coll Cardiol. 2015;65(24):2614–23.
5. Holmes DR, et al. Percutaneous closure of the left atrial appendage versus warfarin therapy for prevention of stroke in patients with atrial fibrillation: a randomised non-inferiority trial. Lancet. 2009;374(9689):534–42.
6. Holmes DR, et al. Prospective randomized evaluation of the Watchman Left Atrial Appendage Closure device in patients with atrial fibrillation versus long-term warfarin therapy: the PREVAIL trial. J Am Coll Cardiol. 2014;64(1):1–12.
7. Korhonen M, et al. Left atrial appendage morphology in patients with suspected cardiogenic stroke without known atrial fibrillation. PLoS One. 2015;10(3):e0118822.
8. Lamassa M, et al. Characteristics, outcome, and care of stroke associated with atrial fibrillation in Europe: data from a multicenter multinational hospital-based registry (The European Community Stroke Project). Stroke. 2001;32(2):392–8.
9. Meier B, et al. EHRA/EAPCI expert consensus statement on catheter-based left atrial appendage occlusion. Europace. 2014;16(10):1397–416.
10. Odell JA, et al. Thoracoscopic obliteration of the left atrial appendage: potential for stroke reduction? Ann Thorac Surg. 1996;61(2):565–9.
11. Ostermayer SH, et al. Percutaneous left atrial appendage transcatheter occlusion (PLAATO system) to prevent stroke in high-risk patients with non-rheumatic atrial fibrillation: results from the international multi-center feasibility trials. J Am Coll Cardiol. 2005;46(1): 9–14.
12. Park JW, et al. Left atrial appendage closure with Amplatzer cardiac plug in atrial fibrillation: initial European experience. Catheter Cardiovasc Interv : Off J Soc Card Angiography Interv. 2011;77(5):700–6.
13. Reddy VY, et al. Left atrial appendage closure with the Watchman device in patients with a contraindication for oral anticoagulation: the ASAP study (ASA Plavix Feasibility Study With Watchman Left Atrial Appendage Closure Technology). J Am Coll Cardiol. 2013;61(25):2551–6.
14. Reddy VY, et al. Percutaneous left atrial appendage closure vs warfarin for atrial fibrillation: a randomized clinical trial. JAMA. 2014;312(19):1988–98.
15. Sick PB, et al. Initial worldwide experience with the WATCHMAN left atrial appendage system for stroke prevention in atrial fibrillation. J Am Coll Cardiol. 2007;49(13):1490–5.

16. Urena M, et al. Percutaneous left atrial appendage closure with the AMPLATZER cardiac plug device in patients with nonvalvular atrial fibrillation and contraindications to anticoagulation therapy. J Am Coll Cardiol. 2013;62(2):96–102.
17. Wang Y, et al. Left atrial appendage studied by computed tomography to help planning for appendage closure device placement. J Cardiovasc Electrophysiol. 2010;21(9):973–82.
18. Wolf PA, et al. Probability of stroke: a risk profile from the Framingham Study. Stroke. 1991;22(3):312–8.
19. Zoni-Berisso M, et al. Epidemiology of atrial fibrillation: European perspective. Clin Epidemiol. 2014;6:213–20.

Closure of Atrial Septal Defect and Patent Foramen Ovale

13

Shakeel Ahmed Qureshi

13.1 Introduction

Secundum atrial septal defects (ASDs) represent 10 % of all congenital heart disease and 40 % of those diagnosed after 40 years of age. The incidence of ASDs is two to three times higher in the female population. There are important gender issues outlined recently in the Dutch population [1]. Whilst adult men with secundum ASDs may have worst survival than the age-matched population and a greater risk of morbidity, female patients have similar long-term survival as the general population.

Because of the left-to-right shunt, ASDs result in an increase in the pulmonary blood flow and an increase in the size of the right heart chambers. This is usually associated with normal pulmonary artery pressure in children and young adults, when the defect occurs in isolation. However, with increasing age, and beyond the second decade of life, progressive elevation in the pulmonary artery pressure and pulmonary vascular resistance may occur. Children and young adults with Down syndrome may develop pulmonary vascular disease at a much younger age. There may be increased tendency to arrhythmias, such as atrial tachycardias or atrial fibrillation or flutter in adults with unoperated atrial septal defects [2, 3]. Whilst men may develop cardiac failure and arrhythmias more frequently, women tend to develop pulmonary hypertension more frequently. Furthermore, when the defect is closed surgically beyond the age of 40 years, almost 60 % of the patients may continue to have persistent atrial arrhythmias [3].

S.A. Qureshi
Department of Paediatric Cardiology, Evelina London Children's Hospital, Westminster Bridge Road, London, UK
e-mail: Shakqureshi@hotmail.com

P. Presbitero et al. (eds.), *Percutaneous Treatment of Cardiovascular Diseases in Women*,
DOI 10.1007/978-3-319-39611-8_13

13.2 Indications for Closure

Ideally closure of atrial septal defects should be performed before the onset of pulmonary hypertension. This means that the defect should be closed preferably in childhood rather than waiting for adult age. However, inevitably there are many undiagnosed and unoperated adult patients, who are referred late for investigation and treatment in the modern era. The Qp/QS of 1.5:1 or more is generally accepted as an indication to close the defect. In adult patients, surgical closure of atrial septal defects in those over the age of 40 years may not confer an improvement in mortality, when compared with medical treatment, but there may be an improvement in their quality of life and a reduction in arrhythmias [4]. Elevation of pulmonary vascular resistance of >5 Wood units and pulmonary hypertension with systolic pulmonary artery pressure of >70 mmHg may be considered relative contraindications, unless detailed assessment with trial occlusion of the defect and response to pulmonary vasodilators and oxygen during cardiac catheterisation indicates reversibility with reduction in the pulmonary artery pressures. In addition, in patients older than 40–50 years of age, left ventricular dysfunction may occur and may present with management difficulties, if the defect is closed without prior medical treatment with diuretics and vasodilators [5]. In adults with an atrial septal defect, the exercise capacity may be reduced with peak oxygen consumption of 50–60 % of predicted values in healthy control subjects [6]. The incidence of arrhythmias increases with increasing age. In particular, atrial flutter and fibrillation have been reported to occur with increasing frequency beyond 40 years of age [7]. Mild to moderate pulmonary hypertension may be common in adults [8]. Pulmonary vascular disease may be present in 5–10 % of adults with atrial septal defects, which have been left untreated, with a higher incidence in females [9]. Even at a younger age, in females, atrial septal defects may need to be assessed carefully and treated early.

13.3 Catheter Closure

Catheter closure of secundum atrial septal defects was first reported in 1974 by King and Mills [10]. Since then many devices have been developed and used in clinical practice, some of which have become obsolete as a result of improvements in technology. However, the continued development of these has widened the indications to close atrial septal defects.

A thorough evaluation is needed before advising closure of atrial septal defects. Transthoracic echocardiography is a simple tool for the diagnosis. It can help to confirm the presence, the size and the location of the defect. Colour Doppler flow assessment is important in confirming a left-to-right shunt. Furthermore, the presence of tricuspid regurgitation and pulmonary regurgitation provides some indications of the presence or absence of pulmonary hypertension. Additional use of three-dimensional imaging may help in evaluating the size of the defect and its surrounding rims [11]. However, in adults, poor acoustic windows due to factors such as obesity may hinder detailed assessment prior to advising closure of the defect. Transoesophageal echocardiography is an essential tool in the diagnosis and detailed assessment of atrial septal defects, providing sufficient information to help make decisions, such as whether the defect is operable, whether device closure is appropriate and indeed whether other treatment should be instituted before closing the defect. Magnetic resonance imaging has established a role in such assessment also [12, 13]. Additional information of the anatomy, such as pulmonary venous drainage, can be assessed more accurately with magnetic resonance imaging, as can baseline Qp/Qs quantification and response to oxygen therapy, if there is concern about pulmonary hypertension. All of these are usually issues specific to the adult patients. There is no role for diagnostic cardiac catheterisation to confirm the diagnosis in the modern era. Cardiac catheterisation should be reserved for the assessment of pulmonary hypertension and to determine operability, and for proceeding with device closure, if this is deemed appropriate for the patient.

Atrial septal defects should be closed, when there is a significant left-to-right shunt, with right heart dilation, and in patients with pulmonary hypertension, if there is evidence of reversibility [14, 15]. Atrial septal defects can also be closed, if the pulmonary vascular resistance is less than 2/3 of systemic vascular resistance (at baseline or after pulmonary vasodilator treatment) together with Qp/Qs of >1.5:1 [14–16]. A baseline right-to-left shunt or pulmonary vascular resistance of eight or more Wood units is generally accepted as a contraindication to closure of the atrial septal defects.

13.4 Benefits of Closing Atrial Septal Defects

There are benefits in closing atrial septal defects in adults, if there are no contraindications mentioned above. Elderly patients may derive symptomatic improvement with closure of the defects, even if there is no impact on longevity [17–19]. Surgical closure of atrial septal defects, in the modern era, is associated with a very low mortality and morbidity. There may be complications postoperatively, such as arrhythmias, bleeding, pericardial and pleural effusions, but these are usually transient. Arrhythmias postoperatively may be more common in the elderly patients, adding to the morbidity [19].

Since the original attempts at catheter closure of secundum atrial septal defects, there has been a great deal of improvement in the design of the devices, some of which have gone out of use, whilst the others have widened the indications. Some of these include Amplatzer septal occluders (St Jude Medical, St Paul, MN, USA), CardioSeal/StarFlex devices (NMT Medical, Inc, Boston, MA, USA), Figulla devices (Occlutech GmbH, Jena, Germany), Cera occluders (Lifetech Scientific, Shenzhen, China) and Helex devices (W L Gore & Associates, Flagstaff, AZ, USA). The technique of catheter closure of atrial septal defects is now well established. Transoesophageal echocardiographic guidance is important. Both cross-sectional and three-dimensional good quality images can be obtained in adolescents and adult patients (Figs. 13.1 and 13.2). The usual approach is from the femoral vein. A catheter is passed through the defect into a pulmonary vein, such as the left upper or

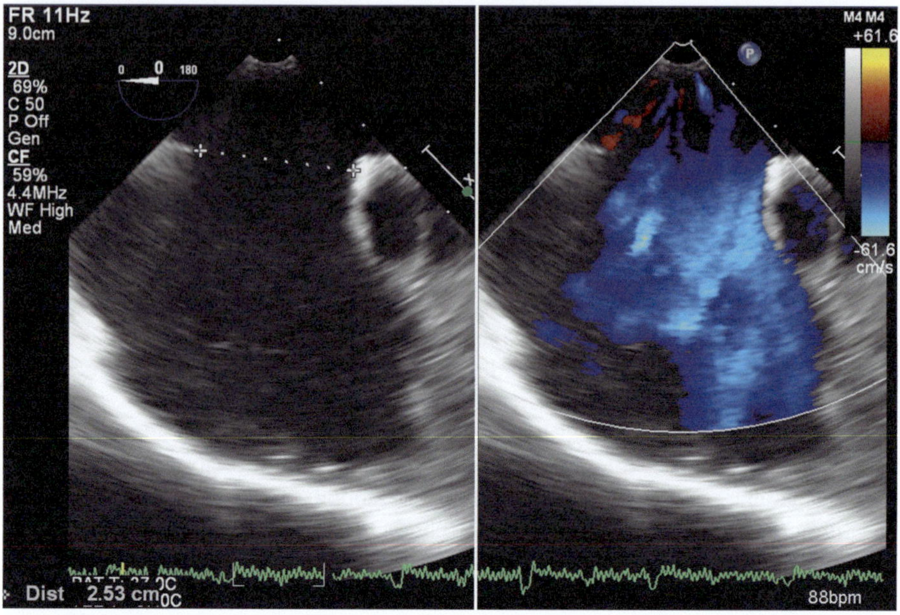

Fig. 13.1 Showing cross-sectional and colour Doppler transoesophageal echocardiographic images of a large atrial septal defect with a deficient aortic rim

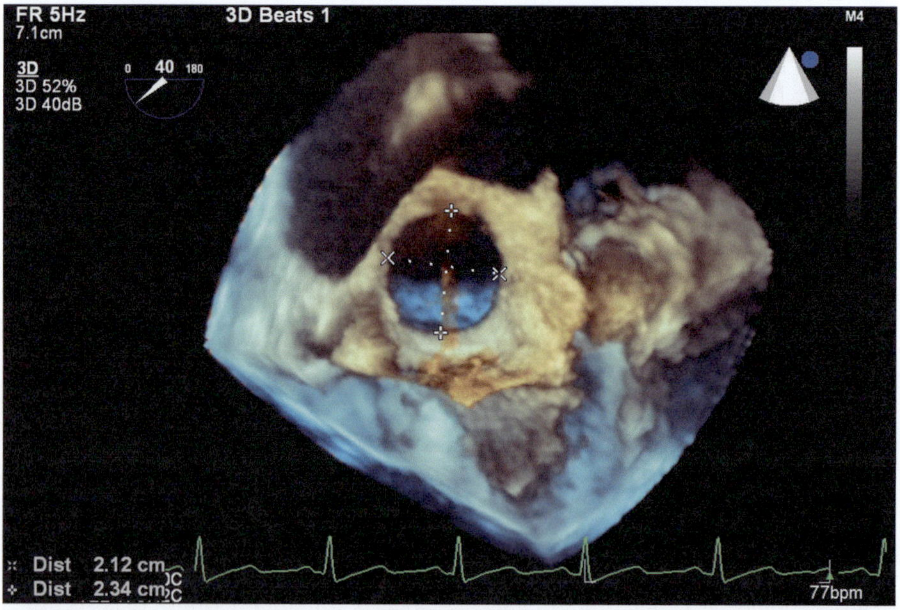

Fig. 13.2 Three-dimensional transoesophageal echocardiographic images with measurements of a central circular shaped atrial septal defect

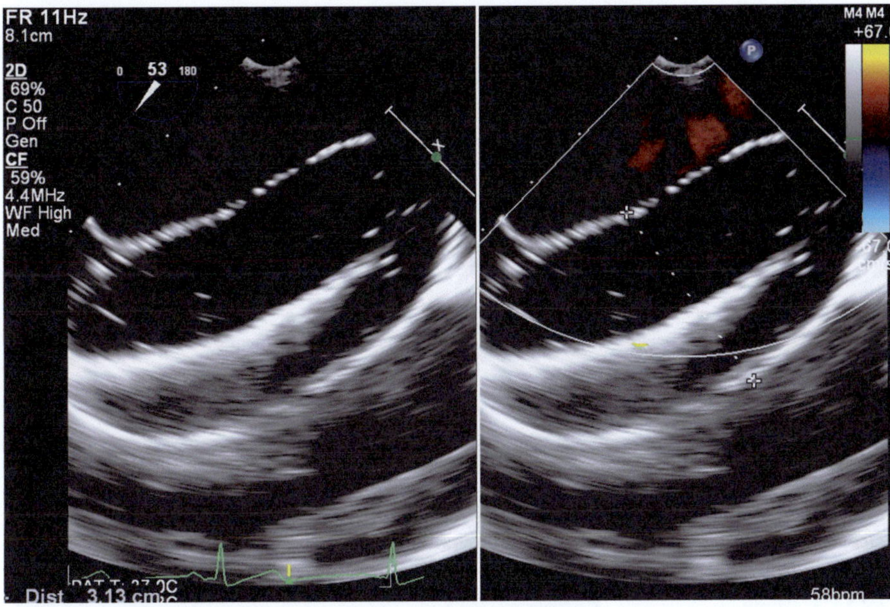

Fig. 13.3 Showing balloon inflated in the atrial septal defect for the purpose of measuring its size and helping to select an appropriate sized device

right upper pulmonary vein. A stiff guidewire is placed in the pulmonary vein. The device may be chosen either with balloon sizing by stop-flow method or without balloon sizing, based on the size of the defect (Fig. 13.3). Once a decision is made on the size of the device, a delivery sheath of appropriate size for the device is passed over the guidewire into the pulmonary vein or the left atrium. The device is passed through the sheath, and under echocardiographic guidance, the left atrial disc is delivered, followed by the right atrial disc across the defect. After a thorough echocardiographic evaluation, the device is released (Figs. 13.4 and 13.5). During the procedure, the patients receive heparin, in order to maintain the activated clotting time at 200–250 s. Subsequently, the patients may be maintained on antiplatelet agents such as aspirin and/or clopidogrel for up to 6 months. In older patients, there may be other co-morbid conditions necessitating the indefinite use of antiplatelet or anticoagulant agents.

Nowadays, catheter closure has become the preferred method of closure in the majority of the patients in the majority of centres [14, 15, 20]. A large study by Butera et al. included over 1000 patients ranging in age from 1 to 80 years, and Amplatzer septal occluder, CardioSeal/StarFlex and Helex devices were used [21]. Post-procedure complications occurred in 1 % of those patients, in whom a device was implanted. These included device embolisation and cardiac erosion.

The patients invariably have an improvement in their symptoms once the atrial septal defect has been closed. In particular, adult patients may report an

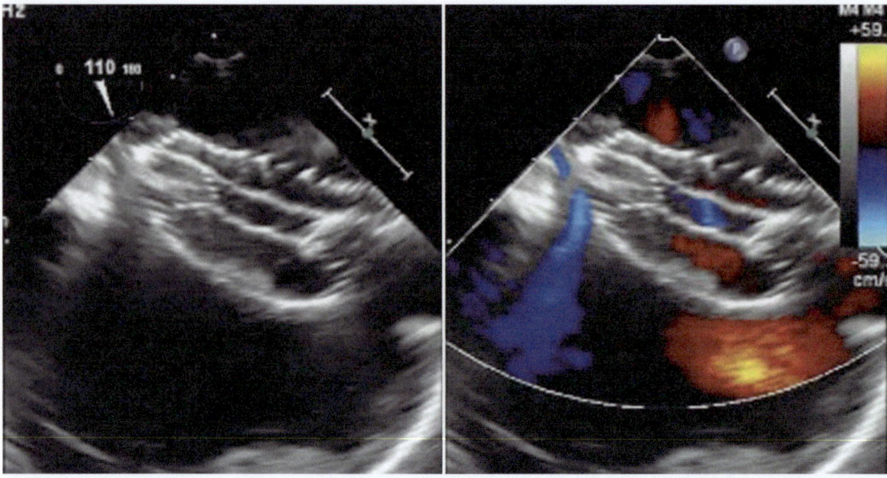

Fig. 13.4 Showing a device correctly deployed and released across a secundum atrial septal defect both on cross-sectional and colour Doppler transoesophageal echocardiogram

Fig. 13.5 Three-dimensional transoesophageal echocardiogram showing a device correctly positioned in an atrial septal defect with deficient aortic rim

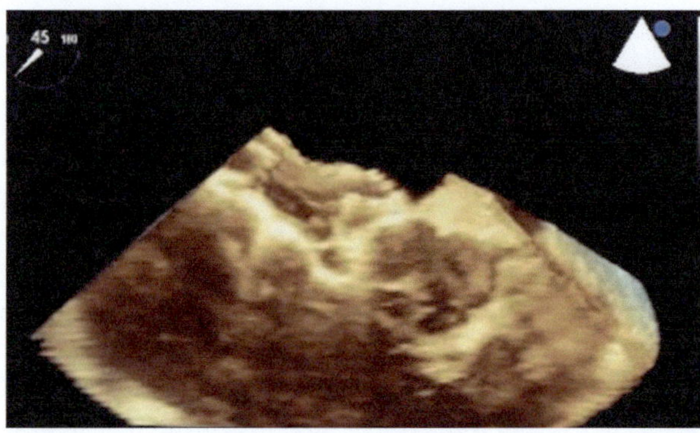

improvement in their effort tolerance [22, 23]; however, right heart dilatation may persist in many patients [24]. In the study by Komar et al., 75 patients, over the age of 60 years, underwent device closure of the defect [23]. A variety of devices were used including the Amplatzer septal occluder, the StarFlex device and the cardiac (Eagan, MN, USA) device. Within 1 month after the closure, there was a significant reduction in the symptoms of breathlessness and palpitations. There was a reduction in the size of the right heart in 89 % of the patients [23]. Another study by Khan et al., in which the age range of the patients was 50–91 years, reported a high procedural success rate, with improvement in symptoms and quality of life and evidence of cardiac remodelling [25].

One of the main concerns in the late middle age or elderly patients undergoing closure is a sudden and rapid increase in the left atrial and pulmonary venous pressures, leading to pulmonary oedema or congestive cardiac failure [5, 26, 27].

The main limitations of device closure include the size of the defect (with the currently available devices, defects greater than 36–38 mm are not suitable) and deficient rims. Although a majority of patients may have a deficient aortic rim, these defects are amenable to catheter closure. However, if there is deficiency of atrioventricular valve or the inferior vena cava rims, then the defects are not suitable for attempting device closure [28]. The results with most devices have been excellent [29–31]. In a multicentre study, technical success was reported in 96 % of the patients, and the closure rate within 24 h of the procedure was 99.6 % with similar results being reported in adult patients also [29–31]. The major complications with device closure are migration of the device after release and cardiac tamponade [32, 33]. Although late complications are rare, they include atrial arrhythmias (especially in adults), thrombus formation on the device, stroke and the most important one of cardiac erosion resulting in tamponade [34–37]. There was no difference between men and women in these complications, especially erosions.

It is important to identify the high-risk patients, such as those with pre-existing other co-morbidities, additional cardiac defects, or left ventricular diastolic dysfunction.

This can be particularly important in the older women with systemic hypertension and a hypertrophied left ventricle. Ewert et al. proposed a method of assessing such patients by trial occlusion of the atrial septal defect by a balloon and measuring the left atrial pressure as well as observing the mitral valve inflow Doppler patterns [27]. These patients may benefit from pretreatment with anti-failure medication, particularly systemic vasodilators, and the use of a fenestrated device for closure of the defect [38, 39]. However, there are no clear guidelines about the cut-off values of pressures and when to use such devices.

13.5 Pregnancy

In females with unoperated atrial septal defects, pregnancy is usually well tolerated and can be allowed to continue. The effect of the increased cardiac output on the volume-loaded right ventricle in patients with left-to-right shunts may be counterbalanced by the decrease in peripheral vascular resistance. There is a small risk of paradoxical emboli, stroke, arrhythmias and, if the defect is very large, heart failure [40]. In the absence of pulmonary hypertension, maternal complications are infrequent [41, 42]. However, Yap et al. reported that pre-pregnancy history of arrhythmias and maternal age older than 30 years were risk factors for maternal cardiac complications [42]. The outcome of the babies from the pregnancies was similar to the general population. In females with atrial septal defects and severe pulmonary hypertension, pregnancy should be avoided, because the maternal mortality may be high [42]. In the study by Bedard et al., maternal deaths occurred soon after delivery and were due to congestive heart failure, thromboembolism, pulmonary hypertensive crisis and sudden cardiac death [43]. It is therefore very important that young women of childbearing with atrial septal defects should undergo thorough evaluation before undertaking a pregnancy, so that their management can be optimised or the defect closed. Percutaneous closure of ASD during pregnancy should be considered only when they are thought to be responsible for neurological events due to paradoxical embolism in the presence of deep vein thrombosis not cured with anticoagulation or in the presence of heart failure.

13.6 Patent Foramen Ovale

Patent foramen ovale (PFO) is usually of no clinical significance as it is found in up to 25 % of the adult population [44]. However, it may be a contributing factor in cryptogenic strokes and migraine. In order to prevent cryptogenic strokes, various studies have been performed to close patent foramen ovale by catheter techniques using a variety of devices. Similarly, studies were performed to assess whether patent foramen closure improved migraine also.

In cryptogenic strokes, it is thought that manoeuvres, which increase the right atrial pressure above the left atrial pressure, causing a right-to-lcft shunt, such as coughing, exercise and performing Valsalva manoeuvre, may increase the propensity to a stroke in patients susceptible to peripheral vein or right atrial thrombosis. Although patent foramen ovale may not be associated with any increased morbidity in the normal population, it has been reported that patients who have had cryptogenic strokes may have an increased prevalence of patent foramen ovale than those in whom the cause of the stroke has been identified, such as atherosclerotic disease [45–48]. The presence of a large patent foramen ovale and atrial septal aneurysm may predispose to a higher occurrence of strokes [49, 50]. Although patients with strokes may be treated with antiplatelet agents or anticoagulants, there may be serious side effects associated with these, such as haemorrhage or inability to tolerate these drugs. This is even more important in young patients [54].

There are also many unresolved issues. In patients more than 55 years of age, careful assessment of the atherosclerotic risk factors is important. If more than three risk factors are present, it is very unlikely that the cause of stroke is venous thromboembolism, and PFO may not be a contributory factor. In these patients, atrial fibrillation needs to be excluded. Implanting a loop recorder for one year to identify episodes of paroxysmal atrial fibrillation before PFO closure may be helpful. A clear indication for PFO closure is stroke during Valsalva manoeuvre in the presence of deep venous thrombosis. Another indication is platypnoea-orthodeoxia syndrome, which is characterised by arterial desaturation worsened by the upright position. It may be due to an atrial deformation caused by factors such as pneumonectomy or ascending aortic aneurysm. In the upright position, stretching of the interatrial septum leads to a permanent opening of the PFO with a large right-to-left shunt. This syndrome may be cured by PFO closure.

It is also debatable whether the closure of PFO as primary prevention of air embolism in divers is useful. It may be useful in professional deepwater (under 40 m) divers.

Migraine may occur in up to 17 % females and 6 % of males and may cause important morbidity to patients [51, 52]. The mechanism of how patent foramen ovale may contribute to migraine is poorly understood. One small randomised study, Migraine Intervention With STARFlex Technology (MIST) trial, with closure of PFO with StartFlex technology, failed to demonstrate complete cessation of migraine six months after PFO closure, compared with medical treatment. Anzola et al. reported the incidence of patent foramen ovale with right-to-left shunting in 48 % of patients who experienced migraine with aura, compared with 23 % in those without aura and 20 % of normal control subjects, possibly identifying a subset of patients, in whom closure of the patent foramen ovale may be beneficial [53]. However, no clear consensus has been reached on the treatment of migraine with closure of PFOs.

13.7 Closing Patent Foramen Ovale

Device closure of PFO is a low-risk procedure; however, there are some rare but important complications, such as device embolisation, erosion, residual shunting through the device or the foramen, arrhythmias and, most importantly, thrombus formation [55]. A variety of devices have been used to close the PFO, and data have been collected and reported, but still some technical issues remain. Lipomatous septum secundum can be a problem, because the device, which embraces this large septum, often leaves residual shunts. Also very long and narrow tunnels can nowadays be dealt with by a separate transeptal puncture to close the defect properly, avoiding distortion of the septum.

Three randomised trials have been performed in patients with cryptogenic stroke to assess the superiority of device closure over medical treatment. In CLOSURE 1, 909 patients were randomised to device closure or medical treatment [56]. In this trial, there was no significant difference between the two groups with regard to the primary end points of death, recurrence of stroke or transient ischaemic attacks. The RESPECT trial comparing medical treatment with device closure using the Amplatzer PFO device (St. Jude Medical, Minneapolis, MN) showed a relative risk reduction of stroke in the patients treated with a device compared with medical treatment, but this was not significant [57]. The 10-year follow-up (mean 5.5 years) results of this trial (presented at TCT 2015) showed that in the intention-to-treat population, the relative risk for recurrent cryptogenic stroke was reduced by 54 % after PFO closure. Furthermore, an additional sensitivity analysis of all-cause stroke in young patients (less than 60 years of age), in whom the strokes are most likely to be cryptogenic, showed a 52 % relative risk reduction. Additional benefit was also seen in a subgroup of patients with a substantial shunt or atrial septal aneurysm, in whom there was a 75 % reduction in cryptogenic stroke risk.

Currently in the patients, who continue to have recurrent strokes despite medical treatment, device closure is an acceptable option. Controversy remains about how to manage patients, who have had a single stroke and have a patent foramen ovale.

Further studies on selected population (young patients with no risk factors) and longer follow-up are required.

References

1. Kuijpers JM, et al. Secundum atrial septal defect is associated with reduced survival in adult men. Eur Heart J. 2015;36(31):2079–86.
2. Roos-Hesselink JW, Meijboom RJ, Spitaels SEC, et al. Excellent survival and low incidence of arrhythmias, stroke and heart failure long-term after surgical ASD closure at young age. A prospective follow-up study of 21–33 years. Eur Heart J. 2003;2003:190–7.
3. Gatzoulis MA, Freeman MA, Siu SC, et al. Atrial arrhythmia after surgical closure of atrial septal defects in adults. N Engl J Med. 1999;340:839–46.
4. Attie F, Rosas M, Granados N, et al. Surgical treatment for secundum atrial septal defect in patients ≥40 years old. A randomized clinical trial. J Am Coll Cardiol. 2001;38:2035–42.
5. Schubert S, Peters B, Abdul-Khaliq H, Nagdyman N, Lange PE, Ewert P. Left ventricular conditioning in the elderly patient to prevent congestive heart failure after transcatheter closure of atrial septal defect. Catheter Cardiovasc Interv. 2005;64:333–7.
6. Van De Bruaene A, Buys R, Vanhees L, Delcroix M, Moons P, Budts W. Cardiopulmonary exercise testing and SF-36 in patients with atrial septal defect type secundum. J Cardiopulm Rehabil Prev. 2011;31:308–15.
7. Berger F, Vogel M, Kramer A, et al. Incidence of atrial flutter/fibrillation in adults with atrial septal defect before and after surgery. Ann Thorac Surg. 1999;68:75–8.
8. Humenberger M, Rosenhek R, Gabriel H, et al. Benefit of atrial septal defect closure in adults: impact of age. Eur Heart J. 2011;32:553–60.
9. Sachweh JS, Daebritz SH, Hermanns B, et al. Hypertensive pulmonary vascular disease in adults with secundum or sinus venosus atrial septal defect. Ann Thorac Surg. 2006;81:207–13.
10. King TD, Mills NL. Nonoperative closure of atrial septal defect. Surgery. 1974;75:383.
11. van den Bosch AE, Ten Harkel DJ, McGhie JS, et al. Characterization of atrial septal defect assessed by real-time three-dimensional echocardiography. J Am Soc Echocardiogr. 2006;19:815–21.
12. Valverde I, Simpson J, Schaeffter T, Beerbaum P. 4D phase-contrast flow cardiovascular magnetic resonance: comprehensive quantification and visualization of flow dynamics in atrial septal defect and partial anomalous pulmonary venous return. Pediatr Cardiol. 2010;31:1244–8.
13. Teo KS, Disney PJ, Dundon BK, et al. Assessment of atrial septal defects in adults comparing cardiovascular magnetic resonance with transoesophageal echocardiography. J Cardiovasc Magn Reson. 2010;12:44.
14. Warnes CA, Williams RG, Bashore TM, American College of Cardiology, American Heart Association Task Force on Practice Guidelines (Writing Committee to Develop Guidelines on the Management of Adults With Congenital Heart Disease), American Society of Echocardiography, Heart Rhythm Society, International Society for Adult Congenital Heart Disease, Society for Cardiovascular Angiography and Interventions, Society of Thoracic Surgeons, et al. ACC/AHA 2008 guidelines for the management of adults with congenital heart disease: a report of the American College of Cardiology/American Heart Association Task Force on Practice Guidelines (Writing Committee to Develop Guidelines on the Management of Adults with Congenital Heart Disease). Developed in collaboration with the American Society of Echocardiography, Heart Rhythm Society, International Society for Adult Congenital Heart Disease, Society for Cardiovascular Angiography and Interventions, and Society of Thoracic Surgeons. J Am Coll Cardiol. 2008;52:e143–263.

15. Baumgartner H, Bonhoeffer P, De Groot NM, Task Force on the Management of Grown-up Congenital Heart Disease of the European Society of Cardiology (ESC), Association for European Paediatric Cardiology (AEPC), ESC Committee for Practice Guidelines (CPG), et al. ESC Guidelines for the management of grown-up congenital heart disease (new version 2010). Eur Heart J. 2010;31:2915–57.
16. Kim YH, Yu JJ, Yun TJ, et al. Repair of atrial septal defect with Eisenmenger syndrome after long-term sildenafil therapy. Ann Thorac Surg. 2010;89:1629–30.
17. Hanninen M, Kmet A, Taylor DA, Ross DB, Rebeyka I, Vonder Muhll IF. Atrial septal defect closure in the elderly is associated with excellent quality of life, functional improvement, and ventricular remodelling. Can J Cardiol. 2011;27:698–704.
18. Nakagawa K, Akagi T, Taniguchi M, et al. Transcatheter closure of atrial septal defect in a geriatric population. Catheter Cardiovasc Interv. 2012;80:84–90.
19. Nyboe C, Fenger-Grøn M, Nielsen-Kudsk JE, Hjortdal V. Closure of secundum atrial septal defects in the adult and elderly patients. Eur J Cardiothorac Surg. 2013;43:752–7.
20. Opotowsky AR, Landzberg MJ, Kimmel SE, Webb GD. Trends in the use of percutaneous closure of patent foramen ovale and atrial septal defect in adults, 1998–2004. JAMA. 2008;299:521–2.
21. Butera G, Romagnoli E, Carminati M, et al. Treatment of isolated secundum atrial septal defects: Impact of age and defect morphology in 1,013 consecutive patients. Am Heart J. 2008;156:706–12.
22. Takaya Y, Taniguchi M, Akagi T, et al. Long-term effects of transcatheter closure of atrial septal defect on cardiac remodeling and exercise capacity in patients older than 40 years with a reduction in cardiopulmonary function. J Interv Cardiol. 2013;26:195–9.
23. Komar M, Przewlocki T, Olszowska M, Sobien B, Podolec P. The benefit of atrial septal defect closure in elderly patients. Clin Interv Aging. 2014;9:1101–7.
24. Veldtman GR, Razack V, Siu S, et al. Right ventricular form and function after percutaneous atrial septal defect device closure. J Am Coll Cardiol. 2001;37:2108–13.
25. Khan AA, Tan J-L, Li W, et al. The impact of transcatheter atrial septal defect closure in the older population: a prospective study. J Am Coll Cardiol Intv. 2010;3:276–81.
26. Masutani S, Taketazu M, Ishido H, et al. Effects of age on hemodynamic changes after transcatheter closure of atrial septal defect: importance of ventricular diastolic function. Heart Vessels. 2012;27:71–8.
27. Ewert P, Berger F, Nagdyman N, Kretschmar O, Dittrich S, Abdul-Khaliq H, Lange P. Masked left ventricular restriction in elderly patients with atrial septal defects: a contraindications for closure? Catheter Cardiovasc Interv. 2001;52:177–80.
28. Valente A, Rhodes JF. Current indications and contraindications for transcatheter atrial septal defect and patent foramen ovale device closure. Am Heart J. 2007;153(suppl):81–4.
29. Everett AD, Jennings J, Sibinga E, et al. Community use of the Amplatzer atrial septal defect occluder: results of the multicenter MAGIC atrial septal defect study. Pediatr Cardiol. 2009;30:240–7.
30. Majunke N, Bialkowski J, Wilson N, et al. Closure of atrial septal defect with the Amplatzer septal occluder in adults. Am J Cardiol. 2009;103:550–4.
31. Jones TK, Latson LA, Zahn E, Multicenter Pivotal Study of the HELEX Septal Occluder Investigators, et al. Results of the U.S. multicenter pivotal study of the HELEX septal occluder for percutaneous closure of secundum atrial septal defects. J Am Coll Cardiol. 2007;49:2215–21.
32. Sadiq M, Kazmi T, Rehman AU, Latif F, Hyder N, Qureshi SA. Device closure of atrial septal defect: medium-term outcome with special reference to complications. Cardiol Young. 2012;22:71–8.
33. Abaci A, Unlu S, Alsancak Y, Kaya U, Sezenoz B. Short and long term complications of device closure of atrial septal defect and patent foramen ovale: meta-analysis of 28,142 patients from 203 studies. Catheter Cardiovasc Interv. 2013;82:1123–38.

34. Divekar A, Gaamangwe T, Shaikh N, Raabe M, Ducas J. Cardiac perforation after device closure of atrial septal defects with the Amplatzer septal occluder. J Am Coll Cardiol. 2005;45:1213–8.
35. Taggart NW, Dearani JA, Hagler DJ. Late erosion of an Amplatzer septal occluder device 6 years after placement. J Thorac Cardiovasc Surg. 2011;142:221–2.
36. Amin Z, Hijazi ZM, Bass JL, Cheatham JP, Hellenbrand WE, Kleinman CS. Erosion of Amplatzer septal occluder device after closure of secundum atrial septal defects: review of registry of complications and recommendations to minimize future risk. Catheter Cardiovasc Interv. 2004;63:496–502.
37. Gaithersburg H. FDA executive summary memorandum. Transcatheter ASD occluders: clinical update and review of events. 2012. http://www.fda.gov/downloads/AdvisoryCommittees/CommitteesMeetingMaterials/MedicalDevices/MedicalDevicesAdvisoryCommittee/CirculatorySystemDevicesPanel/UCM304924. pdf. Accessed 7 Feb 2014.
38. Bruch L, Winkelmann A, Sonntag S, et al. Fenestrated occluders for treatment of ASD in elderly patients with pulmonary hypertension and/or right heart failure. J Interv Cardiol. 2008;21:44–9.
39. Peters B, Ewert P, Schubert S, et al. Self-fabricated fenestrated Amplatzer occluders for transcatheter closure of atrial septal defect in patients with left ventricular restriction: midterm results. Clin Res Cardiol. 2006;95:88–92.
40. Uebing A, Steer PJ, Yentis SM, Gatzoulis MA. Pregnancy and congenital heart disease. BMJ. 2006;332:401–6.
41. Drenthen W, Pieper PG, Roos-Hesselink JW, the ZAHARA Investigators, et al. Outcome of pregnancy in women with congenital heart disease: a literature review. J Am Coll Cardiol. 2007;49:2303–11.
42. Yap SC, Drenthen W, Meijboom FJ, the ZAHARA investigators, et al. Comparison of pregnancy outcomes in women with repaired versus unrepaired atrial septal defect. BJOG. 2009;116:1593–601.
43. Bédard E, Dimopoulos K, Gatzoulis MA. Has there been any progress made on pregnancy outcomes among women with pulmonary arterial hypertension? Eur Heart J. 2009;30:256–65.
44. Hagen PT, Scholz DG, Edwards WD. Incidence and size of patent foramen ovale during the first 10 decades of life: an autopsy study of 965 normal hearts. Mayo Clin Proc. 1984;59:17–20.
45. Lechat P, Mas JL, Lascault G, et al. Prevalence of patent foramen ovale in patients with stroke. N Engl J Med. 1988;318:1148–52.
46. Di Tullio MR, Sacco RL, Sciacca RR, Jin Z, Homma S. Patent foramen ovale and the risk of ischemic stroke in a multiethnic population. J Am Coll Cardiol. 2007;49:797–802.
47. Davis D, Gregson J, Willeit P, Stephan B, Al-Shahi Salman R, Brayne C. Patent foramen ovale, ischemic stroke and migraine: systematic review and stratified meta-analysis of association studies. Neuroepidemiology. 2012;40:56–67.
48. Meissner I, Khandheria BK, Heit JA, et al. Patent foramen ovale: innocent or guilty? Evidence from a prospective population-based study. J Am Coll Cardiol. 2006;47:440–5.
49. Meier B, Lock JE. Contemporary management of patent foramen ovale. Circulation. 2003;107:5–9.
50. De Castro S, Cartoni D, Fiorelli M, et al. Morphological and functional characteristics of patent foramen ovale and their embolic implications. Stroke. 2000;31:2407–13.
51. Stewart WF, Shechter A, Rasmussen BK. Migraine prevalence. A review of population-based studies. Neurology. 1994;44(6 Suppl 4):S17–23.
52. Silberstein SD. Migraine. Lancet. 2004;363(9406):381–91.
53. Anzola GP, Magoni M, Guindani M, Rozzini L, Dalla VG. Potential source of cerebral embolism in migraine with aura: a transcranial Doppler study. Neurology. 1999;52:1622–5.

54. Homma S, Sacco RL, Di Tullio MR, Sciacca RR, Mohr JP. Effect of medical treatment in stroke patients with patent foramen ovale: patent foramen ovale in cryptogenic stroke study. Circulation. 2002;105:2625–31.
55. Tobis J, Shenoda M. Percutaneous treatment of patent foramen ovale and atrial septal defects. J Am Coll Cardiol. 2012;60:1722–32.
56. Furlan AJ, Reisman M, Massaro J, et al. Closure or medical therapy for cryptogenic stroke with patent foramen ovale. N Engl J Med. 2012;366:991–9.
57. Carroll JD, Saver JL, Thaler D, Smalling RW, Berry S, MacDonald LA, et al., editors. Randomized Evaluation of Recurrent Stroke Comparing PFO Closure to Established Current Standard of Care Treatment. Transcatheter Cardiovascular Therapeutics. Miami: Boca Raton; 2012.

Part III

Arrhythmia and Conduction Disease

Ablation of Atrial Fibrillation in Women 14

Stephanie Fichtner

14.1 Epidemiology

Atrial fibrillation (AF) is the most common arrhythmia in elderly persons. The prevalence of AF is 0.95 %, ranging from 0.1 % among adults younger than 55 years to 9 % in persons aged 80 years or older. AF is more common in men than in women (1.1 % versus 0.8 %). In addition AF leads to a significantly increased mortality which is higher in women than in men (odds ratio (OR) 1.9 versus 1.5). Woman presenting with AF are older; their reported quality of life is lower; they have more comorbidities and show an increase of heart failure with preserved ejection fraction compared to men [5]. Because of demographic changes, the number of patients with AF will likely increase 2.5-fold during the next 50 years highlighting the efforts required in stroke prevention and rhythm management [8].

14.2 Adverse Effects of Atrial Fibrillation

In the Framingham Study atrial fibrillation led to a fivefold excess of stroke compared to subjects without any cardiovascular diseases. If atrial fibrillation occurred in addition to coronary artery disease or cardiac failure, atrial fibrillation doubled the stroke risk in men and trebled the risk in women [18]. In a cohort study of 13,559 adults with nonvalvular atrial fibrillation, women had, after multivariable analysis, a significant higher annual rate of thromboembolism off warfarin than did men (3.5 % versus 1.8 %) [7]. Therefore, gender was included in the new $CHADS^2$-Vasc score highlighting the higher incidence of thromboembolism in women [4].

S. Fichtner
Medizinische Klinik und Poliklinik I, LMU Klinikum der Universität München, Munich, Germany
e-mail: stephanie.fichtner@med.uni-muenchen.de

P. Presbitero et al. (eds.), *Percutaneous Treatment of Cardiovascular Diseases in Women*, DOI 10.1007/978-3-319-39611-8_14

14.3 Medication in AF Treatment

14.3.1 Oral Anticoagulation

The most important medication in AF treatment is oral anticoagulation leading to a highly significant reduction in thromboembolism especially in women. In an analysis comparing women and men taking warfarin, warfarin led to a significant reduction in the annual rate of thromboembolism showing no significant differences between genders. In some smaller studies, a higher bleeding risk with warfarin was seen in women; however, in the ATRIA study, major hemorrhage including brain hemorrhage was equally distributed in both genders (1 %). Also in the Stroke Prevention in Atrial Fibrillation (SPAF) study, annual bleeding rates on warfarin treatment showed no differences between women and men [7]. The Canadian Registry of Atrial Fibrillation included patients after first ECG confirmed diagnosis of atrial fibrillation. Compared to men, women were half as likely to receive warfarin and twice as likely to receive acetylsalicylic acid [11].

The direct oral anticoagulants like dabigatran, rivaroxaban, apixaban, and edoxaban showed promising results in large multicenter trials leading to a similar stroke reduction compared to warfarin with significant less bleeding complications. In subgroup analysis of the RE-LY study and ARISTOTLE study, women showed no significant differences in regard to stroke prevention and bleeding complications compared to men [9, 14].

14.3.2 Rhythm Versus Rate Control with Oral Medication

Patients presenting with AF can be managed with either rate or rhythm control. Patients with highly symptomatic AF episodes will more likely receive antiarrhythmic medication for rhythm control, and patients with asymptomatic episodes will more likely receive rate control. In the AFFIRM and RACE trials [13, 19], rate versus rhythm control using cardioversion and antiarrhythmic medication was prospectively tested in big multicenter trials with hard endpoints including mortality, morbidity, hospitalization, and stroke. Unexpectedly, in these trials no advantage for the rhythm control regime could be demonstrated. In the rhythm control, arm hospitalization and adverse drug effects were more common. In the larger AFFIRM trial, no difference between women and men could be detected. However, women randomized to the rhythm control arm in the RACE trial developed more endpoints: mainly heart failure, thromboembolic complications, and significantly more adverse effect on antiarrhythmic medication. In addition, in 62 % in the AFFIRM trial and in only 35 % in the RACE trial stable sinus rhythm could be achieved.

In the Euro Heart Survey on Atrial Fibrillation [5], women received significantly more often digoxin/digitoxin for rate control compared to men. In the last years, doubts about the safety of digoxin have been described. In an analysis of the AFFIRM data, an increased mortality was seen in patients taking digoxin [17].

Since the AFFIRM/RACE trials, the lack of superiority of the rhythm control strategy has been attributed to the negative side effects of the antiarrhythmic medications. Large international studies are now on the way comparing rate versus rhythm control strategies using ablation as the rhythm strategy with hard endpoints like mortality, morbidity, and stroke (CABANA trial, EAST trial). Smaller studies comparing antiarrhythmic medication with ablation showed significantly higher success in achieving sinus rhythm and improving quality of life with the ablation strategy [12].

14.4 Benefit and Risk of Ablation in Women

Pulmonary vein isolation (PVI) (Fig. 14.1) has become a widely used and accepted treatment option in patients with paroxysmal atrial fibrillation (AF) with procedural success rates of 60–80 % and in highly symptomatic patients with persistent AF after failed antiarrhythmic medication with procedural success rates of about 50 % [3, 4].

Interestingly, in a big Medicare analysis including 517,941 patients with AF, women were less likely to have an outpatient visit with an electrophysiologist and also were less likely to undergo catheter ablation for AF [2]. This trend also could be seen in a European survey where women received significantly less electrical cardioversion and significantly less catheter ablation [5].

In a meta-analysis [16] only 21 % of patients who underwent ablation for AF were women. Unfortunately, women had a 20 % greater risk of recurrence of AF after ablation for AF compared to men. The reasons for this phenomenon are not clear, but women were older, already underwent a longer period of antiarrhythmic medication, and had a higher prevalence of coexisting cardiovascular disease when

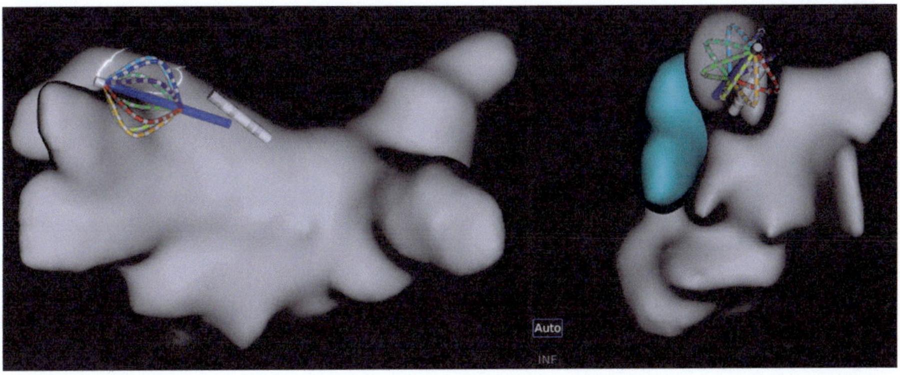

Fig. 14.1 3D anatomy of the left atrium with the Rhythmia System (posterior-anterior- and left lateral view). In both pictures you can see the multipolar mapping catheter (Orion) in the left superior pulmonary vein and the ablation catheter at the ostium of the PV during circumferential pulmonary vein isolation

they underwent the ablation procedure. In addition or because of the treatment delay, women had more nonparoxysmal AF and more non-PV triggers. In a Japanese study [15] including only patients with paroxysmal AF, women were again significant older and also had worse outcome after multiple procedures compared to men. However, women still reached AF-free survival after 5 years of 76.6 % (men 81.3 %). We know from many studies that patients who are older, have longer-lasting episodes of AF, and to have more nonparoxysmal AF have a worse outcome after AF ablation. This could explain the higher recurrence rate after AF ablation in women.

14.4.1 Complications After AF Ablation

The complication rate after AF ablation varies between 4 and 6 %. In several retrospective analyses, female gender was associated with increased complication rate, especially vascular complications [1, 10]. However, in the largest available registry analysis of 93,801 procedures in the United States, no difference in complication rate regarding gender could be detected [6].

Take Home Message
Most importantly, oral anticoagulation is essential in prevention of thromboembolism. Since it does not lead to an increased risk of bleeding events in women, oral anticoagulation should be emphasized more in practice. In addition, AF ablation should be recommended to women more often and at an earlier stage to increase the ablation success and to reduce the amount of women taking antiarrhythmic medication.

References

1. Baman TS, Jongnarangsin K, Chugh A, Suwanagool A, Guiot A, Madenci A, Walsh S, Ilg KJ, Gupta SK, Latchamsetty R, Bagwe S, Myles JD, Crawford T, Good E, Bogun F, Pelosi Jr F, Morady F, Oral H. Prevalence and predictors of complications of radiofrequency catheter ablation for atrial fibrillation. J Cardiovasc Electrophysiol. 2011;22(6):626–31. doi:10.1111/j.1540-8167.2010.01995.x.
2. Bhave PD, Lu X, Girotra S, Kamel H, Vaughan Sarrazin MS. Race- and gender-related differences in care for patients newly diagnosed with atrial fibrillation. Heart Rhythm. 2015. doi:10.1016/j.hrthm.2015.03.031.
3. Calkins H, Kuck KH, Cappato R, Brugada J, Camm a J, Chen S-A, Crijns HJ, Damiano Jr RJ, Davies DW, DiMarco J, Edgerton J, Ellenbogen K, Ezekowitz MD, Haines DE, Haissaguerre M, Hindricks G, Iesaka Y, Jackman W, Jalife J, Jais P, Kalman J, Keane D, Kim YH, Kirchhof P, Klein G, Kottkamp H, Kumagai K, Lindsay BD, Mansour M, Marchlinski FE, McCarthy PM, Mont JL, Morady F, Nademanee K, Nakagawa H, Natale A, Nattel S, Packer DL, Pappone C, Prystowsky E, Raviele A, Reddy V, Ruskin JN, Shemin RJ, Tsao HM, Wilber D. 2012 HRS/EHRA/ECAS expert consensus statement on catheter and surgical ablation of atrial fibrillation: recommendations for patient selection, procedural techniques, patient management and follow-up, definitions, endpoints, and research trial design: a re. Heart Rhythm. 2012;9(4):632–96. doi:10.1016/j.hrthm.2011.12.016.

4. Camm AJ, Kirchhof P, Lip GYH, Schotten U, Savelieva I, Ernst S, Van Gelder IC, Al-Attar N, Hindricks G, Prendergast B, Heidbuchel H, Alfieri O, Angelini A, Atar D, Colonna P, De Caterina R, De Sutter J, Goette A, Gorenek B, Heldal M, Hohloser SH, Kolh P, Le Heuzey JY, Ponikowski P, Rutten FH. Guidelines for the management of atrial fibrillation: the Task Force for the Management of Atrial Fibrillation of the European Society of Cardiology (ESC). Eur Heart J. 2010;31(19):2369–429. doi:10.1093/eurheartj/ehq278.
5. Dagres N, Nieuwlaat R, Vardas PE, Andresen D, Lévy S, Cobbe S, Kremastinos DT, Breithardt G, Cokkinos DV, Crijns HJGM. Gender-related differences in presentation, treatment, and outcome of patients with atrial fibrillation in Europe. A report from the Euro Heart Survey on Atrial Fibrillation. J Am Coll Cardiol. 2007;49(5):572–7. doi:10.1016/j.jacc.2006.10.047.
6. Deshmukh A, Patel NJ, Pant S, Shah N, Chothani A, Mehta K, Grover P, Singh V, Vallurupalli S, Savani GT, Badheka A, Tuliani T, Dabhadkar K, Dibu G, Reddy YM, Sewani A, Kowalski M, Mitrani R, Paydak H, Viles-Gonzalez JF. In-hospital complications associated with catheter ablation of atrial fibrillation in the United States between 2000 and 2010: Analysis of 93 801 procedures. Circulation. 2013;128(19):2104–12. doi:10.1161/CIRCULATIONAHA. 113.003862.
7. Fang MC, Singer DE, Chang Y, Hylek EM, Henault LE, Jensvold NG, Go AS. Gender differences in the risk of ischemic stroke and peripheral embolism in atrial fibrillation: the AnTicoagulation and Risk factors in Atrial fibrillation (ATRIA) study. Circulation. 2005. doi:10.1161/CIRCULATIONAHA.105.553438.
8. Go AS, Hylek EM, Phillips KA, Chang Y, Henault LE, Selby JV, Singer DE. Prevalence of diagnosed atrial fibrillation in adults: national implications for rhythm management and stroke prevention: the Anticoagulation and Risk Factors in Atrial Fibrillation (ATRIA) Study. JAMA. 2001;285(18):2370–5. doi:jcc10004 [pii].
9. Granger CB, Alexander JH, McMurray JJV, Lopes RD, Hylek EM, Hanna M, Al-Khalidi HR, Ansell J, Atar D, Avezum A, Bahit MC, Diaz R, Easton JD, Ezekowitz JA, Flaker G, Garcia D, Geraldes M, Gersh BJ, Golitsyn S, Goto S, Hermosillo AG, Hohnloser SH, Horowitz J, Mohan P, Jansky P, Lewis BS, Lopez-Sendon JL, Pais P, Parkhomenko A, Verheugt FW, Zhu J, Wallentin L. Apixaban versus warfarin in patients with atrial fibrillation. N Engl J Med. 2011;365(11):981–92. doi:10.1056/NEJMoa1107039.
10. Hoyt H, Bhonsale A, Chilukuri K, Alhumaid F, Needleman M, Edwards D, Govil A, Nazarian S, Cheng A, Henrikson CA, Sinha S, Marine JE, Berger R, Calkins H, Spragg DD. Complications arising from catheter ablation of atrial fibrillation: temporal trends and predictors. Heart Rhythm. 2011;8(12):1869–74. doi:10.1016/j.hrthm.2011.07.025.
11. Humphries KH, Kerr CR, Connolly SJ, Klein G, Boone JA, Green M, Sheldon R, Talajic M, Dorian P, Newman D. New-onset atrial fibrillation Sex differences in presentation, treatment, and outcome. Circulation. 2001;103:2365–70.
12. Jais P, Cauchemez B, Macle L, Daoud E, Khairy P, Subbiah R, Hocini M, Extramiana F, Sacher F, Bordachar P, Klein G, Weerasooriya R, Clémenty J, Haissaguerre M. Catheter ablation versus antiarrhythmic drugs for atrial fibrillation: the A4 study. Circulation. 2008;118(24):2498–505. doi:CIRCULATIONAHA.108.772582 [pii] 10.1161/CIRCULATIONAHA.108.772582.
13. Rienstra M, Van Veldhuisen DJ, Hagens VE, Ranchor AV, Veeger NJGM, Crijns HJGM, Van Gelder IC. Gender-related differences in rhythm control treatment in persistent atrial fibrillation: data of the rate control versus electrical cardioversion (RACE) study. J Am Coll Cardiol. 2005;46(7):1298–306. doi:10.1016/j.jacc.2005.05.078.
14. Connolly SJ, Ezekowitz MD, Yusuf S, Eikelboom J, Oldgren J, Parekh A, Pogue J, Reilly PA, Themeles E, Varrone J, Wang S, Alings M, Xavier D, Zhu J, Diaz R, Lewis BS, Darius H, Diener H-C, Joyner CD, Wallentin L, and the RE-LY Steering Committee and Investigators. Dabigatran versus warfarin in patients with atrial fibrillation. N Engl J Med. 2009;361(12):1139–51. doi:10.1056/NEJMoa1404595.
15. Takigawa M, Kuwahara T, Takahashi A, Watari Y, Okubo K, Takahashi Y, Takagi K, Kuroda S, Osaka Y, Kawaguchi N, Yamao K, Nakashima E, Sugiyama T, Akiyama D, Kamiishi T, Kimura S, Hikita H, Hirao K, Isobe M. Differences in catheter ablation of paroxysmal atrial

fibrillation between males and females. Int J Cardiol. 2013;168(3):1984–91. doi:10.1016/j.ijcard.2012.12.101.

16. Vallakati A, Reddy M, Sharma A, Kanmanthareddy A, Sridhar A, Pillarisetti J, Atkins D, Konda B, Bommana S, Di Biase L, Santangeli P, Natale A, Lakkireddy D. Impact of gender on outcomes after atrial fibrillation ablation. Int J Cardiol. 2015;187:12–6. doi:10.1016/j.ijcard.2015.03.341.
17. Whitbeck MG, Charnigo RJ, Khairy P, Ziada K, Bailey AL, Zegarra MM, Shah J, Morales G, Macaulay T, Sorrell VL, Campbell CL, Gurley J, Anaya P, Nasr H, Bai R, Di Biase L, Booth DC, Jondeau G, Natale A, Roy D, Smyth S, Moliterno DJ, Elayi CS. Increased mortality among patients taking digoxin – analysis from the AFFIRM study. Eur Heart J. 2013;34(20):1481–8. doi:10.1093/eurheartj/ehs348.
18. Wolf PA, Abbott RD, Kannel WB. Atrial fibrillation as an independent risk factor for stroke: the Framingham Study. Stroke. 1991. doi:10.1161/01.STR.22.8.983.
19. Wyse DG, Waldo AL, DiMarco JP, Domanski MJ, Rosenberg Y, Schron EB, Kellen JC, Greene HL, Mickel MC, Dalquist JE, Corley SD. A comparison of rate control and rhythm control in patients with atrial fibrillation. N Engl J Med. 2002;347(23):1825–33. doi:10.1056/NEJMoa021328 347/23/1825 [pii].

Biventricular Pacing in Women for Heart Failure

15

Maria Grazia Bongiorni and Francesca Menichetti

Abbreviations and Acronyms

AIV	Anterior interventricular vein
CHF	Chronic heart failure
CRT	Cardiac resynchronization therapy
CS	Coronary sinus
CT	Computed tomography
HF	Heart failure
ICD	Implantable cardioverter–defibrillator
LAO	Left anterior oblique
LBBB	Left bundle branch block
LV	Left ventricle
LVESVi	Left ventricle systolic volume indexed
MCV	Middle cardiac vein
RA	Right atrium
RAO	Right anterior oblique
RV	Right ventricle

15.1 Background

Chronic heart failure (CHF) is one of the most common diseases. Despite optimal modern pharmacological treatment, many CHF patients experience severe and persistent symptoms, and their prognosis remains poor. In selected patients who present with severe left ventricular systolic dysfunction with intra- and interventricular

M.G. Bongiorni, MD (✉) • F. Menichetti, MD
Second Cardiology Department, University Hospital of Pisa, 56100 Pisa, Italy
e-mail: m.g.bongiorni@med.unipi.it

P. Presbitero et al. (eds.), *Percutaneous Treatment of Cardiovascular Diseases in Women*,
DOI 10.1007/978-3-319-39611-8_15

conduction delays, a cardiac resynchronization therapy (CRT) system has been found to improve symptoms, exercise tolerance, quality of life, and outcome.

The CRT was introduced in the 1990s and offered not only atrioventricular synchronization as in dual chamber pacing but also synchronization of the two ventricles. By pacing the region of the left ventricle (LV) with the most delayed activation, it was possible both to improve interventricular synchrony and the synchrony of the LV itself.

When women present with New York Heart Association (NYHA) class II–IV despite adequate medical treatment, low left ventricular (LV) ejection fraction (EF < 35 %), and QRS duration >120–150 m, they are potential candidates for CRT either alone or in combination with an ICD. Yet, the percentage of women undergoing CRT represents only about 20 % of the total CRT population [1]. Despite of clear indications of the guidelines, patient selection optimization for CRT is still an ongoing challenge.

15.1.1 The Women Bias

Epidemiology, treatment, and prognosis of CHF may manifest gender-related differences [2]. Although the overall prevalence of HF in men and women is similar, large clinical trials have consistently shown underrepresentation of women. A gender bias may also occur in the related use of diagnostic resources and achievement of optimal medical treatment [3].

Looking at CHF clinical trials, women are not adequately represented (0–34 % of study population). Many women are not enrolled because they do not have the ejection fraction required by the trials. Underrepresentation is also exacerbated by the exclusion of older patients, as HF predominates in older women. Moreover women, being older, often have multiple health problems that may create additional risks and confuse trial results.

Community-based studies suggest a gender bias in medical treatment and management. Females were less frequently treated with inotropes, spironolactone, amiodarone, nitrates, statins, and antiplatelet agents. At discharge, ACE inhibitors, amiodarone, and spironolactone were less frequently prescribed in females. Women have a relatively low risk of dying during hospital stay but a high probability of being readmitted within a short period of time [2].

15.1.2 CRT Outcomes in Women

In a MIRACLE trial sub analysis, CRT significantly reduced deaths and HF hospitalization in women but not in men highlighting possible differences between genders. On the other hand, some studies reported no differences in CRT response between genders, but in these studies, LV volumes were not normalized to body surface area [4].

In the MADIT-CRT trial, CRT-D has been shown to be associated with a significant reduction in HF or death in mild HF patients with EF ≤30 % and QRS ≥130 ms, and this reduction was more pronounced in women during short-term follow-up [5]. Subsequent study and long-term follow-up of MADIT-CRT revealed that the benefit was restricted to patients with left bundle branch block (LBBB) configuration [6].

A recent sub analysis analyzed the sex-specific benefit of CRT-D to improve long-term outcomes by QRS duration in the mild HF patients with LBBB enrolled in MADIT-CRT [7]. This study had a relatively large proportion of women, almost one-third of the total patient population, and that is much higher than most other clinical trials.

During the median follow-up of 5.6 years, women derived greater clinical benefit from CRT-D compared with ICD only, with a significant 71 % reduction in HF or death and a 77 % reduction in HF alone compared with men, who had a 41 % reduction in HF or death and a 50 % reduction in HF alone. The incremental benefit of CRT-D in women for HF or death and HF alone was consistent with QRS <150 or >150 ms (Fig. 15.1).

15.1.2.1 Reasons for Gender-Specific LV Remodeling Response to CRT

Although we know more about heart failure physiopathology, there is much we do not understand about the physiologic mechanisms that underlie its sex differences.

A different hypertrophy pattern between genders was described, and this was verified also in postinfarction end-stage failing hearts [8]. Moreover, in failing human hearts, a higher myocyte death (necrosis or apoptosis) has been clearly demonstrated in men than in women [9]. Finally, it is well known that inherent physiological sex differences of abnormal conduction exist. It has been suggested that women have shorter QRS duration than men in the absence of any conduction disturbance. Some studies showed that women had significantly shorter baseline QRS durations, but they gained even greater clinical benefit from CRT-D than men, suggesting that women may have more dyssynchrony, at shorter QRS durations, that leads to better response with CRT-D [10].

All these data and observations suggest that gender directly affects physiologic and pathologic myocardial remodeling and that female gender provides a favorable substrate for LV reverse remodeling during CRT.

15.1.2.2 Reasons for Female CRT Undertreatment

In women, the proportion of responders defined on the basis of LVESVi reduction of at least 10 % was significantly higher, and the degree of reverse remodeling was also significantly greater than in men.

Despite this better outcome, women accounted for only 20 % of patients undergoing CRT implantation. This may be due to several factors. Women have less systolic dysfunction than men and are therefore more often treated by generalists. Women are not referred to a hospital as often as men and generally tend to undergo fewer invasive and noninvasive procedures as assessment of LV function.

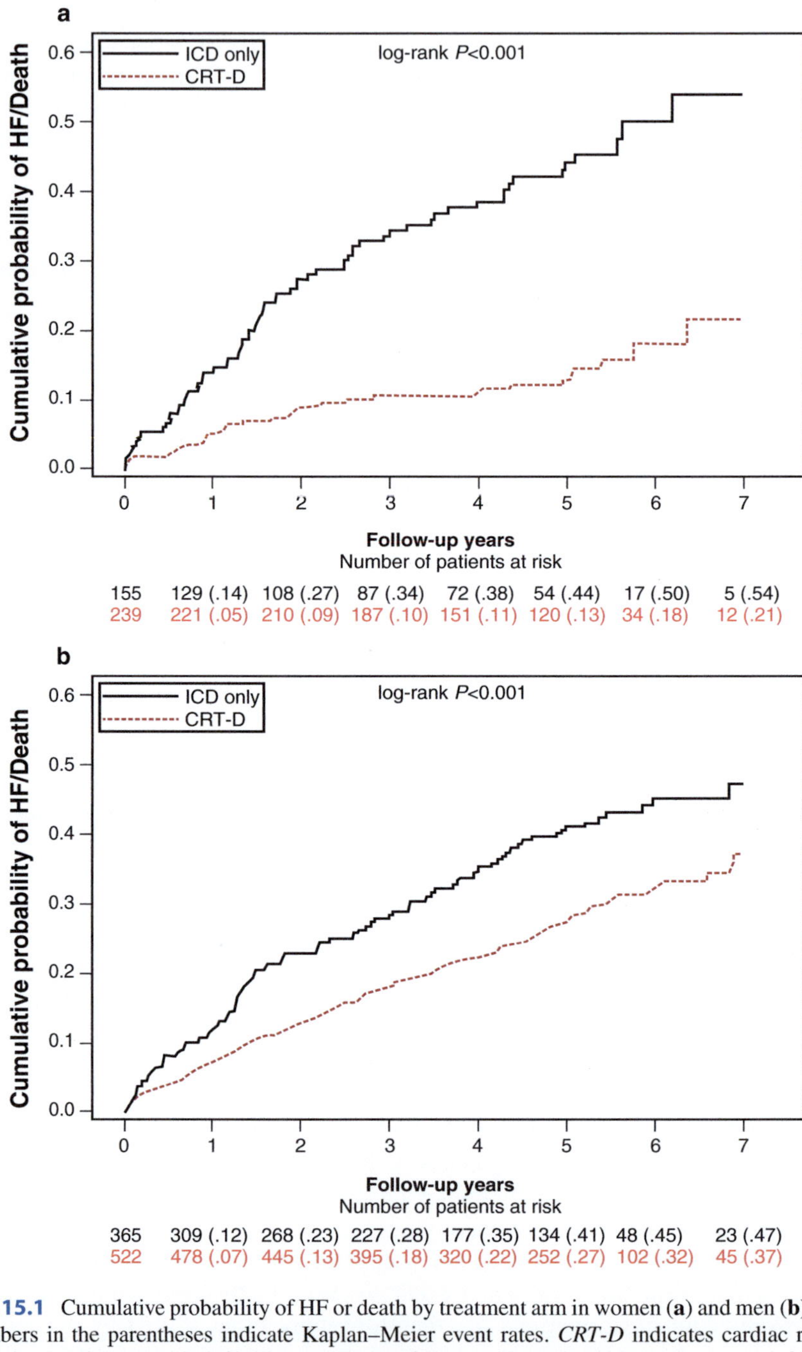

Fig. 15.1 Cumulative probability of HF or death by treatment arm in women (**a**) and men (**b**). The numbers in the parentheses indicate Kaplan–Meier event rates. *CRT-D* indicates cardiac resynchronization therapy with defibrillator, *HF* heart failure, *ICD* implantable cardioverter–defibrillator (Adapted from Biton et al. [7])

Finally fewer women than men received ICDs, despite a similar degree of LV remodeling. This might be related to fewer women who fulfilled the MADIT II criteria and the underutilization of resources in women. On the other hand after the SCD-HeFT [11], there is a clear class I indication for ICD implantation for nonischemic dilated cardiomyopathy that is more common in women.

15.2 Implantation Techniques

15.2.1 Vein Accesses in Women

CRT implantation in women is achieved in a standard fashion, but some specific anatomical features should be taken into account. Because of the smaller vein size in women and the requirement of three leads placement for biventricular pacing—an atrial lead, a right ventricle (RV) lead (defibrillation or pacing), and a left ventricle (LV) pacing lead—it is worthwhile attempting cephalic and subclavian access in these cases. If possible, the right ventricular lead should be placed through a cephalic approach to minimize the potential for subclavian crush of the larger lead. The subclavian vein can then be used for introduction of the atrial lead and a LV lead via the coronary sinus (CS).

15.2.2 Right Ventricle Features in Women

In order to have correct defibrillator lead placement, it is necessary to keep the whole RV-defibrillating coil in the RV. This goal could not be easier to achieve in women patient with small cardiac volumes. The coil must not cross the tricuspid valve leaving a portion of it in the right atrium, avoiding defibrillation capacity deficiency and inappropriate diagnosis of ventricular arrhythmias during atrial tachyarrhythmias. Overcoming this problem may not always be compatible with choosing an optimal RV pacing site, which, for example, may be the mid-septum or another non-apical position. As the septum often bulges into the RV due to huge LV dilatation, the coil may lie partly in the right atrium. The implanter is then forced to select a less optimal site from the hemodynamic point of view in order to achieve effective arrhythmia diagnosis and defibrillation.

15.2.3 Coronary Sinus Anatomy

The CS ostium is partially covered by a Thebesian valve (a remnant of the embryonic right valve) in roughly 60 % of patients. In a small subset of patients, the ostium is completely enclosed by the valve with only small fenestrations allowing venous drainage, thereby presenting a major impediment to CS access. In addition, RA dilation may lead to an abnormally high insertion of the CS ostium, making its

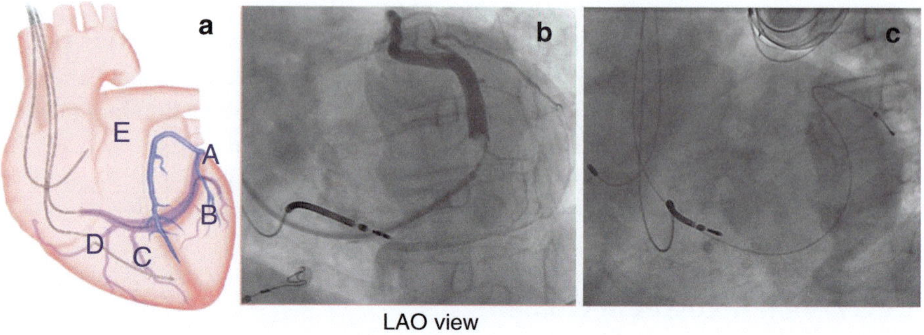

Fig. 15.2 Selecting vein for LV lead placement. The possible targets for the left ventricular lead showed by the scheme in (**a**) free wall are (*A*) lateral (marginal) cardiac vein, (*B*) posterolateral cardiac vein, and (*C*) posterior cardiac vein. Suboptimal lead locations are also (*D*) middle cardiac vein and (*E*) great cardiac vein. In (**b**) an example of CS angiography and in (**c**) the leads' final position are shown

intubation difficult. A second valve (the valve of Vieussens) located at the junction of the great cardiac vein and the vein of Marshall is present in about 8 % of patients [12]. This valve may divert a wire or catheter into the diminutive vein of Marshall, which if not immediately recognized can lead to venous dissection and hemopericardium.

Anatomic studies have shown a median of six veins from the left ventricle draining into the main CS. The nearest branch to the CS ostium is the middle cardiac vein (MCV), which may be covered by a small valve or originate with a separate ostium. The MCV runs in the interventricular groove toward the ventricular apex and is usually not a suitable target for LV lead placement. Three distinct veins drain the lateral wall of the left ventricle (Fig. 15.2). The posterolateral branch, the most prominent and consistent of these veins, usually enters the CS within 1 cm of the ostium. The lateral marginal vein and lateral branches off the anterior interventricular vein (AIV) are variably present. In women with prior myocardial infarction, first-order branches to the lateral wall off the CS are often diminutive or absent.

One of the important elements in a successful implantation is selecting the most appropriate vein to cannulate for CRT lead placement. The best performance for LV pacing is thought to occur in a lateral or posterior–lateral position. This region was accessible from at least two CS tributaries (posterolateral and AIV) in greater than 85 % of patients. In approximately 20 % of patients, the mid-lateral LV wall was also accessible from branches of the MCV.

15.2.4 Coronary Sinus Variability

As proved by several CS angiograms, there is a great variability in CS anatomy (Fig. 15.3), and this matters during the LV lead placement. Rotational venography

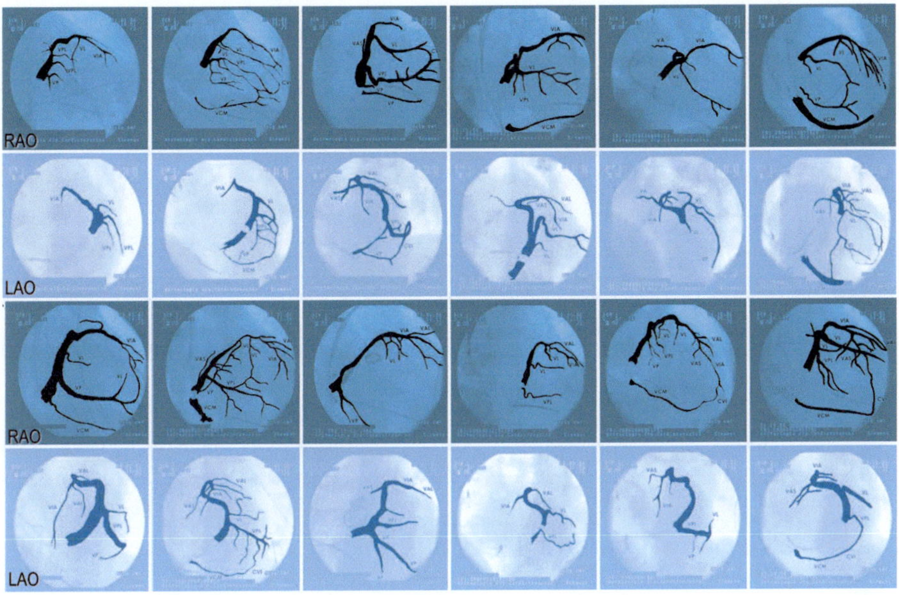

Fig. 15.3 Different angiograms show the great variability in CS anatomy (Adapted from CS venograms. Adapted from CS venograms collection, Bongiorni MG, De Lucia R (with permission))

may provide a more complete assessment of the CS branches to help determine the best viewing angle for target branch access. Multislice computed tomography (CT) scan has been used preprocedure to assess the cardiac vasculature prior to the implant procedure and correlates well with occlusive venograms. In addition, CT may reveal a high CS ostium takeoff and aid in catheter selection for successful CS access [13].

15.2.5 Interventional Approach to LV Lead Placement

The technique for LV lead placement includes the following steps: (1) localization of the CS ostium via contrast puffs through a preformed guide catheter, (2) cannulation of the CS with a sheath advanced over the guide catheter (with or without wire support), and (3) advancement of the LV lead through the delivery guide over an angioplasty wire.

The failure rates for placement of leads via the CS ranged between 7.5 and 10 % [14]. Most of these implant failures are due to difficulty accessing the CS ostium or advancing the pacing lead into an adequate, stable position. Coronary veins are still occasionally inaccessible and, more importantly, may not be present at the optimal stimulation site. In addition, LV lead dislodgement may occur both acutely or in the first few months after implantation in 6 % [15].

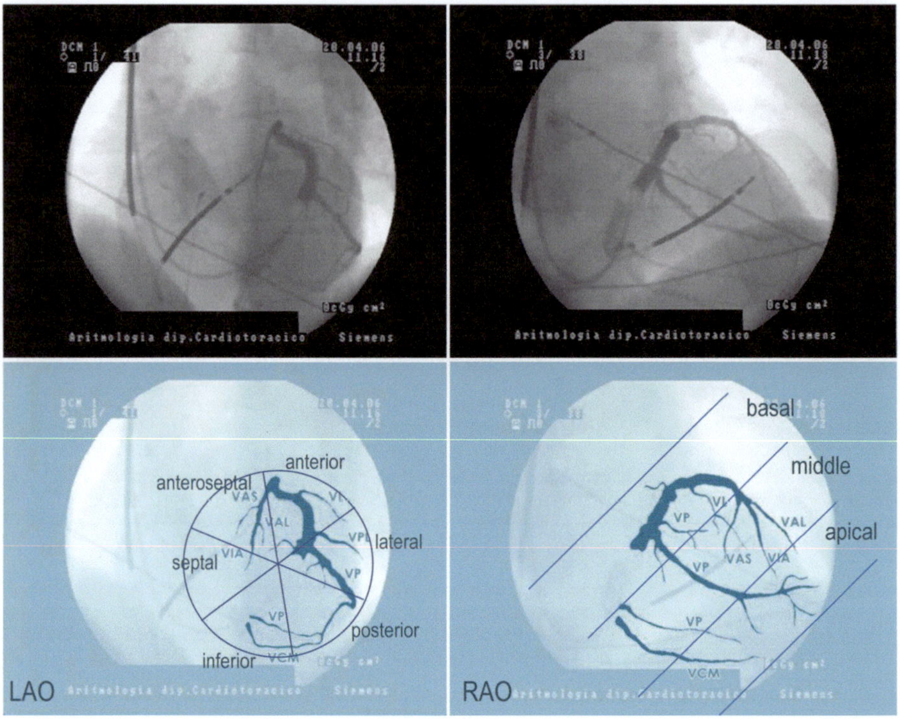

Fig. 15.4 Coronary angiogram (*upper panel*) and its schematic representation (*lower panel*) with LV segments (LAO projection) and regions (RAO projection) (Adapted from CS venograms collection, Bongiorni MG, De Lucia R (with permission))

This issue underlines the need for designing specific implant tools which would allow (1) easier access to the CS, (2) a means of visualizing the CS branches, and (3) maneuverability of the pacemaker lead.

1. The development of preshaped sheaths that follow the curvature of the lateral wall and floor of the RA allows easier access to the CS. In addition, the development of dual, telescoping catheters of various shapes allows improved maneuverability and access to CS side branches [16]. Small injections of contrast through these catheters allow direct visualization of the CS ostium and target branches and speed implant time.
2. Coronary sinus angiography greatly facilitates identification of a suitable branch vessel. Guiding sheaths and balloon catheters specifically designed for this purpose are available. Coronary sinus angiograms, preferably using right anterior oblique (RAO) and left anterior oblique (LAO) projections, should be recorded for reference during lead positioning (Fig. 15.4).
3. The main technique for LV lead placement is "over-the-wire" one. This technique involves probing for the CS ostium with a soft-tipped wire through a preformed sheath followed by advancement of the pacing lead into the target branch

over an angioplasty wire. However, tortuous anatomy may make advancement of the sheath or LV lead using only a wire for support difficult or impossible. If the first target vessel proves inadequate due to instability, poor capture threshold or unacceptable phrenic nerve stimulation, a different implant site should then be tested. Sometimes a sub-cannulation of the target branch with a telescoping support delivery system could act as a stable "rail" to navigate and straighten tortuous anatomy.

15.2.6 Difficult CRT Implantation in Women: Troubleshooting

15.2.6.1 Coronary Sinus Cannulation

The most common reasons for failed LV lead implantation include inability to access the CS ostium, inability to advance the lead into the target branch, and acute lead dislodgement or instability. Several techniques have been reported to overcome these obstacles.

The CS ostium is located in the posteroseptal region of the RA and is accessed by withdrawing the CS guide catheter across the tricuspid valve with counterclockwise torque. With dilated cardiomyopathy and significant right atrial enlargement, however, the ostium may enter more superiorly, making localization or cannulation difficult. Rarely, the CS ostium may enter the atrium in an anomalous fashion. When initial attempts at CS localization fail, a selective coronary angiogram with cine fluoroscopy of the venous phase may help locate a high or unusual ostial insertion.

Once the ostium is located, a prominent Thebesian valve or a steep takeoff due to atrial enlargement may hinder advancement of the catheter into the main body of the CS. When a wire can be placed into the main CS but there is resistance to sheath advancement, several maneuvers may be attempted. With the wire in place, a small, straight hydrophilic catheter can be advanced and used as a "rail" to place the larger diameter sheath beyond the tortuous segment. If the small hydrophilic catheter is advanced but there is still impedance, a larger and rigid sheath can be exchanged through the small sheath to provide additional support.

15.2.6.2 Access Vein Obstruction

Stenosis or total occlusion of the subclavian vein usually occurs as a result of previously implanted leads or surgery. In women this can occur more frequently than men. With proper technique, these stenotic veins can be safely dilated or stented in the large majority of cases, thereby avoiding an implant on the contralateral side or thoracotomy for an epicardial implant. Success is defined as passage of the transvenous lead through the obstruction to its final location.

If the obstruction is not complete, it is first crossed with a guidewire. Once it is confirmed that the guidewire is indeed within the lumen of the superior vena cava (SVC) (and not in a side branch or the azygos vein), a peripheral interventional balloon catheter is advanced over the wire. The balloon is removed while keeping the guidewire in place. A venogram is then performed.

15.2.6.3 Lead Extraction In Order to Enable CRT

When a complete venous obstruction is due to previously placed leads that are no longer in use, it is possible to extract the inoperative lead, then a guidewire is passed through the lumen thus created, and venoplasty is performed to dilate the stenosis sufficiently to allow passage of a sheath and new lead.

Still increasing life expectancy in patients with implanted devices and large number of leads more and more often induce the need to cure the treatment complications or to change especially to cardiac resynchronization therapy (CRT). In order to prevent further complications, the possibility of damaged or redundant leads extraction should be taken into consideration.

15.2.6.4 Coronary Sinus Dissections and Venoplasty

Dissection of the coronary sinus can occur more easily in women than in men, and this is due to a more frailty structure of the vessel. The most common cause of CS dissection is forceful contrast injection after inflating an occlusive balloon for venography but can also occur when the guide catheter tip is lodged against the wall or against a venous valve during forceful contrast injection or due to inexpert manipulation of stiff wires or electrode catheters. Fortunately, the occurrence of tamponade is relatively rare, since the coronary veins form a low pressure system. Deployment of a venous stent is a rapid and safe way of dealing with an ominous dissection in the coronary sinus, especially when blood is documented in the pericardial space. A guidewire is used to negotiate the dissection, and a peripheral stent is advanced to cover the area of the dissection. The stent is then deployed and a venogram obtained to confirm that the dissection has been sealed off.

Sometimes the Thebesian valve may actually be a fenestrated membrane covering the entire CS ostium. When the Thebesian or the Vieussens valves act as impediments to the introduction of the guide catheter, they can be usually negotiated by a hydrophilic-coated guidewire. Then a peripheral balloon of appropriate diameter may be passed over the guidewire and inflated to dilate the valve.

Coronary sinus stenting can also be used to retain conventional passive fixation LV leads in virtually any desired location in a coronary vein.

15.2.6.5 Epicardial Approach for Left Ventricular Lead

To improve CRT in women, a possible alternative approache for LV leads is the transcutaneous epicardial approach, which offers the possibility of positioning the leads anywhere on the surface of the LV. Epicardial placement of LV leads in the coronary veins has three limitations: accessibility to target veins, pacing threshold safety margin, and phrenic nerve stimulation. Some difficulties can also exist with lead fixation and the physical relationship of the stimulation site to the epicardial coronary arteries.

15.3 Future Advancements

New pacing leads have been developed which allow active fixation into the vessel to prevent dislodgement.

A recent trial of an active fixation LV lead has shown promising results [17]. This new model is a bipolar steroid-eluting lead that has a small exposed side helix and can be delivered using a guidewire or a stylet. When the desired vein location is reached, the lead body is rotated clockwise until the helix is fixated. This new tool was specifically designed for stability and precise placement in the coronary sinus vasculature. The first experiences published with this kind of lead were positive.

Additionally, leads with multiple pacing configurations have been developed which may improve thresholds and prevent phrenic nerve capture. The quadripolar model lead is a multipolar LV lead with three ring electrodes in addition to the tip electrode, allowing all four of the electrodes on the lead to act as the cathode and two also as an anode. In addition, the RV coil of the shocking lead may act as an anode thus giving ten possible bipolar and unipolar pacing configurations. Theoretically, problems with phrenic nerve stimulation and high-capture thresholds can be overcome simply by changing the pacing vector.

Recently a new technique was developed for the access to LV endocardium through the interventricular septum. In one of the first experiences described in literature, all patients were anticoagulated and a left ventriculography and coronary angiography were performed to identify LV borders and septal vessels. Subclavian vein access was used for a superior approach ventricular transseptal puncture under fluoroscopic guidance, using a steerable sheath and a standard transseptal needle, radiofrequency needle, or radiofrequency energy delivered through a guidewire. Finally, an active fixation pacing lead is delivered to the endocardial wall of the lateral LV [18].

Another promising technique is to perform an epicardial activation mapping of the left ventricle using a three-dimensional electroanatomic system via all available coronary veins (using the onset of the surface QRS as reference), in order to decide the optimal location for a LV lead [19].

Take-Home Messages

This chapter gives some awareness on gender heart failure biology and CRT women therapy bias due to anatomical differences and procedural characteristics, in spite of their better outcome. Nowadays new tools have greatly improved the efficiency and success rate of LV lead placement. The next great hurdle in CRT is to evolve the LV lead implantation from a strictly anatomically based procedure to a “targeted” implant strategy. Just as cardiothoracic surgeons use an individual patient’s coronary angiography to plan bypass graft placement, electrophysiologists should arm themselves with the best data before and during the procedure to guide proper lead placement for each patient, in order to target then best implant technique for each patient, especially if woman.

References

1. Cleland JGF, Daubert JC, Erdmann E, Freemantle N, Gras D, Kappenberger L, Tavazzi L, for the Cardiac Resynchronization — Heart Failure (CARE-HF) Study Investigators. The effect of cardiac resynchronization on morbidity and mortality in heart failure. N Engl J Med. 2005;352:1539–49.
2. Opasich C, De Feo S, Ambrosio GA, Bellis P, Di Learda A, Di Tano G, Fico D, et al. The 'real' woman with heart failure. Impact of sex on current in-hospital management of heart failure by cardiologist and internists. Eur J Heart Fail. 2004;6:769–79.
3. Sheppard R, Behlouli H, Richard H, Pilote L. Effect of gender on treatment, resource, utilization, and outcomes in congestive heart failure in Quebec, Canada. Am J Cardiol. 2005;95:955–9.
4. Bleeker GB, Schalij MJ, Boersma E, Steendijk P, Van DerWall EE, Bax JJ. Does a Gender difference in response to cardiac resynchronization therapy exist? Pacing Clin Electrophysiol. 2005;28:1271–5.
5. Arshad A, Moss AJ, Foster E, Padeletti L, Barsheshet A, Goldenberg I, Greenberg H, Hall WJ, McNitt S, Zareba W, Solomon S, Steinberg JS. Cardiac resynchronization therapy is more effective in women than in men: the MADIT-CRT (Multicenter Automatic Defibrillator Implantation Trial with Cardiac Resynchronization Therapy) trial. J Am Coll Cardiol. 2011;57:813–20.
6. Zareba W, Klein H, Cygankiewicz I, Hall WJ, McNitt S, Brown M, Cannom D, Daubert JP, Eldar M, Gold MR. Effectiveness of cardiac resynchronization therapy by QRS morphology in the Multicenter Automatic Defibrillator Implantation Trial-Cardiac Resynchronization Therapy (MADIT-CRT). Circulation. 2011;123:1061–72.
7. Biton Y, Zareba W, Goldenberg I, Klein H, et al. MADIT-CRT Executive Committee. Sex differences in long-term outcomes with cardiac resynchronization therapy in mild heart failure patients with left bundle branch block. J Am Heart Assoc. 2015;4(7). pii: e002013. doi:10.1161/JAHA.115.002013.
8. Crebbe DL, Dipla K, Ambati S, et al. Gender differences in postinfarction hypertrophy in end-stage failing hearts. J Am Coll Cardiol. 2003;41:300–6.
9. Guerra S, Leri A, Wang X, et al. Myocyte death in the failing human heart is gender dependent. Circ Res. 1999;85:856–66.
10. Crow RS, Hannan PJ, Folsom AR. Prognostic significance of corrected QT and corrected JT interval for incident coronary heart disease in a general population sample stratified by presence or absence of wide QRS complex: the ARIC Study with 13 years of follow-up. Circulation. 2003;108:1985–9.
11. Bardy GH, Lee KL, Mark DB, Poole JE, Packer DL, Boineau R, Domansi M, Sudden Cardiac Death in Heart Failure Trial (SCDHeFT) Investigators, et al. Amiodarone or an implantable cardioverter defibrillator for congestive heart failure. NEJM. 2005;352:225–37.
12. Habib A, Lachman N, Christensen KN, Asirvatham SJ. The anatomy of the coronary sinus venous system for the cardiac electrophysiologist. Europace. 2009;11 Suppl 5:v15–21.
13. Da Costa A, Gate-Martinet A, Rouffiange P, et al. Anatomical factors involved in difficult cardiac resynchronization therapy procedure: a non-invasive study using dual-source 64-multi-slice computed tomography. Europace. 2012;14:833–40.
14. Tang AS, Wells GA, Talajic M, et al. Cardiac-resynchronization therapy for mild-to-moderate heart failure. N Engl J Med. 2010;363:2385–95.
15. Van Rees JB, de Bie MK, Thijssen J, Borleffs CJW, Schalij MJ, van Erven L. Implantation-related complications of implantable cardioverter-defibrillators and cardiac resynchronization therapy devices: a systematic review of randomized clinical trials. J Am Coll Cardiol. 2011;58:995–1000.
16. Butter C, Gras D, Ritter P, et al. Comparative prospective randomized efficacy testing of different guiding catheters for coronary sinus cannulation in heart failure patients. J Interv Card Electrophysiol. 2003;9:343–51.

17. Yee R, Gadler F, Hussin A, Bin Omar R, Khaykin Y, Verma A, Lazeroms M, Hine DS, Marquard KR. Novel active fixation mechanism permits precise placement of a left ventricular lead: early results from a multicenter clinical study. Heart Rhythm. 2014;11(7):1150–5. doi:10.1016/j.hrthm.2014.04.020. Epub 2014 May 4.
18. Betts TR, Gamble JH, Khiani R, Bashir Y, Rajappan K. Development of a technique for left ventricular endocardial pacing via puncture of the interventricular septum. Circ Arrhythm Electrophysiol. 2014;7(1):17–22. doi:10.1161/CIRCEP.113.001110. Epub 2014 Jan 14.
19. Polasek R, Skalsky I, Wichterle D, Martinca T, Hanuliakova J, Roubicek T, Bahnik J, Jansova H, Pirk J, Kautzner J. High-density epicardial activation mapping to optimize the site for video-thoracoscopic left ventricular lead implant. J Cardiovasc Electrophysiol. 2014;25(8):882–8. doi:10.1111/jce.12430. Epub 2014 May 12.

Part IV

Peripheral Artery Disease

Thoracic and Abdominal Aorta Percutaneous Treatment

16

Roberto Chiesa, Enrico Rinaldi, Luca Bertoglio, Enrico M. Marone, and Domenico Baccellieri

16.1 Introduction

Aortic disease is a potentially serious condition that in many cases can be diagnosed and treated before it becomes dangerous. The most appropriate management is related to the severity, extension, and site of disease and to the specific patient's clinical characteristics and risk factors.

It has been recognized that the "normal aortic diameter" is influenced by a number of factors, including patient age, sex, and body size, location of aortic measurement, method of measurement, and the robustness and type of imaging methods used. The normal aortic diameter for men is larger than that for women, in this regard, the rate of aortic expansion is about 0.9 mm in men and 0.7 mm in women for each decade of life.

For what concerns aortic aneurysms, most of them are caused by degenerative disease resulting in dilatation of the aorta but also several genetic syndromes with a predisposition for aortic aneurysms have been identified. Risk factors for development of aortic aneurysms include hypertension, smoking, and chronic obstructive pulmonary disease. The dichotomy into thoracic (TAA) ad abdominal aortic aneurysms (AAA) is somehow artificial, not only because of the presence of thoracoabdominal aneurysm but also because of the possibility of tandem lesions. In a recent series, 27 % of patients with AAA also presented a TAA, most of whom were women and the elderly. For both the thoracic and the abdominal aorta, an aortic diameter of 5.5 cm is widely recognized as the threshold for interventions [1] in the asymptomatic patients; symptomatic aneurysms should be treated regardless of size if there are no other contraindications, because symptoms often portend rupture.

R. Chiesa (✉) • E. Rinaldi • L. Bertoglio • E.M. Marone • D. Baccellieri
Department of Vascular Surgery, Vita-Salute University, San Raffaele Scientific Institute, Milan, Italy
e-mail: rchiesa@tenaris.com

P. Presbitero et al. (eds.), *Percutaneous Treatment of Cardiovascular Diseases in Women*, DOI 10.1007/978-3-319-39611-8_16

Female gender, smoking, hypertension, and chronic airway disease are associated with an increased risk of small aneurysm rupture. Women are less affected by aneurysms but have a fourfold increased risk of rupture when under surveillance; in fact the risk of rupture is higher in women than in men at similar diameters and women present ruptured AAA on average 10 mm smaller than men. For all these reasons, an aortic diameter of 5.0 cm is recognized as the threshold for interventions for abdominal aortic aneurysms in women [1].

The proportion of women with abdominal aortic aneurysm treated with endovascular aortic repair is lower than for open repair. Unfavorable morphologic features for EVAR in women with AAA and TAA may explain this disproportion [2].

16.2 Materials

16.2.1 Guidewires

A soft guidewire is needed to navigate into the normal aorta or in presence of tortuosities or thrombus, before setting up a stiff guidewire.

We normally use a soft 0.035 in. guidewire (Storq Soft, Cordis Corp. Miami Lakes, FL) with an atraumatic tip segment to avoid intimal trauma or plaque disruption during navigation. It is available in three different configurations (soft, supersoft, and standard) and in three tip configuration (straight, angled, and modified J) with a total length of 180 and 300 cm. This guide incorporates a PTFE coating in the first 10 cm from the tip and then a silicone coating, in order to improve trackability and torqueability.

A stiff guidewire is then exchanged on a diagnostic catheter and it is used to let the endograft advance into the aorta. We normally use a super stiff guidewire with a 0.035 in. diameter (Lunderquist, Cook Medical Inc.), PTFE-coated with a stainless steel core, which is designed to provide maximum support and low surface friction during the endograft deployment.

16.2.2 Introducer Sheat

Introducer sheaths can be used to protect arterial access and lower blood loss when exchanging guidewires and delivering stent grafts. Those are available in different sizes and lengths. Usually a small sheath 6Fr or 7Fr is used once the artery is punctured to let the soft guidewire proceed into the proximal aorta. Those are available both in short or long configuration. They are provided with a valve on the distal end to control blood flow and a high flow conduit to wash the introducer and to perform angiography.

16.2.3 Stent Grafts

A variety of devices are available on the market for both thoracic and abdominal aorta.

Table 16.1 Most commonly used thoracic stent graft in Europe

Thoracic stent grafts	Fabric	Stents	Min Ø	Max Ø	Min Fr	Max Fr
Cook ZenithTX2	Woven polyester	Steel	28	42	20	22
Cook Zenith Alpha	Woven polyester	Nitinol	18	48	16	20
Bolton Relay	Woven polyester	Nitinol	22	46	22	26
Gore TAG	ePTFE	Nitinol	26	45	20	24
Medtronic Valiant	Woven polyester	Nitinol	22	46	22	25
Jotec E-vita	Woven polyester	Nitinol	24	44	20	24

Table 16.2 Most commonly used abdominal stent graft in Europe

Abdominal stent grafts	Fabric	Stents	MB Min Ø	MB Max Ø	MB Min Fr	MB Max Fr
Cook Zenith LP	Woven polyester	Nitinol	22	36	16	17
Medtronic Endurant	Woven polyester	Nitinol	23	36	18	20
Gore Excluder	ePTFE	Nitinol	23	35	14	18
Bolton Treovance	Woven polyester	Nitinol	20	36	18	19
Cordis Incraft	Woven polyester	Nitinol	22	34	14	16
Trivascular Ovation	Woven polyester	Nitinol	20	34	14	15

MB main body

All stent grafts are self-expanding and constrained in a sleeve or sheath. They are mainly made of a metallic nitinol skeleton and covered by a membrane of either polytetrafluoroethylene or polyester. The proximal end for the abdominal and thoracic grafts, and also the distal end for the thoracic graft, can be fully covered or not. A variety of sizes are available, meaning that it is generally possible to treat patients with several different anatomies.

Each stent graft model has an own releasing system with a mechanism that withdraws the delivery sheath and allows the graft to deploy.

Principal thoracic and abdominal stent grafts are summarized in Tables 16.1 and 16.2.

16.2.4 Compliant Balloons

Balloons are currently used to expand vascular stent graft once deployed, to stabilize primary graft and overlap attachment. Several models are available on the market; there are some differences in balloon material which can be found in polyurethane or latex. Diameters have a very wide range from 10 to 46 mm; some models are semicompliant and offer more than one size to adapt to various anatomies; compliant balloon instead can expand to the desired diameter up to 46 mm with only one size.

An alternative type, specific for the thoracic aorta, is represented by a particular compliant tri-lobed polyurethane balloon catheter (Gore Tri-lobe). The lobed design of the balloon catheter allows for inflation without complete blockage of aortic blood flow.

In all these devices, a guidewire lumen allows introduction of a 0.035 in. diameter guidewire for over-the-wire access, and radiopaque markers indicate the balloon edges.

16.3 Endovascular Techniques for Standard Cases

All the procedures are performed in the operating room, using a portable digital C-arm image intensifier with road-mapping capabilities.

Intraoperative trans-esophageal echocardiography (TEE) monitoring is routinely used during all the thoracic procedures. In our experience TEE is useful under many aspects as it allows to double check for the most appropriate landing zone of the endograft (in particular when the LSA origin has to be spared). As a second instance TEE is capable of documenting thrombosis or the presence of slow flow inside the aneurysm sac after deployment of the endograft, thus avoiding repeated angiography and the use of high doses of contrast mcdia [3].

Cerebrospinal fluid drainage has been shown to have a protective role in open surgical repair of DTAs and thoracoabdominal aortic aneurysms, while its role in TEVAR is less defined.

Our current indications for CFSD in TEVAR include:

1. Long coverage (predicted use of more than one endograft)
2. Coverage of high risk area including T10-T12
3. Previous abdominal or thoracic aortic surgery
4. Compromised subclavian and hypogastric arteries supply

In our series, the overall CSFD institution rate was 28 %.

No difference between men and women has been never identified in this field and we use this kind of approach in both male and female patients.

For TEVAR our preferred choice is to perform the endovascular procedure, when not contraindicated, under general anesthesia. In selective cases, depending of the patient general condition and comorbidity, we also perform local anesthesia, avoiding as frequent as possible, spinal anesthesia. The opportunity to perform local or general instead of spinal anesthesia allows us to have early diagnosis of spinal cord injury that may be obtained by early awakening and neurological conditions evaluation.

For EVAR instead, we perform the endovascular procedure preferably under spinal or local anesthesia, but we also perform general anesthesia in selected cases.

Patients are placed in the dorsal decubitus position, and the operative field is prepared and draped. It is mandatory that the operating field is prepared in such a way to allow a laparotomy for access and abdominal aorta and/or iliac arteries control that may be useful in such cases of iliac tortuosity and severe calcifications that could avoid stent graft navigation.

In the last years we started to use totally percutaneous approach for both thoracic and abdominal endovascular procedures.

Percutaneous femoral artery punctures are performed under ultrasound guidance and then the procedures are performed trough a very small skin incision that allows the insertion of the endovascular devices without a direct artery control.

In these cases, percutaneous different closure devices are used at the end of the procedure in order to obtain a valid hemostasis.

This less invasive approach still presents several limitations and could be performed safely only in patients with precise anatomical criteria.

The common femoral artery is normally exposed through a small inguinal incision.

In case of extremely diseased (calcific) bilateral external iliac arteries, or small-caliber vessels, we use the common iliac through a paramedian extraperitoneal approach as the access site; we use to directly puncture the artery through a purse string or we perform a surgical conduit to avoid the extremely diseased iliac axis. In rare cases the abdominal aorta has been used as the access site, with direct puncture and then closure with a purse-string suture. Surgical conduits are mainly used in female patients due to generally smaller access vessels [4] (Fig. 16.1).

At the beginning of the procedure a bolus of heparin (70 IU/Kg) is administered. During thoracic procedures the contralateral femoral artery is percutaneously punctured for diagnostic guidance. We normally use a soft-tip 0.035 in. guidewire (Storq Soft, Cordis Corp. Miami Lakes, FL) to cannulate the aorta and advance up to the thoracic aorta or the aortic arch, and then we exchange it through a catheter with a

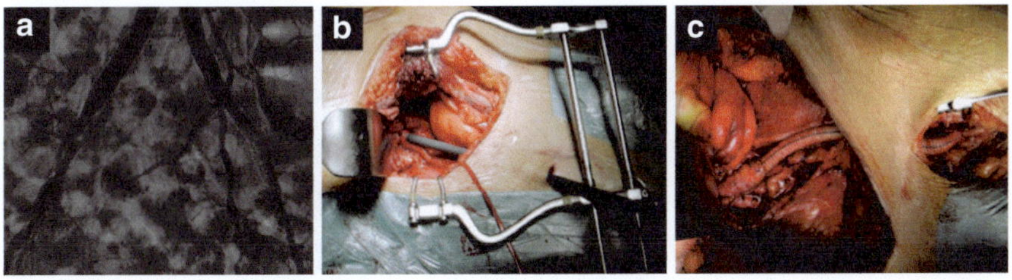

Fig. 16.1 In case of small femoral arteries or diseased external iliac arteries (**a**) a surgical approach to the common iliac artery may be considered (**b**). Otherwise, a surgical conduit could be performed in order to overcome femoral and iliac pathologies (**c**) (in this particular case the conduit is then anastomosed at the end of the endovascular procedure to the femoral artery in an ilio-femoral bypass). These approaches are particularly important in female due to generally smaller access vessels

260-cm long, 0.035-in. precurved super stiff guidewire (Lunderquist, Cook Medical Inc.) under fluoroscopic guidance.

During abdominal procedures instead, both femoral arteries are surgically exposed and purse-string sutures are performed on both of them in order to introduce the main body and, eventually, the ipsilateral limb from one site and the contralateral limb from the other one.

The endograft is passed over the guidewire into the appropriate position under fluoroscopic guidance. During deployment, a mild systemic hypotension is induced pharmacologically by the anesthesiologist with a bolus of fast-acting venous or arterial vasodilators such as nitrates or urapidil.

A rapid right ventricular pacing at a rate of 130–180 beats per minute reduces mean arterial pressure to 40–60 mmHg. The mechanisms involve loss of atrioventricular synchrony and reduction of ventricular filling time, resulting in decreased left ventricular preload, stroke volume, and cardiac output.

Hypotension induced by preload reduction seems to cause less cardiac and aortic stress than other methods. It is well tolerated by the patient and readily undertaken in patients under local anesthesia. Temporary rapid ventricular pacing enables precise deployment of thoracic endovascular stent grafts and safe post-stent ballooning. It also has the advantage of a rapid onset and offset of effect.

In case of very accurate thoracic endograft release, for example, when a thoracic endoprosthesis must be placed close to the supra aortic trunks, we normally use rapid pacing in order to induce hypotension during the release of the endograft [5] (Fig. 16.2).

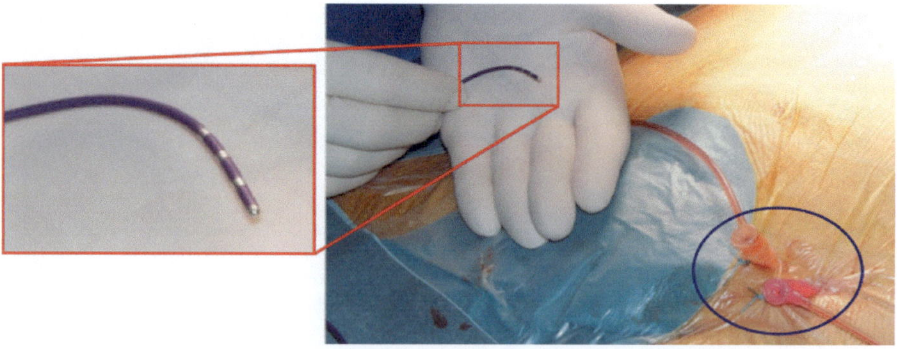

Fig. 16.2 In order to avoid prolonged hypotension during endograft deployment, rapid pacing may be extremely useful and can be safely applied to patients undergoing TEVAR. This adjunct can shorten the operation duration and facilitate precise graft deployment. The pacing catheter is routinely introduced through a femoral venous sheet during TEVAR procedures

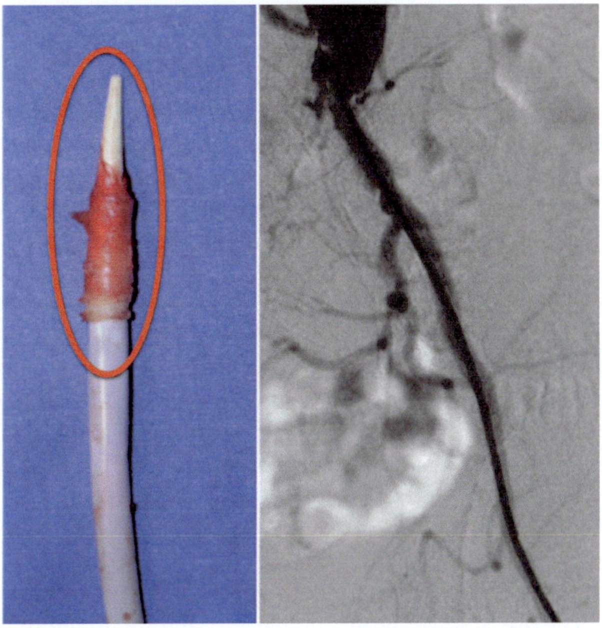

Fig. 16.3 A case of iliac axis avulsion. During endovascular procedure, as many patients eligible for endovascular procedures, especially for TEVAR, may present access contraindications, the higher rates of morbidities are related to the risk of aortoiliac injury, hypotension, and retroperitoneal hematoma that may increase the risk of SCI. Access-related problems are more frequent in the female population

After deployment of the endograft on the selected location, a completion angiogram is performed. Special care is mandatory when removing the introducer sheath, as rupture of the external iliac artery at its origin is more likely to happen with thoracic endografts (Fig. 16.3).

A completion angiography of the iliac axis is routinely performed when iliac arteries small size or severe calcifications are shown on preoperative CT scan.

It is particularly advisable to leave the guidewire in place until the sheath is completely removed in order to perform an emergent endoclamp in case of iliac rupture. Then, the wounds are closed as our standard practice.

16.4 Endovascular Techniques for Complex Cases

How to Navigate in Tortuous Anatomies Extreme tortuosity of the aorta can cause difficulties in endograft deployment. Various maneuvers can help the operator to overcome this problem. An easy solution is to place a stiff guidewire as proximal as possible, (i.e., in the aortic root) to provide more support. If this does not help, a second stiff guidewire can be placed in the aorta from the contralateral femoral access and might help straighten the aorta (double-wire technique).

In extreme situations a brachio-femoral wire conduit (teleferic technique) could be useful to help the navigation through a tortuous aorta. A retrograde percutaneous brachial approach is performed with a 5 F or 6 F 35 cm sheath and a 5 F catheter is used to navigate an angled glide wire (0.035 in.) into the tortuous descending thoracic aorta under fluoroscopic guidance. The wire is then secured through the groin sheath with the help of a goose snare. An exchange catheter is pushed from the groin access cranially trough the brachial access and then the glide wire is exchanged to a 0.035 in. extra-stiff wire. The sheath in the groin is then exchanged to the endograft sheath, which can be advanced into the distal abdominal aorta.

Use of brachio-femoral access wires could help to straighten the most angulated and tortuous aorta. It is important to have at least a 260-cm long wire and constant tension must be placed on both ends of the wire as the graft is advanced through the delivery sheath into the aorta. This technique should be used with a guiding sheath protecting the subclavian vessels to prevent shearing the vessel when traction on the wire is exerted. However, a word of caution must be spent in order to underline that this kind of approach does pose an inherent risk of thromboembolism from the arch vessels and should not be performed if imaging demonstrates atheroemboli in the arch vessels [6].

Access Issues The use of lower profile delivery systems with improved trackability and extra-stiff guidewires has allowed endovascular aneurysm repair in patients with tortuous iliac arteries. However, access problems remain, especially in patients with stenotic and calcified iliac arteries.

A technique is described to help solving access issues, known as "paving and cracking." This technique involves the deployment of a covered stent in the common iliac artery (CIA) and external iliac artery (EIA) to facilitate the introduction of an aortic stent graft through tortuous, narrow, stenosed, or circumferentially calcified iliac arteries.

Both self-expanding and balloon-expandable polytetrafluoroethylene-covered stents can be used. The covered stents are deployed along the length of the diseased iliac arteries, making sure to cover the internal iliac artery bifurcation, as this is typically the site of rupture. The covered stent prevents hemorrhage from the iliac rupture that is likely to follow such excessive dilation. Once the iliac artery has been relined and dilated, the main body of the aortic stent graft is then inserted easily and deployed in the standard fashion [7] (Fig. 16.4).

Another technique is to sewn a Dacron graft, usually a 10-mm, in an end-to-side fashion to the iliac artery through a lower abdominal access. This allows for straight and easy access, as opposed to introducing the device directly into the common iliac artery. Clamping the distal end of conduit and accessing it allows for better control of blood loss. Use of vessel loops and/or umbilical tapes around the conduit can also help to decrease blood loss when the sheath is in place. At completion of the procedure, the graft conduit can be ligated close to the anastomosis or converted to an iliofemoral bypass to allow a simpler delayed intervention in the future.

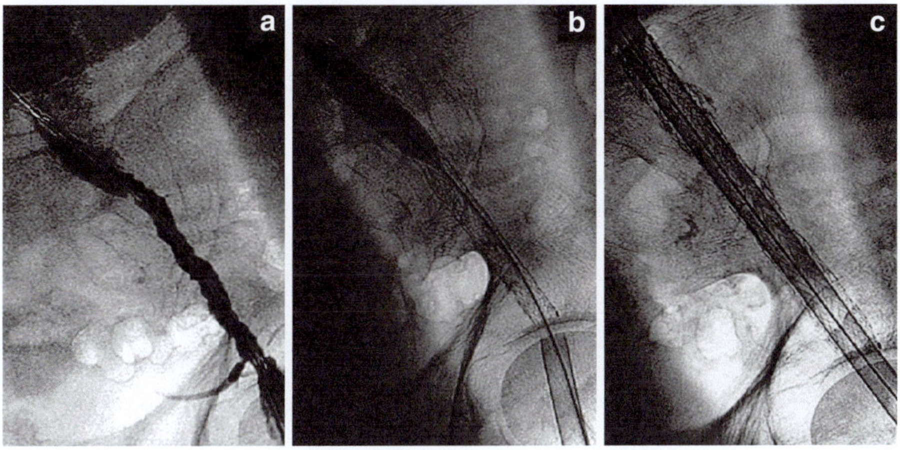

Fig. 16.4 When TEVAR candidates have unfavorable iliac artery anatomy, including a small-caliber iliac artery, iliac artery tortuosity, or occlusive disease, in combination with the need for large-diameter delivery sheaths, the internal endoconduit approach has been introduced as an alternative to the surgical conduit. It could be performed using a standard femoral approach. After an iliac arteriogram (**a**), one or more covered stents are placed across the critical stenotic iliac artery segment, extending proximal and distal to the lesion. Then an angioplasty with a noncompliant balloon is performed in order to obtain a controlled rupture of the iliac artery (**b**). After the endoconduit placement is possible to introduce the endovascular device (**c**)

Surgical and endovascular conduits are more frequently needed in females due to generally smaller access vessels.

16.5 Complications

In spite of the great enthusiasm that endovascular techniques have provoked, it must be remembered that these techniques are by no means completely safe. A significant mortality and morbidity are described in all published series, especially in women.

The 30-day mortality rate for women is three times greater than for men after aortic endovascular procedures. Women have also been shown to be more prone to access-related ischemia, iliac and aortic neck rupture, colonic ischemia, and type 1 endoleak [8].

The reasons for the higher morbidity and mortality are not entirely clear but may be related to smaller access vessels and more hostile anatomical features of the aorta.

Additionally, women are more often found to have prohibitive aortoiliac anatomy which makes them poor candidates for EVAR based on current FDA-approved devices instruction for use.

Damage to Access Vessels Several literature reports have underlined that serious and even fatal problems may arise from introduction of the device from the femoral artery. In particular, rupture or avulsion of the external iliac artery have been reported; this usually becomes dramatically evident only at the time the large introducer sheath used for endograft delivery is withdrawn. We therefore liberally switch to extraperitoneal surgical exposure of the common iliac artery or even the distal aorta if it is difficult to advance the device through the femoral arteries.

Endoleak Endoleak, defined as blood flow within the aneurysm sac, is a serious sequela that may lead to secondary rupture of the aorta.

The classification describes five different types of endoleaks:

- Type 1 endoleaks, proximal or distal, show flow that originates from the stent graft attachment sites.
- Type 2 endoleaks are related to retrograde aortic filling from branch vessels.
- Type 3 endoleaks occur when there is a stent graft structural failure, like fractures or junctional separations of two devices. These endoleaks often result from stent graft disconnection.
- Type 4 endoleaks are caused by stent graft porosity or defects in the fabric.
- Type 5 endoleaks or endotension are also described.

Type I or III are, in the majority of cases, successfully treated with a new graft. In case of secondary procedures failure, surgical conversion could be necessary.

Type II endoleaks could be managed with coil embolization of the branch vessels. Surgical exclusion of the branch arteries is sometimes useful to treat persistent endoleaks. Secondary endoleaks due to migration or dislocation of modular junctions may result from inadequate grip or seal, but also from the inability of the relatively inflexible device to conform to tortuosity of the aorta that may occur after successful exclusion.

In literature, type 1 endoleaks at completion of stenting are generally more frequent in women than men at the end of the procedure, prompting greater use of stents at the aortic neck in order to obtain an adequate proximal sealing and correct the endoleak.

Stroke Cerebrovascular accidents are among the most common and dreaded complications of endovascular therapy of thoracic aortic disease [9]. They are mainly linked to atheromatous embolization into the cerebral arteries caused by devices manipulation. This kind of event could happen with a lower rate also during abdominal procedure; in fact it should be remembered that angiography for diagnostic purposes alone carries a 1–2 % risk of complications. New generation endografts are surely less prone to this complication. This is due to the better flexibility of the grafts and sheaths and to the smaller profiles that result in improved navigability through the access vessels. Greater experience of the operators and an adequate preoperative CT scan play a role both in the selection of candidates with adequate anatomical characteristics and during the procedure itself.

Anyhow, minimal manipulation of the wires and catheters and a meticulous technique are mandatory in the prevention of perioperative stroke.

Paraplegia EVAR allows the avoidance of aortic cross-clamping and its sequelae; however, the intercostal and lumbar arteries covered by the endograft cannot be reimplanted. The reported incidence of both immediate and delayed paraplegia in patients undergoing endovascular procedures of TAAA can be as high as 12% of cases. The coverage of a long thoracic aortic segment has been reported to be a significant risk factor for Spinal Chord Ischemia. Patients who had open AAA repair also appear to be prone to such a risk because of the marginal spinal cord collateral blood supply secondary to the ligation of lumbar arteries performed during the surgical procedure. Also, proximal collateral circulation of the spinal cord may be involved by the occlusion of the left subclavian artery (landing zone 2) that abolishes the contribution to the blood supply provided by the anterior spinal artery, a branch of the ipsilateral vertebral artery.

We reviewed and analyzed our experience with repairs of thoracic aortic pathology to evaluate the incidence and investigate the determinants of spinal cord ischemia in endovascular procedures, identify patients at risk, and assess the role and efficacy of prophylactic adjuncts and therapeutic measures [10]. Our experience addresses the importance of hemodynamic control to prevent postoperative neurologic deficits and encourages aggressive, postoperative care of these patients. In our practice, we now try to maintain a perioperative MAP of >90 mmHg and use CSF drainage in patients deemed at high risk, including those who received AAA repair. In this respect, patients with synchronous thoracic and AAA, which we earlier treated simultaneously for both aneurysms, currently undergo staged procedures to better allow the development of collaterals for spinal cord blood supply. In the case of delayed paraplegia, prompt CSF drainage, if not previously instituted, is also used to keep the CSF pressure <10 mmHg and possibly reverse the deficit.

The risk for paraplegia after endovascular abdominal procedures, as for the stroke, is reduced compared to the thoracic procedures but exists and could be not negligible in particular in case of previously extended thoracic aorta repair.

Infection As follow-up is becoming longer and the reported series larger, new serious complications are emerging and one of the most ominous ones is endograft infection. There are at this time several reports in the literature. This complication does not seem to be specific to a single device. Sometimes it presents as a fatal hemorrhage; however, sometimes the presentation is less dramatic at it may be characterized by fever, pain, dysphagia hematemesis, melena, and septic symptoms. Treatment is very problematic; however, the outcome without treatment is invariably fatal.

Migration Successful long-term aneurysm exclusion requires the durability of proximal and distal fixation sites against the bloodstream forces, the fatigue of the materials, and the morphological behavior of the aneurysm. The Society for Vascular Surgery/American Association for Vascular Surgery (SVS/AAVS) standards defined endograft migration as any movement relative to anatomical therapy. As optimal sealing of a stent graft at the aortic wall still remains an unsolved issue, current technology and techniques cannot definitively prevent stent graft migration or type 1 endoleak due to unfavorable anatomy or late neck dilatation from progression of the degenerative disease. Extensive oversizing of the aortic stent graft at the proximal or distal landing zone has been suggested as a means to increase radial force and improve sealing, but on the other hand, it was associated with an increased risk of stent graft infolding or thrombosis. To address this problem, a variety of fixation methods such as hooks, barbs, free-flows, and longitudinal support devices have been developed. In addition, recently, vascular endostapling systems were developed to achieve better sealing at the proximal neck of the aneurysm and to prevent endograft migration. As the results are not conclusive, all these systems may reduce the reintervention rates after endovascular aneurysm repair.

Conclusions

The endovascular approach represents nowadays a solid alternative to the open repair for many pathologies involving both thoracic and abdominal aorta. However, a smaller proportion of women have been treated nowadays with EVAR and TEVAR compared with open repair and with a slightly higher rate of complications compared with men. The reasons of these mismatches could be explained mainly with peculiar anatomical differences between men and women. In fact, women present generally smaller access vessels and more extensive aortic neck pathology. These aspects could prevent an endovascular approach or could cause complications.

In conclusion, aortic endovascular approach could be performed in women for both thoracic and abdominal aorta but a careful preoperative accurate planning is mandatory in all the cases in order to identify anatomical limitations that could prevent the technical success of the procedure. Future development of endovascular devices should address the complexity of the access vessels and the aortic anatomy, which will benefit all patients with aortic pathology, but especially women.

References

1. Moll FL, et al. Management of abdominal aortic aneurysms clinical practice guidelines of the European society for vascular surgery. Eur J Vasc Endovasc Surg. 2011;41:S1–58.
2. Ouriel K, Greenberg RK, Clair DG, et al. Endovascular aneurysm repair: gender-specific results. J Vasc Surg. 2003;38:93–8.
3. Agricola E, Slavich M, Bertoglio L, et al. The role of contrast enhanced transesophageal echocardiography in the diagnosis and in the morphological and functional characterization of acute aortic syndromes. Int J Cardiovasc Imaging. 2014;30(1):31–8.

4. Tsilimparis N, Dayama A, Perez S, et al. Iliac conduits for endovascular repair of aortic pathologies. Eur J Vasc Endovasc Surg. 2013;45(5):443–8.
5. Nicolaou G, Forbes TL. Strategies for accurate endograft placement in the proximal thoracic aorta. Semin Cardiothorac Vasc Anesth. 2010;14(3):196–200.
6. Kasirajan K. Thoracic endografts: procedural steps, technical pitfalls and how to avoid them. Semin Vasc Surg. 2006;19(1):3–10.
7. Hinchliffe RJ, Ivancev K, Sonesson B, Malina M. "Paving and cracking": an endovascular technique to facilitate the introduction of aortic stent-grafts through stenosed iliac arteries. J Endovasc Ther. 2007;14(5):630–3.
8. Mehta M, Byrne WJ, Robinson H, et al. Women derive less benefit from elective endovascular aneurysm repair than men. J Vasc Surg. 2012;55(4):906–13.
9. Melissano G, Tshomba Y, Bertoglio L, Rinaldi E, Chiesa R. Analysis of stroke after TEVAR involving the aortic arch. Eur J Vasc Endovasc Surg. 2012;43(3):269–75.
10. Chiesa R, Melissano G, Marrocco-Trischitta MM, Civilini E, Setacci F. Spinal cord ischemia after elective stent-graft repair of the thoracic aorta. J Vasc Surg. 2005;42(1):11–7.

Treatment of Peripheral Arteriopathy in Women

17

Marianne Brodmann and Marco De Carlo

17.1 Prevalence and Presentation of PAD in Women

Until recently, peripheral artery disease (PAD) was considered to be more prevalent in men than in women because the diagnosis was based on the presence of typical symptoms, i.e., intermittent claudication (IC) [1]. However, PAD is often asymptomatic or presents with atypical symptoms, and this is particularly frequent in women, leading to an underestimation of PAD prevalence among female subjects. On the contrary, when PAD diagnosis is based on the ankle-brachial index, the actual prevalence of PAD among women is at least the same as in men or even higher. Moreover, women may be hindered by financial and social barriers to accessing and seeking care at an earlier stage [2].

A recent review of population-based studies showed a mean prevalence of PAD of 15.6 % in women and 13.4 % in men, with a larger difference in older age groups [3]. Considering the aging of population and the longer life expectancy of women, an even higher prevalence of PAD among women is expected in the near future. Therefore, the need for proper diagnosis and management of PAD in women is pressing, and we should overcome the gender bias in the diagnosis of this largely underdiagnosed disease. Peripheral and coronary artery disease share most of their risk factors, including smoking, age, diabetes mellitus, hypertension, and dyslipidemia. Among these risk factors, diabetes and smoking are associated with the highest odds ratios for developing PAD (3.0 and 4.0, respectively) [2, 4]. Conflicting data have been reported regarding the association between diabetes and gender in

M. Brodmann, MD
Division of Angiology, Department of Internal Medicine, Karl-Franzens University, Graz, Austria

M. De Carlo, MD, PhD (✉)
Catheterization Laboratory, Cardiothoracic and Vascular Department, Pisa University Hospital, Pisa, Italy
e-mail: marcodecarlo@gmail.com

P. Presbitero et al. (eds.), *Percutaneous Treatment of Cardiovascular Diseases in Women*,
DOI 10.1007/978-3-319-39611-8_17

patients with PAD; in older studies, diabetes was more prevalent among women (16 %) than men (11.9 %) with an abnormal ABI, and in the Framingham Heart Study, diabetes increased the risk of intermittent claudication 3.5 and 8.6-fold in men and women, respectively [2]. On the other hand, in a recent analysis of almost two million hospital admission records for PAD in the United States, women showed a lower prevalence of diabetes than men [5]. Although the risk of developing PAD is proportional to the severity and duration of diabetes, studies evaluating glycemic control in diabetic subjects with PAD failed to find an association between aggressive diabetes treatment and a decrease in adverse cardiovascular events [6]. The presentation of leg symptoms in diabetic women with PAD may be altered by the presence of peripheral neuropathy, further delaying the frequently late diagnosis of PAD in women; the higher prevalence of medial calcinosis in women than in men may also confound diagnosis by falsely raising pressure recordings in the distal vessels.

The atypical presentation of PAD in women often leads to a relevant delay in diagnosis when compared with men, so that women more often present with advanced disease, have a poorer quality of life, and lower extremity function [5, 7]. Among patients with PAD, after controlling for disease severity, age, and comorbidities, women described more physical dysfunction, pain, and mood disturbances than men, leading to lower overall quality of life [8]. The decreased quality of life may be related to depression, which is more prevalent among women and is also associated with worse outcomes after limb revascularization.

17.1.1 Indication of the Procedure in Women

The treatment of PAD has two intents: decrease cardiovascular morbidity and mortality and improve limb-related symptoms, thus improving the quality of life. In fact, in addition to the obvious aim of relieving symptoms, treatment of PAD aims to tackle the two- to threefold higher risk of mortality associated with the presence of either asymptomatic or symptomatic PAD [9].

These goals are achieved by a combination of reduction of risk factors, medical treatment, and revascularization when indicated. Clear indications for revascularization include ischemic rest pain, ischemic ulceration, gangrene, or symptomatic disabling claudication. The decision to pursue or not pursue revascularization in women may be influenced by their higher rate of asymptomatic presentation, and by a gender bias discouraging interventions in women, especially among elderly patients. Men are more likely to undergo an intervention for their PAD than women, even after controlling for potential confounding factors and even when considering only patients with critical limb ischemia (CLI) [4]. However, women often have more advanced disease at the time of presentation, and this may lead to a higher rate of revascularization compared to men, as reported in the US Nationwide Inpatient Sample [5]. Women were older at the time of intervention by an average of 3.5 years; compared to men, women had a small increased likelihood of undergoing endovascular procedures for IC (odds ratio 1.27, 95 %CI 1.25–1.28, $P<0.01$)

and CLI (odds ratio 1.14, 95 % CI 1.13–1.15, $P<0.01$). Similar gender-related differences were reported from the Blue Cross Blue Shield of Michigan Cardiovascular Consortium registry [10]; women were older at the time of revascularization and had higher rates of hypertension and concurrent CAD. Women were more likely to present with CLI as the indication for revascularization (41 vs. 35 %, $P<0.0001$) and to require intervention in two or more arterial beds because of multilevel disease.

To date, no data are available to support gender differences in the indication to revascularization for PAD. As a matter of fact, women are largely underrepresented in PAD revascularization trials, where they account for 20–30 % of participants, while registry data show that women actually represent 40 % of this population [4, 11], so that treatment decision-making is mostly supported by results obtained in men.

17.1.2 Anatomical Special Features of Women for the Procedure

The difference in bodily dimensions between genders leads to a difference in average arterial diameter in the lower limbs. Female iliac artery luminal diameter is smaller in women than in men (6.5 ± 0.5 mm vs. 8.2 ± 0.6 mm; $P<0.001$) [12]. In particular, Timaran et al. reported a common iliac artery diameter of 8.4 mm in men vs. 7.4 mm in women, while the difference in external iliac artery diameters in men was not significant (7.0 mm vs. 6.5 mm) [13]. In the "Safety and Effectiveness Study of EverFlex Stent to Treat Symptomatic Femoral-popliteal Atherosclerosis" (DURABILITY II) trial, the mean diameter of the superficial femoral artery (SFA) was significantly smaller in women than in men (4.4 ± 0.8 mm vs. 5.0 ± 0.9 mm; $P<0.001$) [14]. However, the vessel diameter does not influence the technical success rate of endovascular interventions for PAD, which is comparable between genders both in the iliac and the infrainguinal district. The vessel diameter probably plays a role in the higher rate of vascular access complications observed in women undergoing peripheral vascular interventions (PVI) [15].

17.1.3 Outcomes in Women

There are sex-related differences in revascularization outcomes for women, which may be due to older age, more advanced disease, smaller vessel caliber, and higher rates of comorbidities. Differences in revascularization outcomes for women with IC or CLI were evaluated in the US Nationwide Inpatient Sample from four geographically distinct states [5]. Among women endovascular revascularization was preferred over surgical revascularization, possibly because of smaller arterial diameter and poorer distal runoff; in fact, women were older and had more advanced disease at presentation. The higher risk profile probably explains the increased in-hospital mortality for women across the breadth of revascularization procedures and indications, which persisted after adjustment for age and comorbidities (mortality after endovascular interventions was 0.5 % vs. 0.2 %; OR 1.99; 95%CI, 1.72–2.30; $P<0.01$). Interestingly, women had lower rates of amputation compared to men.

Additional work to understand the sex-related differences in outcomes following percutaneous lower extremity revascularization was done with the Blue Cross Blue Shield of Michigan Cardiovascular Consortium registry [10]. In a propensity-matched analysis, 2346 women were matched to an equal number of men; compared with male patients, women had more advanced disease at the time of presentation, but no sex-related differences for in-hospital death, myocardial infarction, and stroke, or the combined end point of these outcomes were observed. Women showed increased vascular complications and postprocedural transfusions as compared with men; however, the detrimental effect of these complications was compensated by a higher rate of technical success of percutaneous revascularization. These data suggest female patients may benefit to a greater degree with an invasive percutaneous strategy for the management of PAD, particularly if complications can be avoided.

Although data on the association between female gender and diabetes in the general population of patients with PAD are conflicting, such association has been described consistently among patients undergoing PVI. In a series of 385 PVI in patients with claudication (52.2 %) or CLI (47.8 %), DeRubertis and coworkers described a prevalence of diabetes as high as 64 % among women versus 50 % among men ($P=0.025$); as expected, diabetics suffered reduced primary patency at 1 year compared with nondiabetics (53 ± 4 % vs. 71 ± 4 %, $P=0.05$) [16].

While conflicting results have been reported regarding sex effects on survival after PAD revascularization [4, 5], studies have consistently shown that female sex is a risk factor for bleeding complications after percutaneous lower extremity angioplasty [10, 15] and of infections, hematomas, and seromas after lower extremity arterial bypass [17]. In a retrospective analysis of the multicenter Vascular Quality Initiative on 22,226 patients undergoing PVI from August 2007 to May 2013, female sex was found to be an independent predictor of access site complications, together with age >75 years, white race, no prior PVI, nonfemoral arterial access site, >6-Fr sheath size, thrombolytics, arterial dissection, fluoroscopy time >30 min, nonuse of vascular closure device, bedridden preoperative ambulatory status, and urgent indication [15]. In particular, the odds ratio for vascular complications in women was 1.49 (95 % confidence interval: 1.28–1.73); however, 30-day and 1-year survival were similar between genders also in this large cohort of patients undergoing PVI.

Interestingly, no gender-specific differences in the outcome are described also for open surgery on lower limb arteries. Ballotta et al. recently reported a prospective registry of 1333 consecutive patients undergoing primary infrainguinal arterial surgery, comprising 496 women (37.2 %) [18]. Women were older than men (74 vs. 71 years; $P<0.001$) and had a higher incidence of diabetes mellitus (52 % vs. 46 %; $P=0.03$) and surgery for limb salvage (91 % vs. 87 %; $P=0.02$). The major and minor complication rates were comparable between men and women. At 10 years, no differences were observed regarding primary patency rate (47 % in women vs. 49 % in men), secondary patency (61 % vs. 61 %), and limb salvage (93 % vs. 91 %).

Considering the higher risk profile of women at time of intervention, these findings suggest that lower extremity revascularization may be even more effective in women than in men.

17.1.4 Outcome of Endovascular Procedures in the Iliac District

Percutaneous intervention to treat occlusive disease of the iliac arteries has met with mixed results between genders. Timaran et al. [13] reported a decreased primary patency rate at 5 years in women (38 %) compared with men (88 %). In particular, women with external iliac artery (EIA) stents had inferior primary patency rates at 5 years (29 %) compared with women with common iliac artery (CIA) stents (54 %). Decreased EIA patency rates in women may be due to more advanced atherosclerotic lesions that are less amenable to endovascular intervention. However, these results should be interpreted with caution, as absolute numbers were small (36 stents in the EIA). In fact, Orr et al. reported similar primary patency rates between genders after a median follow-up of 13 months, although female iliac arteries were more often occluded before intervention and of smaller diameter [12]. Iliac stenting yielded similar results between genders also in the series of 160 patients described by Abando et al. [19]. More recently, Bechter-Hugl reported comparable primary patency rates up to 7 years of follow-up between women (46.4 %) and men (59.7 %) in a single-center experience on 337 patients (Fig. 17.1) [20]. Younger women (<60 years of age), however, showed significantly worse outcome compared with younger men. The authors concluded that although women are older and present with a more advanced stage of PAD, endovascular revascularization of the iliac arteries is equally effective irrespective of gender.

17.1.5 Outcome of Endovascular Procedures in the Femoropopliteal District

Most contemporary studies describe no significant difference in primary and secondary patency between genders after femoropopliteal endovascular interventions [10, 14, 18, 19, 21–23].

The DURABILITY II trial evaluated the results of primary stenting for femoropopliteal disease; an analysis of the impact of sex on outcome was recently published [14]. Despite presenting at a later age, with more severe claudication, a shorter absolute claudication distance, and smaller vessels than men, women achieved equal patency rates using angioplasty and primary stenting (Fig. 17.2) with similar target lesion revascularization, major adverse event, and mortality rates. However, despite these findings, women subjectively had worse symptoms both before and 1 year after revascularization.

In the most challenging setting of long chronic total occlusions of femoropopliteal arteries, the results of stenting are less favorable, particularly in women. Sakamoto et al. recently described a multicenter series of 352 patients undergoing

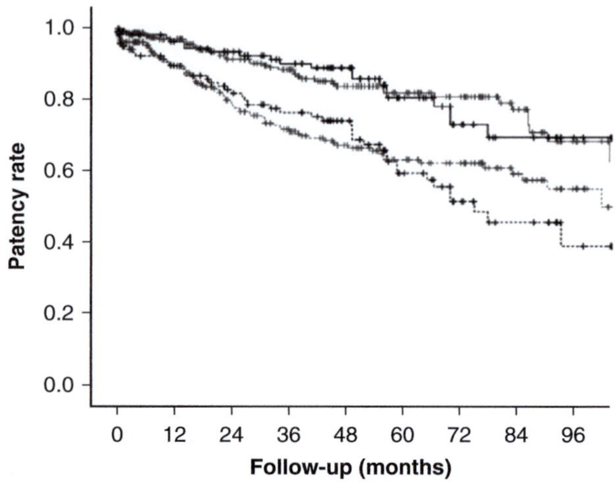

Months	0	12	24	36	48	60	72	84	96

Fig. 17.1 Gender-specific cumulative primary and secondary patency rates after iliac artery stenting. *Black curves* represent the female study population; *gray curves*, the male study population. *Interrupted lines* represent primary patency rates; *solid lines*, secondary patency rates (Reproduced with permission from [20])

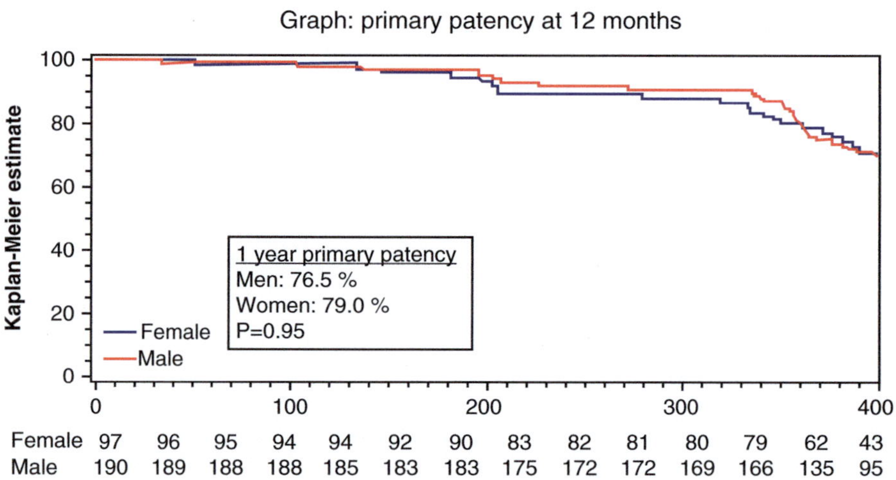

Fig. 17.2 Primary patency for men and women after femoropopliteal stenting (Reproduced with permission from [14])

stent implantation of long femoropopliteal occlusion (mean occlusion length was 194 ± 89 mm); 5-year primary and secondary patency rates were 51.8 % and 79.5 %, respectively, and the rates of freedom from amputation and all-cause death were 96.2 % and 78.4 %, respectively [22]. Female gender (odds ratio, 1.95; $P = 0.005$) and mean stent diameter (odds ratio, 0.77; $P = 0.03$) were predictors of restenosis. Although primary patency was low, the secondary patency rate was acceptable.

The "Local Taxan With Short Time Contact for Reduction of Restenosis in Distal Arteries" (THUNDER) randomized trial investigated the efficacy of a drug-coated balloon (DCB) in the femoropopliteal arteries; no difference was observed between women and men in 6-month late lumen loss both in the control arm (1.61 mm vs. 1.76 mm) and DCB arm (0.37 mm vs. 0.42 mm) [23]. In contrast, 5 years after treatment, the cumulative target lesion revascularization rate was lower in men than in women treated in the DCB group (17 % vs. 38 %). Although absolute numbers of patients are small, this might reflect a gender-related difference in the response to DCB, which may partially be explained by the smaller diameter of femoropopliteal arteries in women. Currently there are no further published data describing an interaction between gender and the results of DCB or drug-eluting stents for PAD.

17.1.6 Outcome of Endovascular Procedures in the Tibial District

Endovascular interventions on BTK vessels in patients with CLI represent the most difficult challenge in the treatment of PAD and results are still far from being fully satisfactory. Recently Domenick et al. reported a gender and age analysis of their single-center experience of 201 patients (40 % female, 39 % aged more than 80 years) undergoing tibial artery angioplasty for CLI [24]. Consistent with previous reports, women were older than men at the time of presentation, but procedural success, comorbidities, and indications for intervention were comparable between sexes and age groups, as well as complications. Limb salvage rate was 88 % and was comparable by gender, while renal insufficiency was an independent predictor of limb loss. Age >80 years was a predictor of impaired wound healing, at variance with sex. Overall primary patency rate was 62 % at 1 year and was similar between genders and age groups, while reintervention rate was 65 % in women vs. 46 % in men ($P=0.03$). Although the exact reasons for the higher reintervention rate are not known, anatomic and socioeconomic factors could account for these findings. Women have smaller arteries than men, and the same degree of intimal hyperplasia after interventions will be more likely to cause a hemodynamically significant restenosis. In addition, women often present at a later stage of disease than their male counterparts.

On the other hand, in a series of 81 patients (53 % women) undergoing percutaneous interventions on BTK vessels, Tye et al. reported statistically higher primary patency rates at 12 and 24 months in women (77.5 % ± 6.9 % and 72.9 % ± 7.8 %) than in men (58.7 % ± 9.3 % and 45.2 % ± 9.9 %; $P=0.03$) [25]. Women also had statistically better secondary patency rates than men at 12 and 24 months (90.4 % ± 4.8 % and 85.1 % ± 6.8 % in women vs. 76.0 % ± 8.1 % and 58.5 % ± 10.8 % in men; $P=0.03$). Female gender remained an independent predictor of superior patency even after controlling for gender-related differences in lesion anatomic complexity. There were no significant differences in limb salvage rates and overall survival rates at 12 and 24 months between genders. Importantly, in this series women were not older than men and had less advanced disease (chronic total occlusion rate 25.4 % in women vs. 25.4 % in men; $P=0.03$). These results suggest that a timely diagnosis and the use of endovascular procedures may lessen the gap in gender-related treatment outcomes and postoperative complications seen after open arterial reconstructions for CLI.

Take-Home Messages

Lower extremity peripheral arterial disease is prevalent in women and associated with an increased risk of cardiovascular events and mortality. Women are more likely than men to have asymptomatic disease or atypical symptoms. Women undergoing vascular procedures for PAD are older and have more advanced disease than men. Although procedural success rates are similar between genders, women suffer from higher restenosis rates, particularly for more complex lesions, and require reintervention more often as compared with men. In addition, women also suffer a higher rate of vascular access complications. Smaller vessel diameter may partially explain these sex-specific differences. Amputation rates have declined steadily over the last decades, and women now have lower rates than men. In-hospital mortality for both men and women also continues to decline, but still women have an increased risk of cardiovascular complications, possibly because of their older age.

In order to successfully impact the burden of PAD and associated ischemic heart disease risks, we must increase the awareness of this disease. An improve in outcomes requires highlighting the sex-based differences in PAD to the multidisciplinary group of physicians involved in PAD diagnosis and management, including primary care, cardiology, vascular medicine, interventional radiology, and vascular surgery specialists.

References

1. Higgins JP, Higgins JA. Epidemiology of peripheral arterial disease in women. J Epidemiol. 2003;13(1):1–14.
2. Egorova N, Vouyouka AG, Quin J, et al. Analysis of gender-related differences in lower extremity peripheral arterial disease. J Vasc Surg. 2010;51(2):372–8e.371.
3. Vavra AK, Kibbe MR. Women and peripheral arterial disease. Womens Health (Lond Engl). 2009;5(6):669–83.
4. Hirsch AT, Allison MA, Gomes AS, et al. A call to action: women and peripheral artery disease: a scientific statement from the American Heart Association. Circulation. 2012;125(11):1449–72.
5. Lo RC, Bensley RP, Dahlberg SE, et al. Presentation, treatment, and outcome differences between men and women undergoing revascularization or amputation for lower extremity peripheral arterial disease. J Vasc Surg. 2014;59(2):409–18.e403.
6. UKPDS Group. Tight blood pressure control and risk of macrovascular and microvascular complications in type 2 diabetes: UKPDS 38. BMJ. 1998;317(7160):703–13.
7. Moussa ID, Jaff MR, Mehran R, et al. Prevalence and prediction of previously unrecognized peripheral arterial disease in patients with coronary artery disease: the Peripheral Arterial Disease in Interventional Patients Study. Catheter Cardiovasc Interv. 2009;73(6):719–24.
8. Oka RK, Szuba A, Giacomini JC, Cooke JP. Gender differences in perception of PAD: a pilot study. Vasc Med. 2003;8(2):89–94.
9. Fowkes FGR, Rudan D, Rudan I, et al. Comparison of global estimates of prevalence and risk factors for peripheral artery disease in 2000 and 2010: a systematic review and analysis. Lancet. 2013;382(9901):1329–40.

10. Jackson EA, Munir K, Schreiber T, et al. Impact of sex on morbidity and mortality rates after lower extremity interventions for peripheral arterial disease: observations from the Blue Cross Blue Shield of Michigan Cardiovascular Consortium. J Am Coll Cardiol. 2014;63(23):2525–30.
11. Hoel AW, Kayssi A, Brahmanandam S, Belkin M, Conte MS, Nguyen LL. Under-representation of women and ethnic minorities in vascular surgery randomized controlled trials. J Vasc Surg. 2009;50(2):349–54.
12. Orr JD, Leeper NJ, Funaki B, Leef J, Gewertz BL, Desai TR. Gender does not influence outcomes after iliac angioplasty. Ann Vasc Surg. 2002;16(1):55–60.
13. Timaran CH, Stevens SL, Freeman MB, Goldman MH. Predictors for adverse outcome after iliac angioplasty and stenting for limb-threatening ischemia. J Vasc Surg. 2002;36(3):507–13.
14. Tadros RO, Faries PL, Rocha-Singh KJ, et al. The impact of sex on angioplasty and primary stenting for femoropopliteal occlusive disease: results of the DURABILITY II trial. Ann Vasc Surg. 2014;28(1):1–9.
15. Ortiz D, Jahangir A, Singh M, Allaqaband S, Bajwa TK, Mewissen MW. Access site complications after peripheral vascular interventions: incidence, predictors, and outcomes. Circ Cardiovasc Interv. 2014;7(6):821–8.
16. DeRubertis BG, Pierce M, Ryer EJ, Trocciola S, Kent KC, Faries PL. Reduced primary patency rate in diabetic patients after percutaneous intervention results from more frequent presentation with limb-threatening ischemia. J Vasc Surg. 2008;47(1):101–8.
17. Greenblatt DY, Rajamanickam V, Mell MW. Predictors of surgical site infection after open lower extremity revascularization. J Vasc Surg. 2011;54(2):433–9.
18. Ballotta E, Gruppo M, Lorenzetti R, Piatto G, DaGiau G, Toniato A. The impact of gender on outcome after infrainguinal arterial reconstructions for peripheral occlusive disease. J Vasc Surg. 2012;56(2):343–52.
19. Abando A, Akopian G, Katz SG. Patient sex and success of peripheral percutaneous transluminal arterial angioplasty. Arch Surg. 2005;140(8):757–61.
20. Bechter-Hugl B, Falkensammer J, Gorny O, Greiner A, Chemelli A, Fraedrich G. The influence of gender on patency rates after iliac artery stenting. J Vasc Surg. 2014;59(6):1588–96.
21. DeRubertis BG, Vouyouka A, Rhee SJ, et al. Percutaneous intervention for infrainguinal occlusive disease in women: equivalent outcomes despite increased severity of disease compared with men. J Vasc Surg. 2008;48(1):150–8.
22. Sakamoto Y, Hirano K, Iida O, et al. Five-year outcomes of self-expanding nitinol stent implantation for chronic total occlusion of the superficial femoral and proximal popliteal artery. Catheter Cardiovasc Interv. 2013;82(3):E251–6.
23. Tepe G, Schnorr B, Albrecht T, et al. Angioplasty of femoral-popliteal arteries with drug-coated balloons: 5-year follow-up of the THUNDER trial. JACC Cardiovasc Interv. 2015;8(1 Pt A):102–8.
24. Domenick N, Saqib NU, Marone LK, Rhee RY, Makaroun MS, Chaer RA. Impact of gender and age on outcomes of tibial artery endovascular interventions in critical limb ischemia. Ann Vasc Surg. 2012;26(7):937–45.
25. Tyc A, Han DK, Tadros RO, et al. Percutaneous intervention for infrageniculate arterial disease in women may be associated with better outcomes when compared to men. J Vasc Surg. 2013;57(3):706–13.

Gender Differences in CAS

18

Marco Borghesi, Luca Dozza, Roberto Nerla, Antonio Micari, Chiara Grattoni, Fausto Castriota, and Alberto Cremonesi

18.1 General Considerations

18.1.1 Carotid Artery Disease

Ischemic stroke is now the third most common cause of death in the Western world [1] (Fig. 18.1). In addition, the morbidity related to cerebrovascular disease is particularly disabling, because it causes neurological deficits leading to a loss of autonomy and disability in performing normal daily activities, due to enormous costs for the national health system and society [2]. The incidence of stroke was 0.2 % per year in the general population but rises significantly in the presence of multiple risk factors [3].

Annually in the United States, there are more than 700,000 new cases of stroke. Of these, it is estimated that 15–20 % depends on the carotid occlusive disease, and about 70–80 % of these events occurs as the first manifestation of the disease, but there have been earlier clinical symptoms related to transient cerebral ischemia. In Italy a stroke affects about 6.5 % of the population over 65, and a percentage between 20 and 40 % of ischemic stroke is correlated with the presence of carotid artery stenosis in extracranial district. Therefore, carotid stenosis, symptomatic and asymptomatic, remains a significant cause of stroke and the subsequent morbidity and mortality related to it. It is estimated that the incidence of asymptomatic carotid disease in the general population is not negligible, averaging between 2 and 8 %. Advanced age is a strong risk of increased incidence of disease. In fact, if in patients aged <65 years the incidence is about 0.5–1 %, this increases to 2.7 % in patients aged > 65 years and reaches 10 % in patients aged > 80 years. There is also the strong correlation of asymptomatic carotid disease in the presence of classic risk factors

M. Borghesi • L. Dozza • R. Nerla • A. Micari • C. Grattoni • F. Castriota • A. Cremonesi (✉)
Maria Cecilia Hospital – Gvm Care & Research, Cotignola, Ravenna, Italy
e-mail: cremonesi.a@gmail.com

P. Presbitero et al. (eds.), *Percutaneous Treatment of Cardiovascular Diseases in Women*, DOI 10.1007/978-3-319-39611-8_18

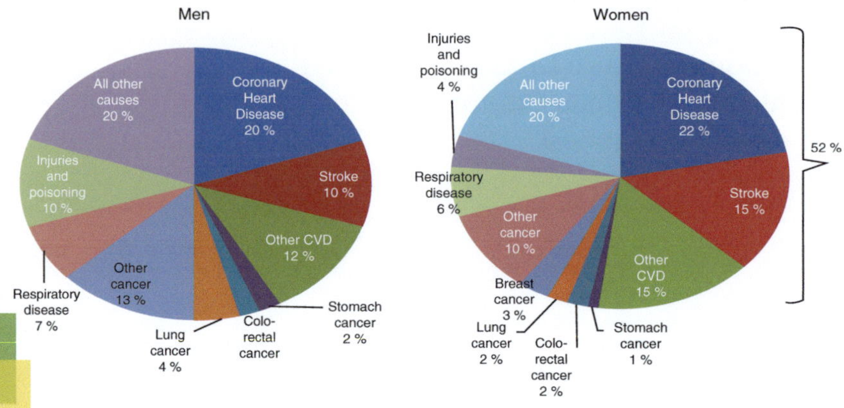

Fig. 18.1 Deaths by cause in men and women, Europe (European Cardiovascular Disease Statistics, 2012)

for cardiovascular disease (dyslipidemia, diabetes, cigarette smoking, high blood pressure) [4].

Carotid stenosis is considered the most common cause of acute ischemic cerebrovascular events. The treatment of extracranial carotid stenosis is therefore of great importance in the prevention of cerebrovascular disease [5].

18.1.2 Carotid Artery Revascularization

Since the carotid endarterectomy (CEA) was described in 1954 as a treatment for stroke prevention, this procedure was subjected, to determine its effectiveness and duration, in various large-scale randomized clinical trials like the European Carotid Surgery Trial (ECST) [6] and the North American Symtomatic Carotid Endarterectomy Trial (NASCET) [7] which showed that the surgical removal of plaque by endarterectomy is superior to medical therapy in preventing stroke in patients with symptomatic carotid stenosis disease criticism. For asymptomatic carotid disease, it is useful to refer to the data derived by ACAS (Asymptomatic Carotid Atherosclerosis Study) [8], the first large randomized trial that compared medical treatment to surgical treatment. This study demonstrated a risk of ipsilateral stroke at 5 years, respectively, of 5.1 % in the surgical arm and 11 % in the medical therapy arm ($p=0.004$). The study, therefore, showed a relative risk reduction of 53 % with a greater benefit in men (66 %) compared to females (17 %). The ACST (Asymptomatic Carotid Surgery Trial) [9] has finally confirmed the role of the superiority of surgery compared to medical therapy alone in the treatment of asymptomatic carotid disease. In this randomized study, the risk of stroke at 5 years was 6.4 % in the treatment arm CEA against 11.8 % in the group treated with medical therapy alone (p <0.0001). This has led to consider the CEA treatment of reference (gold standard) in symptomatic or asymptomatic carotid disease. It should be noted, however, that some of the patients with carotid stenosis was excluded from these trials because it was considered "high-risk surgery." Moreover all these reference works are dated and were conducted without the modern medical therapy.

18.1.2.1 Carotid Artery Stenting

In recent decades the endovascular treatment of carotid stenosis has developed considerably, guided by the success achieved in the coronary district, since the latter has some advantages such as less invasiveness, the absence of risk of injury of cranial nerves, no need for general anesthesia, and reduced hospitalization time. After the first carotid angioplasty performed by Mathias in 1977 [10], the endovascular techniques have rapidly developed, especially after the introduction of the self-expandable stent. In 1996, Dietrich et al. reported the first large series of patients, suffering from symptomatic and asymptomatic carotid stenosis, treated with angioplasty and carotid stenting [11]. In 1997, Yadav et al. reported the results of the first study carried out on the basis of a defined protocol and having an independent neurological assessment [12]. In that series, in which most of the 126 patients included could not be treated by TEA, on the basis of the exclusion criteria of NASCET, it has been reported a technical success of 100 % and a rate of stroke and death equal to 2.4 %. These results have led to a rapid spread of such a procedure, so that Wholey and colleagues reported in 2000 over 5000 procedures of carotid stenting in the world [13].

18.1.2.2 CEA Versus CAS

In 2001 the results of the first trial that compared CAS to CEA was published. The CAVATAS (Carotid and Vertebral Artery Transluminal Angioplasty Study) evaluated patients with high-grade carotid stenosis, treated by carotid angioplasty, with or without stenting and without any cerebral protection or by CEA. The incidence of stroke or death at 30 days and in the follow-up was almost the same. CAS, compared with CEA, however, demonstrated a lower incidence of cranial nerve injury. An increased incidence of severe restenosis at follow-up 1 year, however, was observed after CAS (14 % vs. 4 %) [14].

The trial SAPPHIRE (Stenting and Angioplasty with Protection in Patients at High Risk for Endarterectomy) evaluated patients at high surgical risk, with asymptomatic stenosis > 80 % or symptomatic > 50 %, who underwent CAS with cerebral protection system (Fig. 18.2) or endarterectomy. In this study, the protected CAS was even superior compared to surgery. Indeed, while the results were similar in regard to mortality and stroke (3.1 % vs. 3.3 %), CAS was superior considering the incidence of myocardial infarction (1.9 % vs. 6.6 %) and overall incidence of stroke, MI and death 4.4 % in patients undergoing CAS versus an incidence of 9.9 % in patients undergoing CEA [15, 16].

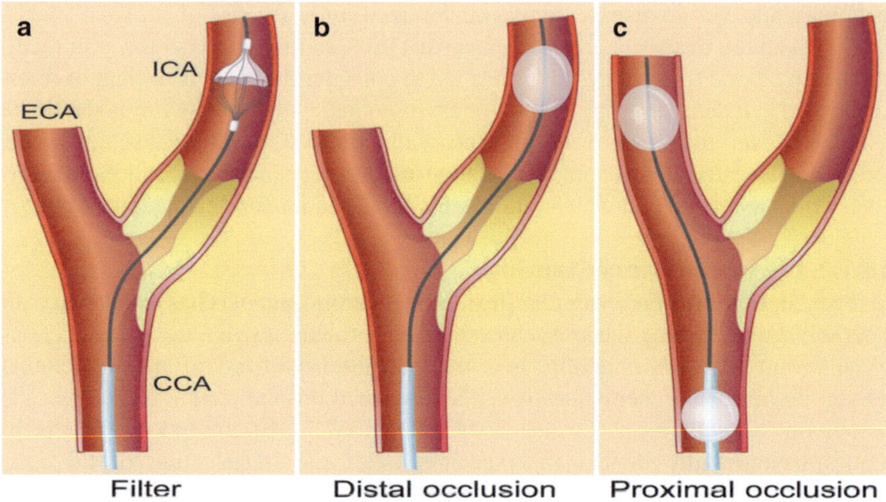

Fig. 18.2 Types of cerebral protection devices: (**a**) Filter positioned distal to the lesion of ICA. (**b**) Protection Balloon inflated distally to the lesion of ICA. (**c**) One Balloon inflated in the external Carotid artery and one inflated in the common Carotid artery in order to interrupt the anterograde flow in the ICA

Three other randomized trials have instead reported results favorable to CEA: study SPACE (Stent-protected Percutaneous Angioplasty of the Carotid vs. Endarterectomy), which evaluated CAS (with cerebral protection) versus CEA in 1214 patients with symptomatic carotid stenosis>70 % [17]; trial EVA-3S (Endarterectomy Versus Angioplasty in Patients with Symptomatic Severe Carotid Stenosis), which has randomized 527 patients with symptomatic carotid stenosis>60 %, undergoing protected CAS or CEA [18]; and finally the study CAVATAS 2-ICSS (International Carotid Stenting Study), which has evaluated 1713 patients at high surgical risk with symptomatic carotid stenosis>70 % underwent to protected CAS or CEA [19]. On the basis of these trials, and of various independent works conducted by vascular surgeons, for many years the gold standard for the treatment of carotid artery disease remains CEA, and CAS has been indicated only for patients not eligible to surgery.

In 2010, however, were published the final data of the CREST (Carotid Revascularization Endarterectomy versus Stent Trial), a multicenter randomized trial which compared TEA and protected CAS in symptomatic and asymptomatic patients at high risk (carotid stenosis >50 % for the symptomatic and >70 % for asymptomatic). In this study, conducted on 2502 patients, the primary end point (stroke, MI, death from any cause in the perioperative period and ipsilateral stroke within 4 years of follow-up) showed no significant differences between the two procedure (7,2 % versus 6,8 %, $p=0.51$) [20].

The impact of technology on the results of CAS was then confirmed by more recent studies in which endovascular procedures, all performed with the routine use of stents dedicated and cerebral protection system, have shown a lower incidence of stroke and death, comparable with the best results reported for the surgical treatment (43). Although CAS has proven safe and effective method in asymptomatic and symptomatic patients at high surgical risk, still it remains unsolved and debated the correct strategy for asymptomatic patients at low risk, particularly in the population of octogenarians and women.

18.1.2.3 "Tailored CAS"

The "tailored approach" to CAS consists of the planning of a specific endovascular strategy for a specific patient. This approach depends on an in-depth knowledge of all characteristics of the endovascular equipment (guiding catheters, guiding sheaths, guide wires, embolic protection devices, balloons, and stents) to precisely match the most suitable device to a specific vascular anatomy, carotid lesion, or cerebral circulation pattern as well as to the patient clinical presentation. Our group in 2009 published the results of the "tailored-CASE registry" which analyzed the use of the "tailored approach" in 1.523 procedures. A procedural success rate of 99.6 % was achieved. The 30-day all-stroke and death rates were 1.2 % and 2.7 % for the asymptomatic and symptomatic patient groups, respectively. The highest-risk population, the symptomatic patients aged more than 80 years, had a 30-day all-stroke and death rate of 4.5 %. Based on those findings, the use of the "tailored approach" by experienced operators seems to be a valuable tool to increase the overall CAS safety [21].

18.1.3 Gender Differences in Cardiovascular Diseases

The awareness of the different realities of the female begins when Bernadine Healy, in 1991, wrote a famous editorial in the prestigious *New England Journal of Medicine* entitled "The Yentl syndrome," commenting on two studies that reported how women with coronary artery disease were generally cared less and receive less aggressive interventions than men [22]. The article was clearly defiant by the first woman to head the US National Institute of Health and had huge coverage in scientific world as well as the media.

In the last two decades, several studies have investigated the gender differences in clinical manifestations and prognosis of cardiovascular disease. The results of these studies showed some important differences related to gender. In fact, while the effects of gender, age, and culture on the health of man and woman have been extensively studied, what is still missing is a similar focus on the impact that gender differences have on the pathophysiology and, therefore, on the treatment of the most common social diseases, including cardiovascular disease.

This difference is particularly marked in cerebrovascular diseases where women show a higher mortality and morbidity than men (Fig. 18.3). Of the estimated 795,000 new or recurrent stroke each year in the USA, 53.3 % appears in women and 61 % of the disease-related mortality is the prerogative of the female sex.

Stroke in women kills twice than breast cancer and it is estimated that one in five women will have a stroke in their lifetime. Even the risk factors are more common in women or are specific to women. Hypertension, diabetes, atrial fibrillation, migraine with visual aura, and depression are more common in women. In addition,

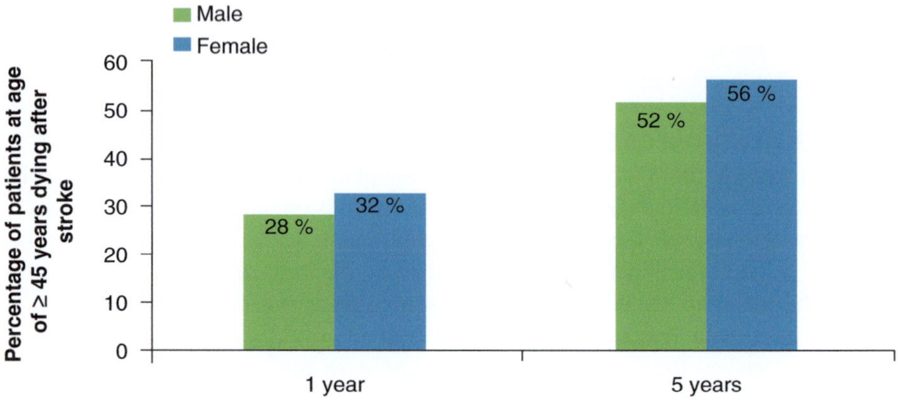

Fig. 18.3 (Source: Roger et al. [23])

pregnancy, preeclampsia, use of contraceptives, postmenopausal hormone replacement therapy, and gestational diabetes are specific risk factors for cerebrovascular events in female sex. The damage produced by a cigarette in a woman is equivalent to that produced by five cigarettes in man, and diabetes increases the risk of vascular disease from three to five times in woman.

In a study published in 2009, Petrea RE et al. explored gender differences in the incidence and severity of stroke in the Framingham Heart Study, based on the data from a follow-up of 56 years. In the population of participants in the Framingham original (5119 of which 2829 women) and in the offspring cohort (4957 of which 2565 women), the authors observed 1136 strokes (638 in women) during follow-up. Women were statistically older at the time of stroke and had an increased rate of stroke over the age of 85, but minor in the other ages. Furthermore, from 3 to 6 months after the stroke, women were significantly more disabled [24].

18.1.3.1 Gender Differences in Carotid Artery Revascularization

The influence of sex on the rise in the risk of stroke and perioperative death during carotid revascularization has been well described for CEA. The Asymptomatic Carotid Atherosclerosis Study (ACAS) was the first study that showed a nonsignificant trend toward an increased risk of stroke and death in women underwent to CEA [25]. The European Carotid Surgery Trial (ECST) found a significantly increased periprocedural risk for women with symptomatic stenosis compared to men (11.1 % vs. 6.4 %, $p=0.002$) [26]. Schulz and Rothwell have speculated that this effect may be caused by the anatomy of the internal carotid arteries that in women may have a diameter of up to 40 % smaller than those of men, making the surgical procedure technically most challenging [27]. These data could have led to “undertreat” women in clinical practice, particularly if asymptomatic.

In 2009, Howard et al. submitted an analysis of the lead-in phase of CREST comparing the results of 1564 patients (in which only 26.5 % were symptomatic) underwent CAS distinct by gender. There was no significant difference in the rate of periprocedural stroke and death between women and men (4.2 % vs. 4.5 %). Taking into account the symptomatic status, the difference between symptomatic and asymptomatic women (5.6 % vs. 4.1 %) was smaller than it was for men (5.9 % vs. 3.5 %). After adjustment for demographic factors (age and race), vascular characteristics (reference diameter, lesion length, percent stenosis), and cardiovascular risk factors (hypertension, hypercholesterolemia, diabetes, and smoking), gender differences were not statistically significant [28].

In 2011, Howard et al. presented the results of CREST comparing CAS and CEA according to gender. The composite primary end point of MI, stroke, or death during the periprocedural period or ipsilateral stroke within 4 years did not differ significantly by sex. The primary end point occurred in 6.2 % of men treated with CAS compared to 6.8 % treated with CEA. The rates for women were 8.9 % in the stenting group versus 6.7 % in the surgical group. Regarding periprocedural events only, the rate of complications was 4.3 % in the male CAS group compared with 4.9 % in the male surgical group. Among women, the rate in the CAS group was 6.8 % compared with 3.8 % in the CEA group [29]. The result of CREST has definitely changed the knowledge about the superior of CEA over CAS and about a more conservative treatment of carotid stenosis in women, even if the debate is still open.

18.2 Women and Carotid Artery Disease: The "Maria Cecilia Hospital" Experience

Maria Cecilia Hospital has gained a renowned experience in percutaneous treatment of carotid artery disease. As a single high-volume center performing CAS, we performed a large number of procedures using a "tailored" approach according to patient's and lesion's characteristics.

18.2.1 CAS Procedures: Our Common Practice

We retrospectively collected all CAS procedures performed in the Department of Diagnostics and Interventional Cardio-Angiology at Maria Cecilia Hospital (Group GVM Care & Research) of Cotignola between March 2012 and January 2015.

A total number of 516 procedures of CAS in 461 patients with symptomatic or asymptomatic carotid stenosis $\geq$ 70 % were identified, and demographic data, risk factors, cardiovascular and neurological history, as well as clinical status at presentation were collected. In addition, for each patient a systematic review of the angiography of supra-aortic vessels performed before the procedure considering anatomical features like aortic arch type (Fig. 18.4), arch bovine type, and vascular tortuosity (Fig. 18.5) was defined according to the criteria of Weibel and Fields.

All carotid stenting procedures were performed by an interventional cardiologist with extensive experience in carotid revascularization using the concept of "tailored CAS."

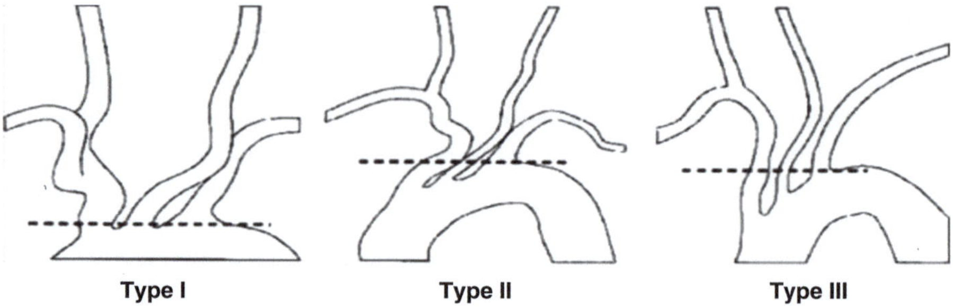

Fig. 18.4

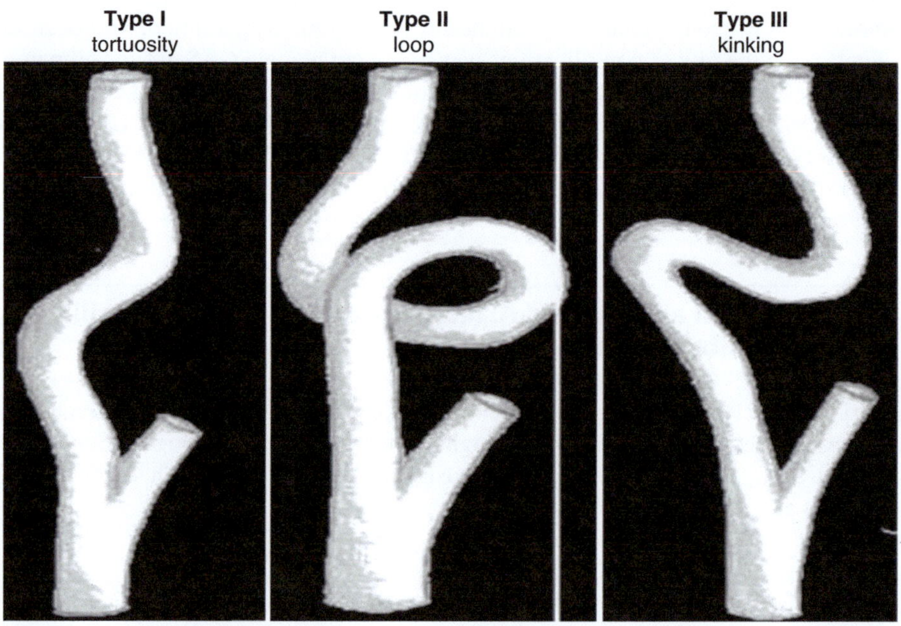

Fig. 18.5

The different types of stents used included Xact Carotid Stent System (Abbott Vascular), Monorail Carotid Wallstent Endoprothesis (Boston Scientific), Cristallo Ideale (Platform Invatec, Medtronic), RoadSaver (Terumo), ViVEXX (VIVA), and noncarotid stents (off-label use).

In 98.4 % of cases, access was transfemoral, while in seven cases it was transradial. A guide catheter of appropriate shape and a hydrophilic standard guidewire 0.035 inch (Terumo Corporation) were used. A distal filter (EPI FilterWire, Boston Scientific, Nanterre, France, Spider, ev3, Irvine, USA) or a proximal cerebral protection system (Mo.Ma system, Invatec, Roncadelle, Italy) was used for cerebral protection.

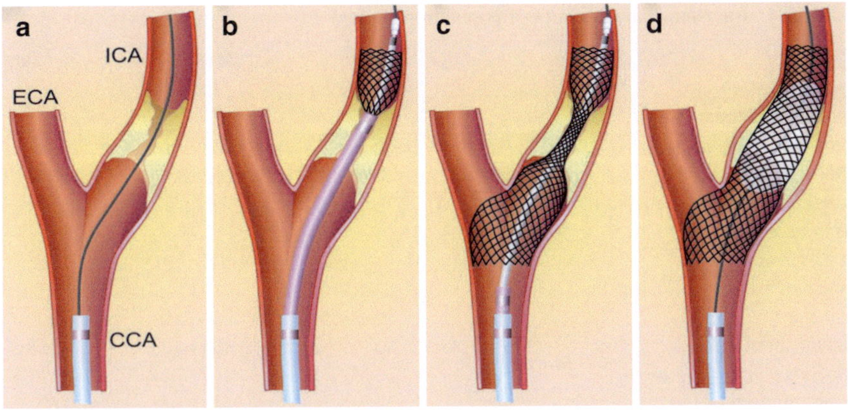

Fig. 18.6 A self expanding stent is released (**a–c**) and then a postdilatation with a baloon inflaten within the stent is performed (**d**)

In every case, a self-expanding stent was released at the level of the carotid bifurcation, without predilatation if possible, and then was performed a postdilatation with an appropriate balloon (Fig. 18.6).

Hemostasis was achieved by positioning device closure system Angio-Seal (St. Jude Medical) in 79.5 % of cases, Perclose ProGlide (Abbott Vascular) in 4.1 % of cases, or by manual compression in the remaining 16.3 % of cases.

18.2.2 CAS Procedures: Our Data About Gender Differences

A total of 435 procedures were included in the study, 165 (37.9 %) of these were performed on female individuals. The baseline characteristics of the study population are shown in Table 18.1. The two populations were homogeneous for age, BMI, and cardiovascular risk factors, with the exception of smoking where it is interesting to note that although men with a history of smoking status are prevalent (49.4 % vs. 31.8 %, $p=0.0003$), in the subgroup of current smokers, women do prevail (19.1 % vs. 14.2 %, $p=0.19$). Women had more frequently at least moderate renal dysfunction (45.9 % vs. 34.4 %, $p=0.03$), while in men a history of ischemic heart disease (48.2 % vs. 31, 2 %, $p=0.00099$) as well as evidence of peripheral vascular disease (19.2 % vs. 12.1 %, $p=0.07$) was significantly more prevalent. No difference instead was recorded between the two groups on the clinical status at presentation, although TIA was more frequent in the group of men (9.5 % vs. 1.9 %, $p=0.005$).

Despite ultrasound data on the percentage of stenosis and the peak systolic velocity in the two groups that were homogeneous, the presentation of carotid disease was most severe in males being more frequent a bilateral stenosis of the internal carotid arteries (43.9 % vs. 30.3 %, $p=0.0066$) and an occlusion of the internal carotid artery contralateral to the critical one (5.6% vs. 0.6%, $p=0.02$). Finally, in

Table 18.1 Baseline characteristics of population studied

	Females	Males	*p* value
Population (%)	165 (39.7)	270 (62.1)	
Baseline characteristics			
Age (years)	72.6 ± 7.9	73.4 ± 8.1	0.31
BMI	26.5 ± 4.3	26.7 ± 3.7	0.54
Creatinine clearance (mL/min)	66.7 ± 24.3	70.9 ± 24.6	0.09
Risk factors (%)			
Hypertension	136 (86.6)	205 (81.0)	0.18
Dyslipidemia	120 (76.4)	189 (74.7)	0.78
Diabetes	45 (28.7)	76 (30.0)	0.85
Current smoking	30 (19.1)	36 (14.2)	0.19
Previous smoker (>1 anno)	20 (12.7)	89 (35.2)	<0.001
Family history of IHD	24 (15.3)	44 (17.4)	0.67
Kidney disease (ClCr <60 mL/min)	72 (45.9)	87 (34.4)	0.03
Obesity	31 (19.8)	42 (16.6)	0.50
Clinical history (%)			
IHD	49 (31.2)	122 (48.2)	<0.001
PAD	19 (12.1)	49 (19.4)	0.07
AVS	9 (5.7)	25 (9.9)	0.19
Previous CEA/CAS	40 (24.4)	66 (24.4)	1.00
Clinical presentation (%)			
Symptoms	33 (21.0)	69 (27.3)	0.19
Stroke	16 (10.2)	18 (7.1)	0.36
TIA	3 (1.9)	24 (9.5)	0.005
Other	14 (8.9)	27 (10.3)	0.24
CEA restenosis	14 (8.5)	10 (3.7)	0.06
ISR	4 (2.4)	3 (1.1)	0.51
Contralateral ICA occlusion	1 (0.6)	15 (5.6)	0.02
Ultrasound data			
ICA stenosis (%)	79.5 ± 8.0	80.6 ± 8.7	0.32
PSV (m/s)	3.0 ± 1.6	2.8 ± 1.3	0.20

AVS aortic valve stenosis, *BMI* body mass index, *CAS* carotid artery stenting, *CEA* carotid endarterectomy, *ICA* internal carotid artery, *IHD* ischemic heart disease, *ISR* intra-stent restenosis, *PAD* peripheral artery disease, *PSV* peak systolic velocity, *TIA* transient ischemic attack

female group a restenosis of a previous intervention of CEA (8.5 % vs. 3.7 %, $p = 0.06$) was found more frequently.

The anatomical characteristics of the treated lesions are reported in Table 18.2. In women, there was a more frequent finding, albeit not significant, of type 2 (20 % vs. 17 %), type 3 (15.2 % vs. 9.6 %), and bovine type (17 % vs. 15.6 %) aortic arch variants. A significant and relevant difference was found in the presence of supra-aortic vessels tortuosity between the two groups (44.9 % in women vs. 21.9 % in men, $p = 0.0001$) (Fig. 18.7).

The analysis of the characteristics of the plaque showed that the most represented lesion in both groups was the fibro-calcific one. However, heavily calcified plaques were observed more frequently in women (12.1 % vs. 6.3 %), while

Table 18.2 Vascular anatomy and lesion's features

	Females	Males	*p* value
Anatomical features (%)			
Type 1 aortic arch	107 (64.8)	198 (73.3)	0.12
Type 2 aortic arch	33 (20.0)	46 (17.0)	0.12
Type 3 aortic arch	25 (15.2)	26 (9.6)	0.12
Bovine-type aortic arch	28 (17.0)	42 (15.6)	0.80
Vascular tortuosity	74 (44.9)	59 (21.9)	<0.001
Plaque characteristics (%)			
Soft	28 (17.0)	38 (14.1)	
Fibrous	96 (58.2)	141 (51.2)	
Calcific	20 (12.1)	17 (6.3)	0.07
Complex	21 (12.7)	74 (27.4)	<0.001
Characteristics (%)			
Length (mm)	20.1 ± 9	21.8 ± 9.1	0.05
Ipsilateral CCA/ECA involvement (%)	38 (23.1)	61 (22.6)	1.00

CCA common carotid artery, *ECA* external carotid artery

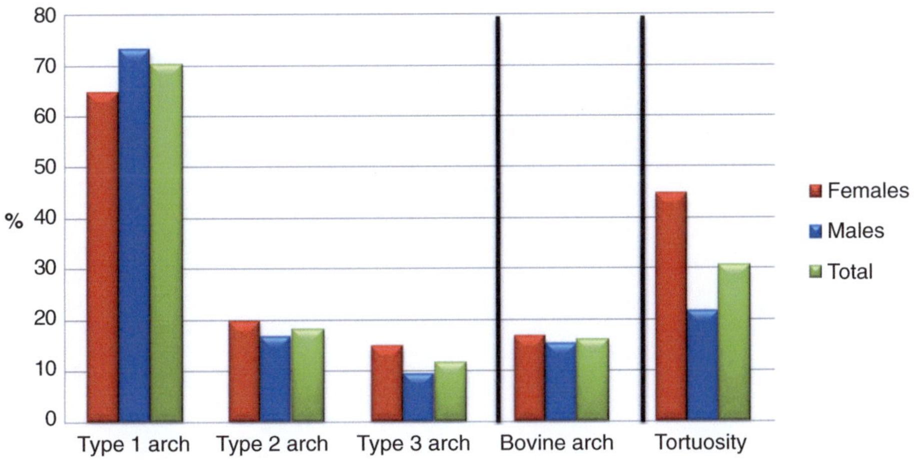

Fig. 18.7 Gender and vascular anatomy

complex plaques were significantly more common in men (27.4 % vs. 12.7 %, $p=0$, 0025). Finally there was a statistically significant difference between men and women in the length of the lesion (Fig. 18.8).

Procedural technical features are reported in Table 18.3. In the group of women, it was more common to use a distal device for cerebral protection (47.3 % vs. 34.1 %, $p=0.01$), while no significant difference was found in the involvement of common carotid artery or ipsilateral external carotid artery in obstructive disease (which represented one of the major limitations in the use of a proximal cerebral protection systems).

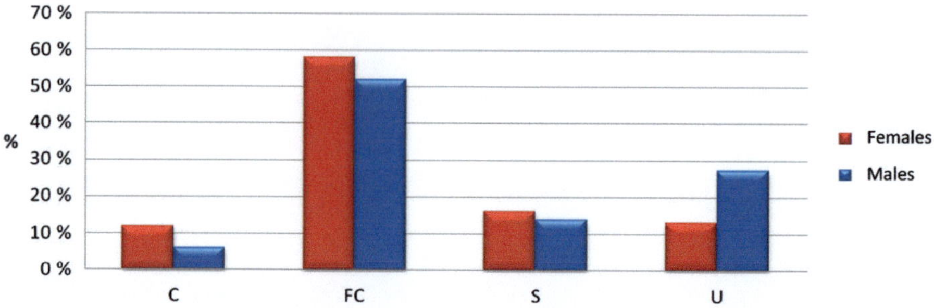

Fig. 18.8 Gender and plaque type (*C* calcific, *FC* fibro-calcific, *S* soft, *U* ulcerated)

Table 18.3 Procedural data

	Females	Males	*p* value
Access site (%)			
Transfemoral	162 (98.2)	266 (98.5)	1.00
Transradial	3 (1.8)	4 (1.5)	
Cerebral protection system (%)			
Proximal occlusion	87 (52.7)	176 (65.2)	0.01
Distal filter	78 (47.3)	92 (34.1)	0.01
Technique (%)			
Direct stenting	131 (79.4)	227 (84.1)	0.27
Predilatation	34 (20.6)	43 (15.9)	
Cutting balloon	8 (4.8)	8 (3.0)	0.45
Stent type (%)			
Xact	83 (50.3)	131 (48.5)	1.00
Carotid Wallstent	34 (20.6)	87 (32.2)	0.017
Cristallo	42 (25.4)	37 (13.7)	0.017
RoadSaver	4 (2.4)	7 (2.6)	
ViVEXX	0 (0.0)	4 (1.5)	
Balloon only	1 (0.6)	2 (0.7)	
Technique complications (%)			
Cross-access site	5 (3.0)	11 (4.1)	0.77
Cross-cerebral protection system	2 (1.2)	0 (0.0)	0.28
Embolic material	18 (10.9)	33 (12.2)	0.80
Plaque prolapse	3 (1.8)	4 (1.5)	1.00
Access closure (%)			
Angio-Seal	133 (80.6)	213 (78.9)	0.15
Perclose ProGlide	3 (1.8)	15 (5.6)	
Manual compression	29 (17.6)	42 (15.6)	
Procedural time (min) (mean+/−sd)	58.0 (23.5)	53.7 (18.0)	0.03
Amount of contrast medium (mL) (mean+/−sd)	180.9 ± 44.7	183.1 ± 49.2	0.64

In both groups a direct stenting was performed in most cases; however, in women predilatation was required more frequently (20.6 % vs. 15.9 %, $p = 0.27$). The stent Xact Carotid Stent System (Abbott Vascular) was the one most

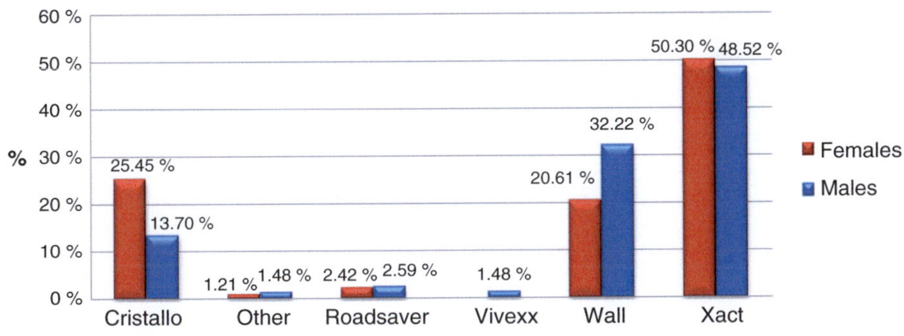

Fig. 18.9 Gender and stent type

commonly used in both groups, while the stent Cristallo Ideale (Platform Invatec, Medtronic), which is usually the preferred choice in case of severe internal carotid artery tortuosities, was used much more in women than men (25, 4 % vs. 13.7 %, $p=0.009$). Conversely, the Monorail Carotid Wallstent Endoprothesis (Boston Scientific) was used more in men than in women (32.2 % vs. 20.6 %, respectively; $p=0.0017$) (Fig. 18.9).

21 % of women were symptomatic, with no statistically significant differences in age, BMI, and creatinine clearance compared to asymptomatic ones. Basal clinical features only differed in smoking habit (33.3 % in the symptomatic group vs. 15.3 % in the asymptomatic group, $p=0.04$). Asymptomatic women showed a trend (not statistically significant) to have diabetes mellitus (32.3 % vs. 15.6 %, $p=0.06$) and a history of ischemic heart disease, peripheral vascular disease, and aortic valve stenosis (52.4 % vs. 36.1 %, $p=0.74$). Symptomatic women more frequently received a Carotid Wallstent (39.4 % vs. 16.1 %, $p=0.02$), and there was a trend toward a more frequent use of proximal cerebral protection system (63.6 % vs. 50.8 %, $p=0.26$) compared to the asymptomatic group. Instead no statistically significant differences were found in the vascular anatomy and in the characteristics of the plaque between the two groups.

In the group of men, asymptomatics were 27.3 %, with no statistically significant differences in age, BMI, and creatinine clearance compared to symptomatic ones. As in women, asymptomatic men had a slight tendency (not statistically significant) to have diabetes mellitus (32.1 % vs. 24.6 %, $p=0.32$). Compared to symptomatic ones, the asymptomatic group had a more frequent history of ischemic heart disease (56 % vs. 27.5 %, $p=0.0001$), while the presence of a history of peripheral vascular disease and aortic valve stenosis was similar in the two groups. There were no statistically significant differences between symptomatic and asymptomatic groups in the analysis of anatomical features, plaque characteristics, and intraprocedural data.

Comparative analysis of the two subgroups of symptomatic patients according to sex showed that the most frequent clinical presentation in men was TIA (34.8 % vs. 10.7 %, $p=0.03$), while in women it was stroke (46.4 % vs. 26.1 %,

Table 18.4 Procedural success and adverse events

	Females	Males	*p* value
Procedural success (%)			
Angiography	165 (100.0)	267 (98.9)	0.45
Ultrasound	158 (95.8)	257 (95.2)	0.97
Major adverse events (%)			
Total	14 (8.5)	13 (4.8)	0.18
MACCE	3 (1.8)	5 (1.8)	1.00
Death	0 (0.0)	0 (0.0)	1.00
AMI	1 (0.6)	0 (0.0)	0.80
Major stroke	1 (0.6)	3 (1.1)	0.99
Minor stroke	1 (0.6)	2 (0.7)	1.00
TIA	2 (1.2)	4 (1.5)	1.00
CIN	5 (3.0)	2 (0.7)	0.15
Bleeding	5 (3.0)	2 (0.7)	0.15
Pseudoaneurysm	2 (1.2)	3 (1.1)	1.00
Minor adverse events (%)			
Total	40 (24.4)	36 (13.3)	0.005
Hypotension	9 (5.4)	6 (2.2)	0.13
Hematoma not complicated	7 (4.2)	3 (1.1)	0.11
Anemia (GUSTO 1)	13 (7.9)	7 (2.6)	0.006
Increased in serum creatinine (>25 % baseline)	11 (8.1)	20 (7.4)	0.90

AMI acute myocardial infarction, *CIN* contrast-induced nephropathy, *MACCE* major adverse coronary or cerebrovascular events, *TIA* transient ischemic attack

$p=0.09$). Of note, the frequency of use of the proximal cerebral protection system and the type of stent deployed were similar in the two groups.

As shown in Table 18.4, the primary end point of procedural success was achieved in 98.9 % cases in men group and in 100 % of cases in the group of women. No statistically significant differences between the two groups were found either in the composite end point of all relevant adverse events (8.5 % in women group vs. 4.8 % in men group) or in major adverse cardiovascular and cerebrovascular events (including death from any cause, periprocedural myocardial infarction, major or minor stroke). No peri- and postprocedural death was observed. There was only one case of acute myocardial infarction readily treated with percutaneous angioplasty. The rate of stroke was 1.8 % in the group of men and 1.2 % in the women group and, considering only the cases of major stroke, respectively, 1.1 % and 0.6 %. Bleeding and clinically relevant CIN occurred, respectively, in 3.2 % and in 3.7 % of cases in the whole population, with a trend, although not statistically significant, toward greater frequency in women. Hematoma complicated by pseudo-aneurism formation at femoral access site was detected in 2.3 % of cases in the whole population, equally distributed between males and females. Figure 18.10 summarizes the gender differences in the incidence of periprocedural adverse events.

A statistically significant difference between the two groups was found in the duration of the procedure, longer in women than in men (23.5 ± 58 min vs. 53, 7 min ± 18, $p=0.03$), while we did not find any differences in the amount of contrast medium used during the procedure.

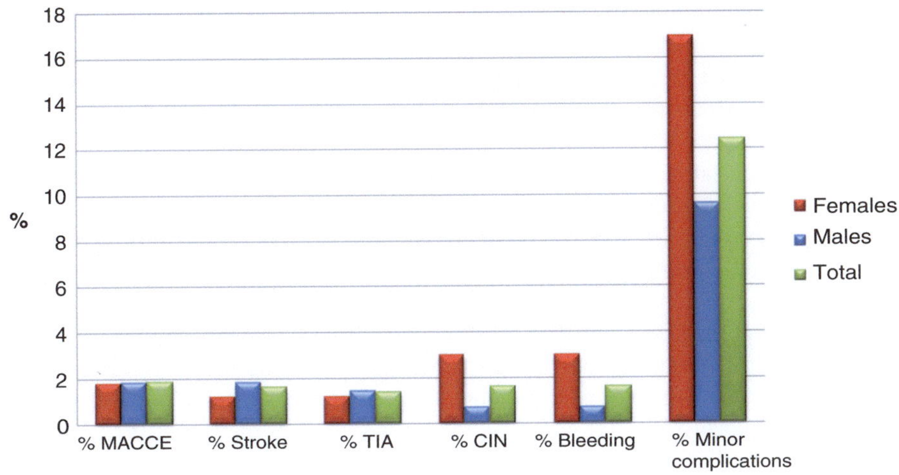

Fig. 18.10 Gender and complications

Finally, the percentage of patients who had minor complications justifying a longer hospital stay for medical observation was higher in female patients than in male ones (24.2 % in women vs. 13.3 % in men, $p=0.024$). In the women group, a postprocedural drop in hemoglobin was more common (7.9 % vs. 2.6 %, $p=0.0061$), as well as an increase in serum creatinine levels (6.7 % vs. 1.2 %, $p=0.0065$), symptomatic hypotension (5.4 % vs. 2.2 %, $p=0.13$), and the evidence of uncomplicated hematoma (4.2 % vs. 1.1 %, $p=0.11$).

18.3 What We Have Learnt About Gender Differences in CAS

The first studies that have directly compared CAS with CEA have undoubtedly shown the superiority of the latter, for the presence of high rates of stroke and death in patients treated endovascular [30, 31]. However, most of these papers refer to a period in which the carotid stenting was performed without the use of a cerebral protection system. The subsequent development of various cerebral protection systems has shown a reduction of the rate of neurological morbidity up to a level which does not significantly differ from that of CEA [32, 33]. In particular, the system of proximal occlusion with reversal flow Mo.Ma (Invatec), whose effectiveness and safety has been tested in the study ARMOUR [34], requires a longer operator's training but provides better results and should represent the first choice, when possible [35, 36]. Similarly, stents used had predominantly an open cell design, now largely replaced by closed cell stents or the new generation of hybrid stent which ensures a better coverage of the plaque, especially in complex lesions at risk of embolization [37]. In addition for some time, the patient population studied in clinical trials on carotid stenting was almost exclusively "high surgical risk," by age and comorbidities and then of course at increased risk of adverse events. Finally, in these clinical trials, women were generally underrepresented and generally older and with more comorbidities, which explains, at least in part, the worse outcome detected in many works in comparison with CEA. These findings led to a tendency to a less aggressive treatment for women, especially in asymptomatic ones, as compared to men, which was firstly questioned by a work of Goldstein et al. [38] and then denied by the CREST study.

In our series, all CAS procedures were performed using a cerebral protection system and minimizing the "manipulation" of the plaque (direct stenting in 82.3 % of cases), also using the last type of stents available (closed cell stent or hybrids in 97.7 % of cases). Women were almost 40 % of the population studied. In fact, male and female populations were extremely homogeneous, both for demographic characteristics that for risk factors. The only major difference was the major presence of at least moderate renal dysfunction in women and ischemic heart disease in men. The percentage of symptomatic patients at presentation was also similar in both groups particularly for what concerns the stroke (10.2 % of women vs. 7.1 % of men).

In this context, the procedural success was higher than 99 %, and the overall rate of permanent neurological complications, disable stroke, or death, which are the real hard end points, amounted to 0.6 % in women and 1,1 % in men, with no significant difference in gender and far below the maximum limits generally accepted for surgical treatment (3 % for asymptomatic patients and 6 % for symptomatic patients) [39]. These results were achieved despite proven more complex vascular anatomy in women than men, due to the frequent presence of tortuosity of supra-aortic vessels and the tendency to have a more "difficult" aortic arch anatomy (type 3 or bovine arch), which resulted in a longer procedural time but not in any change in clinical outcome. Women, however, showed more inherent fragility in the analysis of the postprocedural course, due to more frequent adverse events, even if judged clinically not relevant, which have justified an extension of the hospital stay for clinical observation.

Based on the results obtained in this study, therefore, CAS is an effective and safe procedure, in the hands of expert operators, irrespective of gender distinctions.

By the way, the debate on the best option between drug therapy and CAS in primary prevention of stroke in a fragile population, as the one represented by women with symptomatic carotid artery disease, remains open [40]. Eventually, the final data of the ACST-2, the largest trial ever conducted in order to compare CEA to CAS in asymptomatic patients, will likely provide important information in this respect [41].

In conclusion, CAS is effective and safe in both sexes. In spite of the presence of significant gender's differences in vascular anatomy that might influence procedural technique and time, in the hands of an experienced operator in a high-volume center where it is applied the modern concept of "tailored CAS" where the procedure is planned on the characteristics of the individual patient [42], this would not affect the rate of procedural success or periprocedural adverse events, even in a group of asymptomatic women. This particular setting should be considered as a more challenging population which, however, could benefit even more from a properly planned and performed procedure of CAS.

References

1. Sarti C, Rastenyte D, Cepaitis Z, Tuomilehto J, Sarti C, Rastenyte D, Cepaitis Z, Tuomilehto J. International trends in mortality from stroke, 1968 to 1994. Stroke. 2000;31:1588–601.
2. Murray CJ, Lopez AD, Murray CJL, Lopez AD. Global mortality, disability and the contribution of risk factors. Global burden of the disease study. Lancet. 1997;349:1436–42.
3. Marini C, Baldassarre M, Russo T, De Santis F, Sacco S, Ciancarelli I, Carolei A, Marini C, Baldassarre M, Russo T, De Santis F, Sacco S, Ciancarelli I, Carolei A. Burden of first-ever ischemic stroke in the oldest old. Evidence from a population-based study. Neurology. 2004;62:77–81.
4. Cremonesi A, Liso A, Furgieri A. Estevao Carvalho de Campos Martins, Fausto Castriota. Carlo Setacci G Ital Cardiol. 2009;10(10):671–6.
5. Marmont MG, Poulter NR. Primary prevention of stroke. Lancet. 1992;339:344–7.
6. Randomised trial of endarterectomy for recently symptomatic carotid stenosis: final results of the MRC European Carotid Surgery Trial (ECST). Lancet. 1998;351(9113):1379–87.
7. Ferguson GG, Eliasziw M, Barr HW, Clagett GP, Barnes RW, Wallace MC, Taylor DW, Haynes RB, Finan JW, Hachinski VC, Barnett HJ. The North American Symptomatic Carotid Endarterectomy Trial: surgical results in 1415 patients. Stroke. 1999;30(9):1751–8.
8. Young B, Moore WS, Robertson JT, Toole JF, Ernst CB, Cohen SN, Broderick JP, Dempsey RJ, Hosking JD. An analysis of perioperative surgical mortality and morbidity in the asymptomatic carotid atherosclerosis study. ACAS Investigators. Asymptomatic Carotid Atherosclerosis Study. Stroke. 1996;27(12):2216–24.
9. Halliday A, Mansfield A, Marro J, Peto C, Peto R, Potter J, Thomas D, MRC Asymptomatic Carotid Surgery Trial (ACST) Collaborative Group. Prevention of disabling and fatal strokes by successful carotid endarterectomy in patients without recent neurological symptoms: randomised controlled trial. Lancet. 2004;363(9420):1491–502.
10. Mathias K. A new catheter system for percutaneous transluminal angioplasty (PTA) of carotid artery stenoses. Fortschr Med. 1977;95(15):1007–11.
11. Diethrich EB, Ndiaye M, Reid DB. Stenting in the carotid artery: initial experience in 110 patients. J Endovasc Surg. 1996;3(1):42–62.
12. Yadav JS, Roubin GS, Iyer S, Vitek J, King P, Jordan WD, Fisher WS. Elective stenting of the extracranial carotid arteries. Circulation. 1997;95(2):376–81.
13. Wholey MH, Wholey M, Mathias K, Roubin GS, Diethrich EB, Henry M, Bailey S, Bergeron P, Dorros G, Eles G, Gaines P, Gomez CR, Gray B, Guimaraens J, Higashida R, Ho DS, Katzen B, Kambara A, Kumar V, Laborde JC, Leon M, Lim M, Londero H, Mesa J, Musacchio A, Myla S, Ramee S, Rodriquez A, Rosenfield K, Sakai N, Shawl F, Sievert H, Teitelbaum G, Theron JG, Vaclav P, Vozzi C, Yadav JS, Yoshimura SI. Global experience in cervical carotid artery stent placement. Catheter Cardiovasc Interv. 2000;50(2):160–7.
14. Endovascular versus surgical treatment in patients with carotid stenosis in the Carotid and Vertebral Transluminal Angioplasty Study (CAVATAS): a randomized trial. Lancet. 2001;357:1729–37.
15. Yadav JS. Carotid stenting in high-risk patients: design and rationale of SAPPHIRE trial. Cleve Clin J Med. 2004;71:S45–6.
16. Gurm HS, Yadav JS, Fayad P, Katzen BT, Mishkel GJ, Bajwa TK, Ansel G, Strickman NE, Wang H, Cohen SA, Massaro JM, Cutlip DE, SAPPHIRE Investigators. Long-term results of carotid stenting versus endarterectomy in high-risk patients. N Engl J Med. 2008;358(15):1572–9.
17. SPACE Collaborative Group; Ringleb PA, Allenberg J, Brückmann H, Eckstein HH, Fraedrich G, Hartmann M, Hennerici M, Jansen O, Klein G, Kunze A, Marx P, Niederkorn K, Schmiedt W, Solymosi L, Stingele R, Zeumer H, Hacke W. 30 day results from the SPACE trial of stent-protected angioplasty versus carotid endarterectomy in symptomatic patients: a randomised non-inferiority trial. Lancet. 2006;368(9543):1239–47.

18. Mas JL, Chatellier G, Beyssen B, Branchereau A, Moulin T, Becquemin JP, Larrue V, Lièvre M, Leys D, Bonneville JF, Watelet J, Pruvo JP, Albucher JF, Viguier A, Piquet P, Garnier P, Viader F, Touzé E, Giroud M, Hosseini H, Pillet JC, Favrole P, Neau JP, Ducrocq X, EVA-3S Investigators. Endarterectomy versus stenting in patients with symptomatic severe carotid stenosis. N Engl J Med. 2006;355(16):1660–71.
19. International Carotid Stenting Study investigators; Ederle J, Dobson J, Featherstone RL, Bonati LH, van der Worp HB, de Borst GJ, Lo TH, Gaines P, Dorman PJ, Macdonald S, Lyrer PA, Hendriks JM, McCollum C, Nederkoorn PJ, Brown MM. Carotid artery stenting compared with endarterectomy in patients with symptomatic carotid stenosis (International Carotid Stenting Study): an interim analysis of a randomised controlled trial. Lancet. 2010;375(9719):985–97.
20. Brott TG, Hobson 2nd RW, Howard G, Roubin GS, Clark WM, Brooks W, Mackey A, Hill MD, Leimgruber PP, Sheffet AJ, Howard VJ, Moore WS, Voeks JH, Hopkins LN, Cutlip DE, Cohen DJ, Popma JJ, Ferguson RD, Cohen SN, Blackshear JL, Silver FL, Mohr JP, Lal BK, Meschia JF, CREST Investigators. Stenting versus endarterectomy for treatment of carotid-artery stenosis. N Engl J Med. 2010;363(1):11–23.
21. Cremonesi A, Gieowarsingh S, Spagnolo B, et al. Safety, efficacy and long-term durability of endovascular therapy for carotid artery disease: the tailored-carotid artery stenting experience of a single high-volume centre (tailored-CASE Registry). EuroIntervention. 2009;5:589–98.
22. Healy B. The Yentl syndrome. N Engl J Med. 1991;325(4):274–6.
23. Roger VL, Go AS, Lloyd-Jones DM, Adams RJ, Berry JD, Brown TM, Carnethon MR, Dai S, de Simone G, Ford ES, Fox CS, Fullerton HJ, Gillespie C, Greenlund KJ, Hailpern SM, Heit JA, Ho PM, Howard VJ, Kissela BM, Kittner SJ, Lackland DT, Lichtman JH, Lisabeth LD, Makuc DM, Marcus GM, Marelli A, Matchar DB, McDermott MM, Meigs JB, Moy CS, Mozaffarian D, Mussolino ME, Nichol G, Paynter NP, Rosamond WD, Sorlie PD, Stafford RS, Turan TN, Turner MB, Wong ND, Wylie-Rosett J, American Heart Association Statistics Committee and Stroke Statistics Subcommittee. Heart disease and stroke statistics--2011 update: a report from the American Heart Association. Circulation. 2011;123:e18–209.
24. Petrea RE, Beiser AS, Seshadri S, Kelly-Hayes M, Kase CS, Wolf PA. Gender differences in stroke incidence and poststroke disability in the Framingham heart study. Stroke. 2009;40(4):1032–7.
25. Young B, Moore WS, Robertson JT, et al.; for the ACAS investigators. An analysis of perioperative surgical mortality and morbidity in the Asymptomatic Carotid Atherosclerosis Study. Stroke. 1996;27:2216–24.
26. Messé SR, Kasner SE, Mehta Z, et al.; for the European Carotid Trialists. Effect of body size on operative risk of carotid endarterectomy. J Neurol Neurosurg Psychiatry. 2004;75:1759–61.
27. Schulz U, Rothwell PM. Sex differences in carotid bifurcation anatomy and the distribution of atherosclerotic plaque. Stroke. 2001;32:1525–31.
28. Howard VJ, Voeks JH, Lutsep HL, et al.; for the CREST Investigators. Does sex matter? Thirty-day stroke and death rates after carotid artery stenting in women versus men. Results from the carotid revascularization endarterectomy versus stenting trial (CREST) lead-in phase. Stroke. 2009;40:1140–47.
29. Howard VJ, Lutsep HL, Mackey A, et al.; for the CREST investigators. Influence of sex on outcomes of stenting versus endarterectomy: a subgroup analysis of the Carotid revascularization Endarterectomy Versus Stenting Trial (CREST). Lancet Neurol. 2011;10:530–7.
30. Jordan Jr WD, Voellinger DC, Fisher WS, Redden D, McDowell HA. A comparison of carotid angioplasty with stenting versus endarterectomy with regional anesthesia. J Vasc Surg. 1998;28(3):397–402; discussion 402–3.
31. Naylor AR, Bolia A, Abbott RJ, Pye IF, Smith J, Lennard N, Lloyd AJ, London NJ, Bell PR. Randomized study of carotid angioplasty and stenting versus carotid endarterectomy: a stopped trial. J Vasc Surg. 1998;28(2):326–34.

32. Yadav JS, Wholey MH, Kuntz RE, et al. Protected carotid-artery stenting versus Endarterectomy in high-risk patients. N Engl J Med. 2004;351:1493–501.
33. Bush RL, Kougias P, Guerrero MA, Lubbe DF, Zhou W, Lumsden AB, Lin PH. A comparison of carotid artery stenting with neuroprotection versus carotid endarterectomy under local anesthesia. Am J Surg. 2005;190(5):696–700.
34. Ansel GM, Hopkins LN, Jaff MR, et al. Safety and effectiveness of the INVATEC MO.MA proximal cerebral protection device during carotid artery stenting: results from the ARMOUR pivotal trial. Catheter Cardiovasc Interv. 2010;76:1–8.
35. Criado E, Doblas M, Fontcuberta J, Orgaz A, Flores A, Lopez P, Wall Phillip L. Carotid angioplasty with internal carotid artery flow reversal is well tolerated in the awake patient. J Vasc Surg. 2004;40:92–7.
36. Hornung M, Bertog SC, Franke J, Id D, Grunwald I, Sievert H. Evaluation of proximal protection devices during carotid artery stenting as the first choice for embolic protection. EuroIntervention. 2015;10(11):1362–7.
37. Hart JP, Peeters P, Verbist J, Deloose K, Bosiers M. Do device characteristics impact outcome in carotid artery stenting? J Vasc Surg. 2006;44(4):725–30; discussion 730–1.
38. Goldstein LJ, Khan HU, Sambol EB, Kent KC, Faries PL, Vouyouka AG. Carotid artery stenting is safe and associated with comparable outcomes in men and women. J Vasc Surg. 2009;49(2):315–23; discussion 323–4.
39. Moore WS, Barnett HJ, Beebe HG, Bernstein EF, Brener BJ, Brott T, Caplan LR, Day A, Goldstone J, Hobson 2nd RW, et al. Guidelines for carotid endarterectomy. A multidisciplinary consensus statement from the ad hoc Committee, American Heart Association. Stroke. 1995;26(1):188–201.
40. Abbott AL. Medical (nonsurgical) intervention alone is now best for prevention of stroke associated with asymptomatic severe carotid stenosis: results of a systematic review and analysis. Stroke. 2009;40(10):e573–83.
41. ACST-2 Collaborative Group; Halliday A, Bulbulia R, Gray W, Naughten A, den Hartog A, Delmestri A, Wallis C, le Conte S, Macdonald S. Status update and interim result from The Asymptomatic Carotid Surgery Trial-2 (ACST-2). Eur J Vasc Endovasc Surg. 2013;46(5):510–8.
42. Stabile E, Garg P, Cremonesi A, Bosiers M, Reimers B, Setacci C, Cao P, Schmidt A, Sievert H, Peeters P, Nikas D, Werner M, de Donato G, Parlani G, Castriota F, Hornung M, Mauri L, Rubino P. European Registry of Carotid Artery Stenting: results from a prospective registry of eight high volume EUROPEAN institutions. Catheter Cardiovasc Interv. 2012;80(2):329–34.

Part V

Complex Clinical Scenarios

Percutaneous Treatment During Pregnancy

19

Patrizia Presbitero and Giacomo Giovanni Boccuzzi

Cardiac conditions that need percutaneous intervention during pregnancy are very rare because usually they are diagnosed and treated before pregnancy. However, as a result of the hemodynamic changes (Fig. 19.1) and hypercoagulability state of pregnancy, some previously undiagnosed conditions can be unmasked or can rapidly deteriorate even in previously stable women.

19.1 Indications for Intervention

1. Worsening of cardiac conditions that had previously been missed or underestimated and became symptomatic: this can occur particularly in mitral and aortic valve disease. The pressure gradient across a narrowed valve may increase greatly during pregnancy because of the rise in cardiac output. As a result of the high metabolic state of pregnancy, a possible acceleration of the disease process with progressive calcification can occur either in the native or, even more often, in bioprosthetic cardiac valves (either porcine or bovine). These conditions have to be closely followed clinically and with echocardiography in order to optimize the time for possible interventional treatment.
2. Occurrence of sudden life-threatening complications such as acute myocardial infarction due to coronary artery disease or coronary dissection. In a recent review comprising 103 pregnant women with acute myocardial infarction, atherosclerosis was the underlying cause in 40% of infarctions, and coronary dissection was responsible for 27% of the cases [1]. In these cases, it is very important not to delay intervention because the fetal risk is related to the maternal state.

P. Presbitero, M.D, FESC, EAPCI Member (✉)
Clinical and Interventional Cardiology Unit, Humanitas Hospital, Rozzano, Milan, Italy
e-mail: patrizia.presbitero@humanitas.it

G.G. Boccuzzi, MD, FESC, EAPCI Member
Ospedale San Giovanni Bosco, Unità Operativa di Cardiologia, Turin, Italy

P. Presbitero et al. (eds.), *Percutaneous Treatment of Cardiovascular Diseases in Women*,
DOI 10.1007/978-3-319-39611-8_19

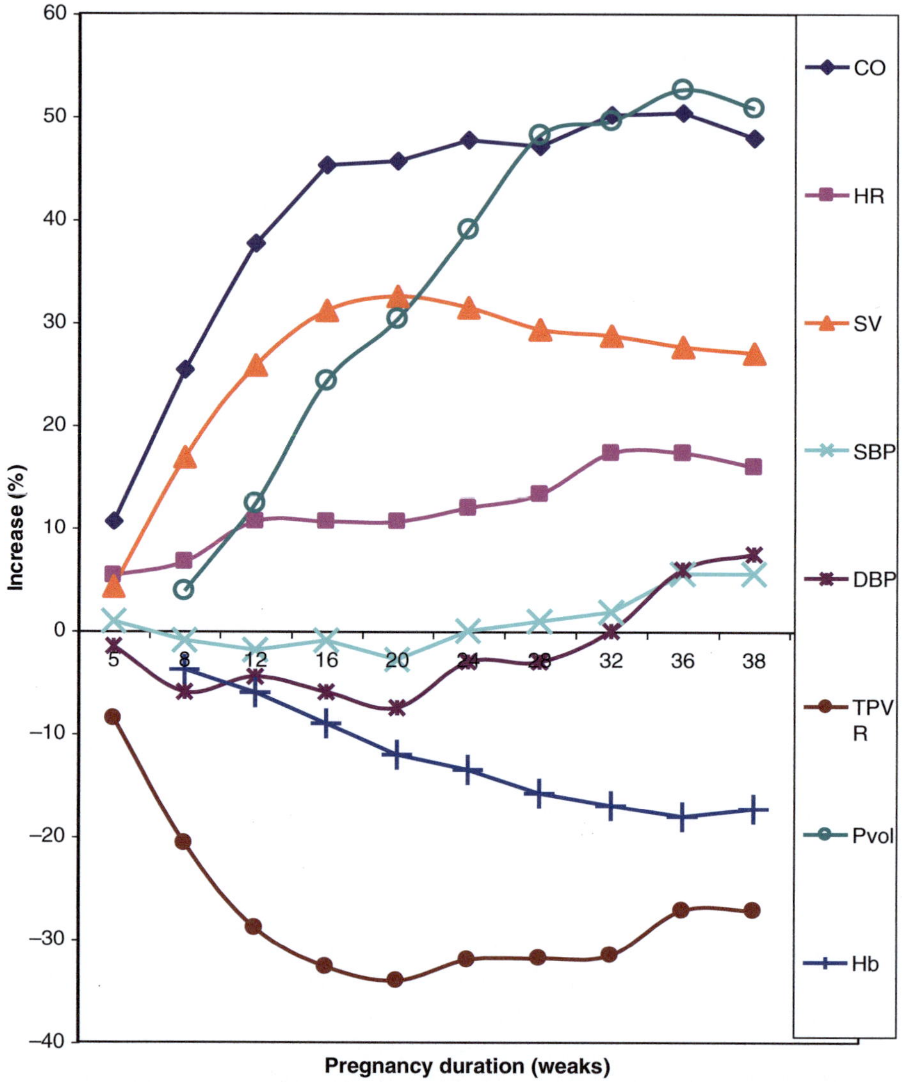

Fig. 19.1 Changes in cardiac output (*CO*), stroke volume (*SV*), plasma volume (*PV*), total peripheral vascular resistance(*TPVR*), heart rate (*HR*), blood pressure (*SBP* systolic blood pressure, *DBP* diastolic blood pressure), and hemoglobin concentration (*Hb*) during pregnancy

19.2 Radiation Exposure

Over the last 30 years, interventional cardiology has emerged as a new therapeutic tool and an effective alternative to surgical therapy in several cardiac diseases, particularly valve stenosis and coronary artery disease. There is a lot of worry about the "real" fetal risk of radiation and contrast medium. The ionizing radiation can have harmful effects, which are cell death, teratogenic effects, carcinogenesis and genetic effects (mutations); however, these effects are not observed with the doses that are needed for the majority of diagnostic and therapeutic procedures. The effects of radiation on the fetus depend on the maternal radiation dose and gestational age at which the exposure occurs. The maximal permissible dose of radiation to the pregnant woman has been set at 50 mGy (www.bt.cdc.gov/radiation/prenatalphysician.asp). The effect of radiation during pregnancy can be divided into three main phases. Irradiation during the preimplantation period (0–9 days) tends to cause death rather than anomalies. The effect appears to be "all or none." The incidence of spontaneous embryo resorption during the first 2 weeks of gestation is approximately 25 %, and a dose of 100 mGy is estimated to increase the number by 0–1 %. During the period of active organogenesis (9–42 days), radiation causes severe structural anomalies. A dose of 2000 mGy will produce a 100 % incidence of congenital abnormalities, whereas a dose of 100 mGy results in 1 % increase in malformations over a baseline of 5–10 %. During the second and third trimester, risks are primarily related to the development of childhood leukemia and other malignancies. It has been estimated that a dose of 10 mGy increases the risk of childhood cancer by two cases per 100,000 births to a total of six cases in 100,000 live births. It has been calculated that the radiation dose to the mother for the most frequently performed cardiac percutaneous intervention (mitral balloon valvuloplasty and coronary angioplasty) are <20 mGy. Even though the risks are small, the interventional procedures have to be performed with forethought and care to minimize the radiation levels using the ALARA principle (as low as reasonably achievable). Maneuvers to minimize radiation are: (1) use echo guidance when possible, (2) place the source as distant as possible from the patient and the receiver as close as possible to the patient, (3) use only low-dose fluoroscopy as we learned from the total chronic occlusion procedures, (4) favor anteroposterior projections, (5) avoid direct radiation of the abdominal region, (6) collimate as tightly as possible to the area of interest, (7) minimize fluoroscopy time, and (8) let the procedure be done by experienced cardiologist. Abdominal shielding (placement of lead apron between the patient and the table) is recommended, although this lowers the dose to the fetus by only 2 %, paying particular attention to avoid the presence of lead in the field of the primary beam (systems automatically adjust the emitted radiation via an automatically modulatory system allowing a constant image quality; in these conditions, the presence of lead would increase scattered radiation). The best time for performing percutaneous intervention procedures is considered to be the fourth month, during which period organogenesis has been completed, the fetal thyroid is still inactive, and the volume of the uterus is still small so that there is greater distance between the fetus and the chest than in the following months. Monitoring and recording of radiation exposures is important to enable future assessment of possible effects on the fetus. These data should be included in the patient's medical record or the procedure report [2].

19.3 Percutaneous Mitral Balloon Valvotomy

Mitral valve stenosis, almost always of rheumatic origin, is the most common (90 %) and important cardiac valvular problem during pregnancy, particularly in developing countries. Most of the women with severe, but also those with moderate, mitral valve stenosis have worsening of their symptoms in the second or third trimester of pregnancy. Percutaneous balloon mitral valvotomy (PBMV) or valve repair/replacement during pregnancy should be considered in patients with moderate or severe mitral valve stenosis and persistent symptoms despite optimal medical therapy. Open mitral valvotomy or valve replacement during pregnancy is rarely necessary and has virtually disappeared from the surgical repertoire because young women have pliable valves without too much calcification that are suitable for percutaneous balloon valvotomy. This technique has been taken over from surgical closed mitral valvotomy which has been carried out safely with excellent results since the 1950s. PBMV, since the initial description by Inoue in 1984, has been shown to be successful in large studies of patients with symptomatic mitral stenosis. The mechanism of PBMV –commissural splitting – is similar to that of surgical valvotomy. This procedure has given good results, especially in young patients with noncalcified, thin valves without subvalvular thickening or significant mitral regurgitation. Dilatation of the stenotic mitral valve results in immediate hemodynamic improvement.

The mitral gradient generally decreases from 33 to 50 % of its initial value, and the cross-sectional area doubles. Both pulmonary capillary wedge pressure and pulmonary artery pressure decrease immediately, with the latter dropping further during the week after valvuloplasty. There are potential complications associated with this procedure, including atrial perforation resulting from transseptal puncture, cardiac tamponade, arrhythmias, embolism, mitral regurgitation, and hypotension. Mortality in the more recent series is reported to be 0.5 % [3]. Mitral regurgitation is the most common complication; in published reports its incidence varies from 0 to 50 %. Severe regurgitation is, however, uncommon and will occur only when there is structural damage to the mitral valve. The development or increase in the grade of mitral regurgitation is predicted by the presence of regurgitation and the severity of stenosis before the procedure. In patients with pliable valves, the development of mitral regurgitation is less frequent. Creation of a significant atrial septal defect secondary to septal dilatation has been reported to vary from 5 to 20 % and is hemodynamically insignificant in all patients. The long-term effect of these shunts is unknown, but it seems that most atrial septal defects close within 24 h.

Since 1988, more than 300 women are reported to have had PBMVs in pregnancy. In women with severe mitral stenosis and well-documented immediate clinical and hemodynamic results, the mean gradient across the stenotic mitral valve declined from the mean value of 21 to 5 mmHg, and the mitral valve area increased from the mean value of 0.9 to 2.1 cm^2. There have been no reports of serious maternal complications and only two fetal deaths. The reported incidence of mitral regurgitation is low, and in most cases it was only trivial or mild [4].

Balloon inflation generally causes transient maternal hypotension and a transient decrease in fetal heart rate. Both parameters return to baseline within a few seconds of balloon deflation, with no serious fetal distress noted. During balloon mitral valvolotomy, the supine position is necessary. This may cause maternal hypotension that can be alleviated by intravenous fluid infusion. The recumbent position causes pressure of the gravid uterus on the pelvic vessels, which may obstruct the passage of catheters. In the pregnant patient, the procedure has been performed with both the single and the double-balloon technique. Nowadays the use of single-balloon catheter is the preferred choice. Transesophageal ultrasonography or even simple transthoracic ultrasonography can be used during PBMV in order to minimize radiation exposure.

At the present, percutaneous mitral commissurotomy is preferably performed after 20 weeks gestation. It should only be considered in women with NYHA class III/IV and/or estimated systolic PAP 50 mmHg at echocardiography despite optimal medical treatment, in the absence of contraindications and if patient characteristics are suitable. In asymptomatic patients with mitral stenosis, the risk of maternal death during pregnancy and delivery is very low. However, the deterioration in hemodynamic conditions can be expected and emergency valvotomy may become necessary. A simple "rule of thumb" is an increase of one NYHA functional class any time during pregnancy. In these cases a "prophylactic" percutaneous mitral valvotomy should be considered, provided that there is a satisfactory echocardiographic score (<8).

Balloon mitral valvotomy in the pregnant patient is technically a complex procedure that needs to be done quickly by an expert team. As a result of the possibility of a need for subsequent emergency surgery, it should be done only in centers that have extensive experience with this procedure and have a cardiac surgery department on-site.

19.4 Percutaneous Aortic Balloon Valvotomy

Severe aortic valve stenosis is rare during pregnancy because both the congenital bicuspid form is more commonly found in men and patients are normally treated before conception either with percutaneous or surgical valvotomy. During pregnancy, as results of the increase in the cardiac output, the transvalvular gradient may double its basal value, and clinical deterioration can develop. Intervention is indicated only in severe symptomatic aortic valve stenosis, and the echocardiographic features alone are not enough to decide on management.

Percutaneous aortic balloon valvotomy is a procedure in which one or more balloon are placed across the stenotic aortic valve and inflated. The aim is to relieve the stenosis, presumably by separation of the fused commissures or fracturing calcified deposits within the valve leaflets. Early changes after successful valvotomy include a moderate reduction in transvalvular pressure gradient and a dramatic improvement in symptoms. However, the post procedure valve area rarely exceeds 1.0 cm^2. Some cases of balloon aortic valvotomy during pregnancy have been reported in the literature with significant reduction of valve gradient, hence enabling the pregnancy to continue. As it is only a palliative procedure, allowing deferral of valve replacement until delivery and postpartum period, the aim, particularly in the case of thick and calcified aortic valves, is just to obtain a modest increase in the aortic valve area, avoiding important aortic insufficiency. Balloon size of aortic annulus of 1:1 is recommended. In women with significant aortic regurgitation as well as in those with heavily calcified valves, surgery should be considered, knowing that cardiopulmonary bypass carries a risk of maternal and fetal mortality rates of 1.5 % and 9.5 %, respectively [5].

19.5 Acute Myocardial Infarction

It is well known that the incidence of acute myocardial infarction (AMI) is decreasing in the Western countries as is its mortality. However, the young women population is the only one which shows a contrary trend with an increasing incidence of AMI. It is probably related to childbearing at an older age, increasing cigarette smoking and diabetes in women (Fig. 19.2) [6]. Fortunately it remains a rare event occurring in 1 in 20,000–30,000 deliveries with a mortality rate ranging from 21 to 37 % in past series to 7 % in the most recent ones owing improvement in diagnosis and treatment strategies.

Most commonly it happens during the third trimester or in the peripartum and puerperal period and more often in multigravidas.

There are three main etiologies for the development of AMI during pregnancy, and risk factors, clinical presentations, and treatments vary according to them. (1) Coronary atherosclerotic lesions are present in 20–43 % of pregnancy-related AMI cases. In these cases risk factors are similar to the one observed in the

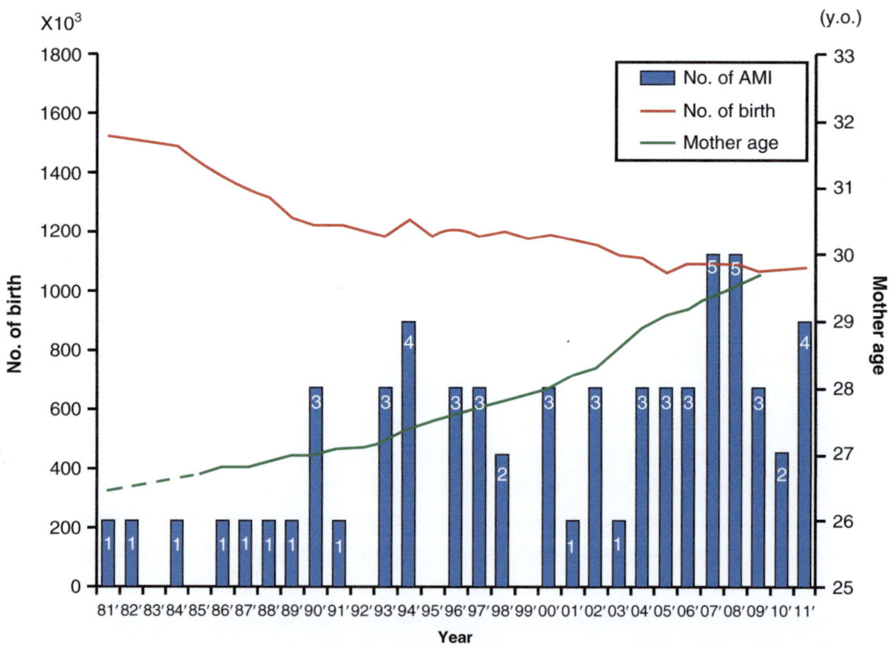

Fig. 19.2 Relationship between mother's age, which is increasing in the last 30 years, and the incidence of myocardial infarction (To the courtesy of Satoh H)

general coronary artery disease population: family history of coronary disease, familial hyperlipoproteinemia, low levels of high-density lipoprotein (HDL), high levels of low-density lipoprotein (LDL), diabetes mellitus, maternal obesity, smoking, hypertension, and previous use of oral contraceptives, and at least two of them are invariably present in a pregnant woman with AMI that is caused by atherosclerotic plaque. The presentation peak in the third trimester (42 % of all cases of atherosclerosis) and the age of the mother are more advanced than in the others etiology [7]. (2) Spontaneous coronary artery dissection (SCAD) is present in 15–35 % of the cases mostly in young otherwise healthy women and occurs in late pregnancy (near term) or within 3 months postpartum. An increase risk is present in case of multiparity. The arterial wall changes (smooth muscle cell proliferation, impaired collagen synthesis, alterations in the protein, and acid mucopolysaccharide content of the media which can weaken the arterial wall) under hormonal influence associated with hemodynamic changes are the basis of the pathogenesis of aortic as well as coronary dissection. It most commonly affects the left anterior descending coronary artery often extending in the left main and in the circumflex artery. The clinical presentation in this case can be severe hemodynamic compromise with a high risk of maternal and fetal adverse outcomes.

(3) Thrombus/emboli is found to be an important cause of AMI during pregnancy (around 30 %) in the more contemporary group [7]. The increased risk of thrombosis during pregnancy is a result of profound alterations in the coagulation and fibrinolytic system. Thrombus can be formed in loco or be a result of emboli coming from the various sources such as the left atrial appendage during atrial fibrillation, prosthetic valves, mitral stenosis, and left ventricle in peripartum cardiomyopathy. Paradoxical embolism comes from the venous system in patients with a patent foramen ovale (it is well known that pregnancy is associated with a fourfold increase in venous thrombosis) (Fig. 19.3).

Coronary angiography is recommended as the first step in patients with AMI allowing a correct diagnosis of the etiology and consequently of the therapeutic strategy. Sometimes other imaging modality such as IVUS or OCT can help particularly in case of coronary dissection to confirm the diagnosis and to evaluate the extension of the disease (Fig. 19.4).

As it is described in the previous paragraph, right radial approach does not carry, in experienced hands, more radiation dose to the mother and to the fetus than femoral approach, and it should be the preferred one in these young patients.

Primary percutaneous coronary angioplasty represents, now days, the treatment of choice in any case of acute occlusion of a main coronary vessel during pregnancy, and the risks of angioplasty in pregnancy are similar to those in nonpregnant patients [8].

The atherosclerotic lesions are treated as in nonpregnant patients. However, in the dissected vessel, the location and extent of the dissection can guide the treatment strategy. Distal lesions are managed conservatively with heparin, antiplatelet therapy, and beta-blockers, even if some of these patients can have

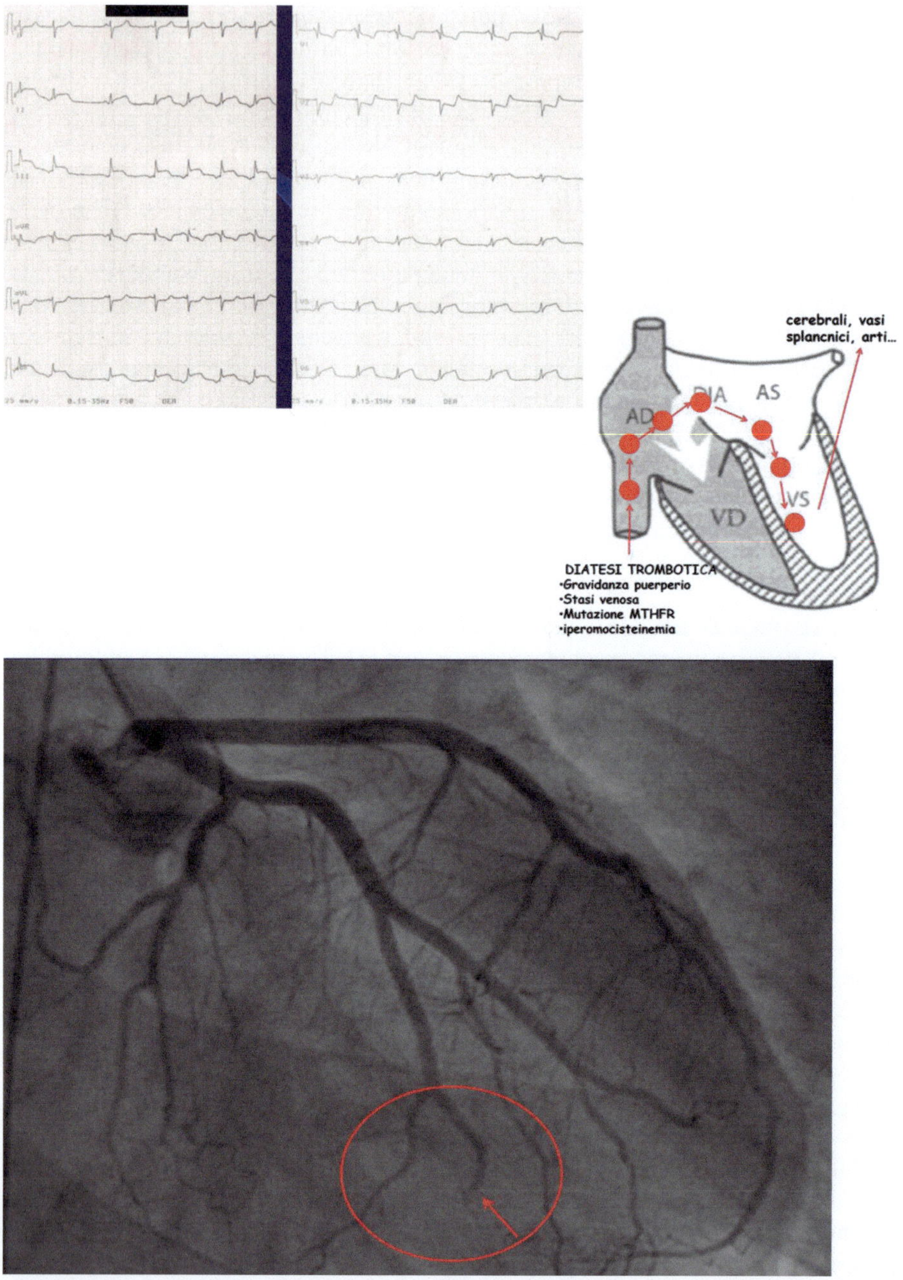

Fig. 19.3 Twenty-six-year-old woman presenting a 6 months pregnancy with dyspnea and chest pain. Evidence of occluded distal marginal branch due to paradoxical embolism through a large patent foramen ovale from deep venous thrombosis (To the courtesy of Dr. Ferdinando Varbella)

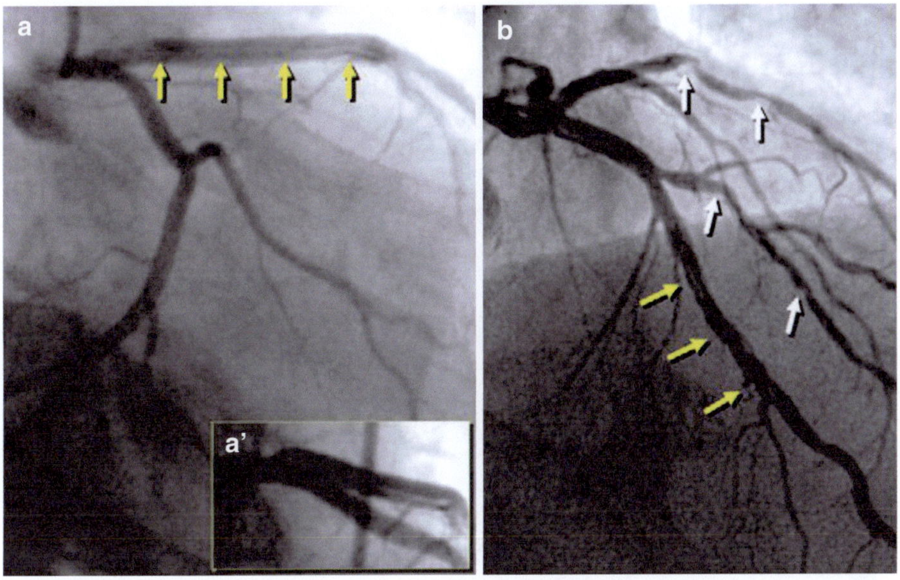

Fig. 19.4 Left anterior descending coronary dissection is well seen at angiography by a translucent appearance (*yellow arrows*) in the middle of the vessel

recurrent ischemia due to extension of dissection and have to be treated with PTCA later. Medium or proximal lesions are treated with PTCA: IVUS or OCT has to guide the procedure either to be sure to be in the true lumen (guidewire have to be positioned very distally), to decide the dimension and length of stenting, and to assess the results (Fig. 19.5). Long and/or multiple stents are often needed because with short stents, intramural hematoma can propagate extending the dissection anterogradely or retrogradely and also because multiple dissections can be present at the same time.

Bare-metal stents were indicated in the guidelines of the European Society of Cardiology in order to avoid prolonged antiplatelet therapy because incidence of cesarean section in patients with heart diseases is relatively high, and this drug regimen can lead to hemorrhagic complications at delivery [2]. However, the third generation of drug-eluting stents allowed a shorter dual antiplatelet treatment, and, taking into account that the extension of stenting in the dissected vessels is quite high, often with bifurcation stenting, DES use can be considered also in this setting. Use of bioresorbable vascular scaffold (BVS) has never been reported in a PTCA in a pregnant patient but was already reported in a dissected vessel with good results [9]: due to extensive stenting in the middle portion of the main dissected coronaries, it could be a nice option, but we need more data before recommending them.

The use of intra-aortic balloon pump or the Impella device to improve left ventricular output and coronary perfusion is also considered safe [10] in patients presenting in low output. In fact it is not an uncommon late presentation because

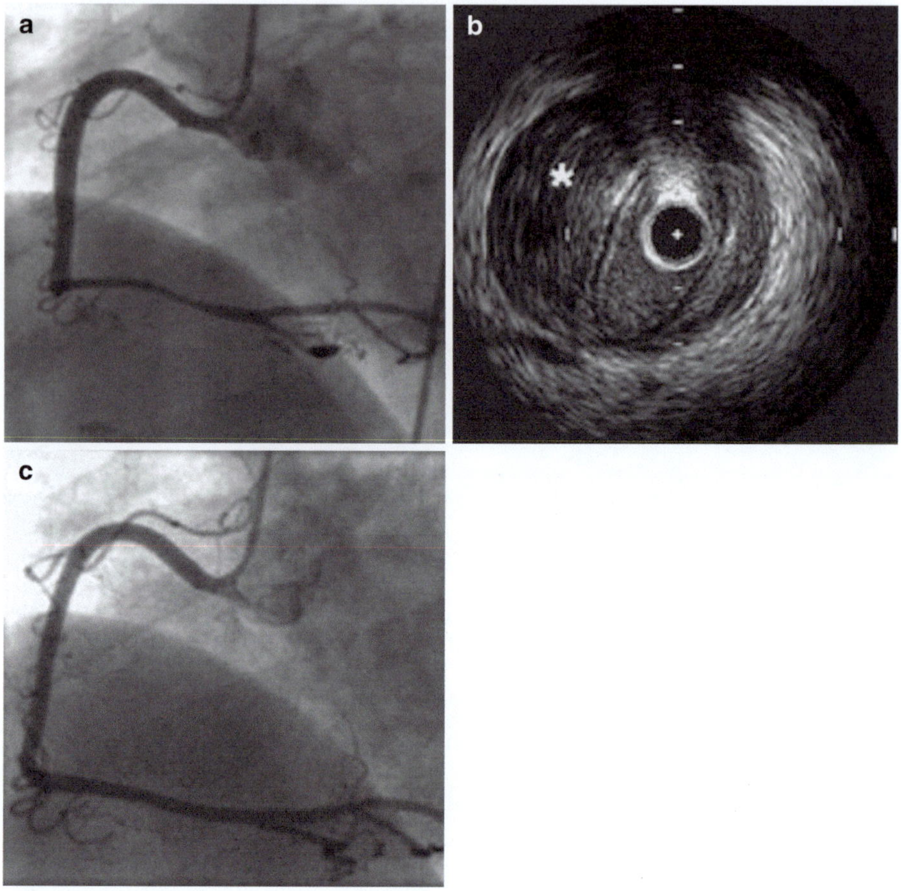

Fig. 19.5 (**a**) Distal coronary artery shows a tight stenosis. (**b**) IVUS shows an intimal flap of a dissection as a cause of the stenosis. (**c**) Good result after stenting

the symptoms and signs can be mistaken for the normal manifestations of pregnancy and because there is a low index of suspicion. Rapidly irreversible myocardial damage in these patients is the result of lack of preconditioning ischemia and is responsible of the clinical presentation in shock in some patients. Heparin and dual antiplatelets during the procedure are used at usual dosage, and in case of important coronary thrombosis, the intracoronary use of IIb–IIIa inhibitors should be considered as adjunctive therapy even if only limited data are available. Bypass grafting should be available for failed PTCA or for complications such as extensions of dissection in the ascending aorta or stenting the false lumen resulting in coronary occlusion. The most important objective in a young pregnant woman with AMI is avoidance of treatment delay. Mortality in the contemporary group is 6 %, and cardiac function is very much dependent from the reperfusion time with two reported heart transplant in late-treated women [7].

19.6 Congenital Heart Disease

Even if many patients, particularly with complex congenital heart diseases operated in infancy, have some residual anomalies or sequelae, they very rarely need interventions during pregnancy, because they are evaluated and screened before pregnancy.

Mild, moderate, and even moderately severe right ventricular outflow tract obstruction are very well tolerated during pregnancy, as shown in some reports in which no deaths and low incidence of complications have been reported. However, severe pulmonary valve stenosis, for some reason not treated during childhood and even moderate forms with impaired right ventricular function and/or symptoms, may require percutaneous pulmonary balloon valvuloplasty during pregnancy. Percutaneous pulmonary valvotomy with splitting of the valve commissures has been shown to be safe and effective with no mortality reported and low morbidity [11]. The valve gradient was halved and the pregnancy continued uneventfully. As happens outside pregnancy, arrhythmias, transient right bundle-branch block, and a mild, clinically irrelevant pulmonary regurgitation can occur during and after the procedure.

Severe pulmonary regurgitation either in native right ventricular outflow or in a conduit is normally treated before pregnancy in order to optimize the cardiac status before the important right ventricular overload induced by the pregnancy itself. But if an unplanned pregnancy occurs in a sick patient, a case report showed a successful percutaneous pulmonary valve replacement, a well-established strategy for patients with severe pulmonary valve disease of degenerated conduits in pulmonary atresia or tetralogy of Fallot [12]. Minimizing the radiation dose with fluoroscopy only above the diaphragm, collimation to a minimum field, and a fluoroscopy frame rate at 2 frames per second, the dose area production to the patient was recorded as 437 micro Gy/m^2.

Aortic coarctation is a condition normally repaired before pregnancy. If this condition is discovered during pregnancy, percutaneous angioplasty should be avoided because, being the mechanism of aortic enlargement after percutaneous dilatation stretching and tearing of the aortic wall, the risk of dissection is high.

Most patients with ASDs tolerate pregnancy without difficulty in the absence of pulmonary hypertension: The effect of the increased cardiac output on the volume-loaded right ventricle in patients with left to right shunts may be counterbalanced by the decrease in peripheral vascular resistance. A large left to right intracardiac shunt rarely causes congestive heart failure during pregnancy. Percutaneous closure of

ASD or PFO should be considered only when they are responsible of neurological events due to paradoxical embolism in presence of deep vein thrombosis not cured with anticoagulation.

Take-Home Messages

Percutaneous interventions during pregnancies have similar indications as outside pregnancy; however, strict parameters apply to this subgroup of patient because of the risks connected to the treatment. In the presence of a sick mother, the fetal age has to be taken into account in order to evaluate the right timing to undertake these procedures, before or after delivery. Technical issues are also similar but with additional cautions due to the need to keep the radiation exposure as low as possible. For this reason additional instrumentations like OCT/IVUS and TE echo have to be available in the catheterization lab.

References

1. Roth A, Elkayam U. Acute myocardial infarction associated with pregnancy. J Am Coll Cardiol. 2008;52:171–80.
2. Regitz-Zagrosek V, Blomstrom Lundqvist C, Borghi C, et al. ESC guidelines on the management of cardiovascular diseases during pregnancy of the European Society of Cardiology. Eur Heart J. 2011;32:3147–97.
3. Henriquez DD, Roos-Hesselink JW, Schalij MJ, et al. Treatment of valvular heart disease during pregnancy for improving maternal and neonatal outcome. Cochrane Database Syst Rev. 2011:CD008128.
4. Esteves CA, Munoz JS, Braga S, et al. Immediate and long-term follow-up of percutaneous balloon mitral valvuloplasty in pregnant patients with rheumatic mitral stenosis. Am J Cardiol. 2006;98(6):812–6.
5. Sliwa K, Johnson MR, Zilla P, Roos-Hesselink JW. Management of valvular disease in pregnancy: a global perspective. Eur Heart J. 2015;36(18):1078–89.
6. Satoh H, Sano M, Suwa K, et al. Pregnancy-related acute myocardial infarction in Japan: a review of epidemiology, etiology and treatment from case reports. Circ J. 2013;77(3):725–33.
7. Lameijer H, Kampman MA, Oudijk MA, Pieper PG. Ischaemic heart disease during pregnancy or post-partum: systematic review and case series. Neth Hear J. 2015;23(5):249–57.
8. Sahni G. Chest pain syndromes in pregnancy. Cardiol Clin. 2012;30(3):343–67.
9. Basavarajaiah S, Naganuma T, Qadir M. Use of bioresorbable vascular scaffold in acute dissection: insights from optical coherence tomography. JACC Cardiovasc Interv. 2016;9(1):e5–9.
10. Ginwalla M, Pillai D, Gandhi S. Use of intra-aortic balloon counterpulsation during emergent cesarean section in a pregnant patient with myocardial infarction. J Invasive Cardiol. 2010;22(6):E104–6.
11. Oakley C. Acyanotic congenital heart disease. In: Heart disease in pregnancy. London: BMJ Publishing group. 1997. pp. 19–51.
12. Ormerod O. Percutaneous pulmonary valve replacement during pregnancy. Circulation. 2014;129:e373–5.

Left Ventricular Assist Devices

20

Christina Baum, Alexander M. Bernhardt,
and Renate B. Schnabel

The therapy regimen of acute and chronic heart failure consists of medical therapy, causal cardiac surgery and, as ultima ratio, heart transplantation or mechanical circulatory support (MCS). MCS comprises diverse technologies for short- and long-term hemodynamic support.

Because of growing organ shortage (www.eurotransplant.org) and technical progress, ventricular assist devices (VAD) are gaining importance not only as bridge-to-transplant but also as destination therapy. In contrast to the growing use of implantable devices, large-scale data on everyday clinical practice and outcomes are rare. In particular, gender aspects in indication, timing, device choice and adverse event rates of available and continuously refined devices have not been in the focus of investigations. Most information can be derived from registries such as INTERMACS (Interagency Registry for Mechanically Assisted Circulatory Support) [1] and EUROMACS (European Registry for Patients with Mechanical Circulatory Support) [2]. They are joint efforts to collect available evidence in a standardized fashion. Both registries provide most comprehensive data in men and women across countries to date.

The indication of MCS depends on the INTERMACS level, which determines the necessity and the time frame for the implantation of an assist device. Seven levels are defined, whereas level 1 characterizes the critical cardiogenic shock with increase of lactate and beginning organ failure. At this level, an assist device should be implanted within the next few hours. Further gradations are made up to level 7, which describes a reduced ejection fraction in a clinical stable condition without need for VAD implantation. In principle, there are four indications for the implantation of a short-term or long-term device (Table 20.1). The type of the implanted device depends on the respective indication.

C. Baum, MD (✉) • A.M. Bernhardt, MD • R.B. Schnabel, MD, MSc
University Heart Center Hamburg, Hamburg, Germany
e-mail: c.baum@uke.de

P. Presbitero et al. (eds.), *Percutaneous Treatment of Cardiovascular Diseases in Women*,
DOI 10.1007/978-3-319-39611-8_20

Table 20.1 Indications of mechanical circulatory support

Indication	Device	Reason of implantation
Bridge-to-decision	vaECMO, Impella, TandemHeart	Cardiogenic shock (INTERMACS Level 1); need for further evaluation before implantation of a long-term device (e.g., evaluation of neurological outcome after cardiopulmonary resuscitation)
Bridge-to-recovery	vaECMO, Impella, TandemHeart	Postcardiotomy syndrome, reperfusion syndrome after heart transplantation, acute myocardial infarction or myocarditis
Bridge-to-transplantation	VAD	Hemodynamic instability with secondary organ failure (e.g., renal insufficiency) despite inotropic therapy *Cave*: Device-associated sensitization by preformed antibodies increases risk of antibody-mediated rejection after heart transplantation
Destination therapy	VAD	End-stage heart failure (NYHA state IV, ejection fraction < 30 %) with recurrent cardiac decompensation despite best medical therapy and presence of contraindications for heart transplantation

vaECMO veno-arterial extracorporeal membrane oxygenation; *VAD* ventricular assist device

20.1 Percutaneous Assist Device Support

In the emergency setting of cardiogenic shock, acute decompensated heart failure and large myocardial infarctions, percutaneously implantable short-term devices are used frequently in the cardiac catheterization laboratory. The ease of use of modern devices suggests a benefit in high-risk percutaneous coronary intervention and other procedures. But evidence on meaningfully improved outcomes is limited [3].

The intra-aortic balloon pump (IABP) has long been the only representative of this group with a broad range of indications of its adjunctive use in heart failure and cardiogenic shock. Recently, the 2013 STEMI guidelines have downgraded the IABP from a I to a IIa recommendation [4], because of no mortality benefit with or without IABP at 30 days after myocardial infarction induced cardiogenic shock in the Intra-aortic Balloon Support for Myocardial Infarction with Cardiogenic Shock (IABP-SHOCK II) trial [5]. The IABP is increasingly replaced by the veno-arterial extracorporeal membrane oxygenation (vaECMO), the Impella pump (Abiomed) or the Tandem Heart (CardiacAssist). The cannulas of the vaECMO are implanted through the femoral artery and vein. An extracorporeal centrifugal pump generates high blood flow rates without load relieve of the left ventricle. An external oxygenator ensures gas exchange. Complications are severe bleeding, hemorrhagic stroke, peripheral and central embolisms and infections [6]. Until now, there are no recommendations from the ACC/AHA concerning timing of implantation [4].

The TandemHeart device has, comparable to the vaECMO, an external centrifugal pump. The inflow cannula is placed transseptally in the left atrium and the outflow cannula in the femoral artery. A flow of 3.5–4.5 l/min can be generated. Complications include pericardial tamponade, major bleeding, aortic regurgitation, critical limb ischemia, arrhythmias and iatrogenic atrial septal defect [7]. The TandemHeart can be a good option in patients with severe aortic stenosis. A higher cardiac index but no mortality benefit at 30 days was shown after randomization to IABP or TandemHeart [8]. The Impella pump is introduced via the femoral artery and directed via the aortic valve. The axial flow pump delivers non-pulsatile blood flow to the ascending aorta, which results in load relieve of the left ventricle. Currently, three Impella systems (Impella 2.5, 5.0 and CP) with different maximum flow rates are used. The Impella–EUROSHOCK-registry evaluates the Impella 2.5 device in patients with cardiogenic shock after acute myocardial infarction. Men tended to have a higher 30-day mortality, which did not reach statistical significance [9]. Due to the wide flow range and the possibility of fast and atraumatic implantation, the Impella is also used for hemodynamic stabilization in elective high-risk coronary procedures despite convincing evidence of a net benefit [10]. The most commonly reported complications are limb ischemia, vascular injury, bleeding and hemolysis [11]. The Impella LP 2.5 versus IABP in Cardiogenic Shock (ISAR-SHOCK) trial found a slightly higher cardiac index at 30 min in the Impella group compared to the IABP group, but no differences in mortality rates at 30 days were seen [12].

Despite the hemodynamic improvement seen with Impella and TandemHeart in comparison to IABP, no study has shown a survival benefit yet. Therefore, there is actually only a class IIb recommendation for alternative left ventricular assist devices in patients with severe cardiogenic shock [4]. The majority of individuals, in whom percutaneous ventricular assist devices are used, are male. The distribution of generally two-thirds or more male patients, however, most likely only mirrors the underlying disease distribution since it resembles coronary artery disease and acute heart failure samples [8, 13]. Data considering gender aspects in percutaneous assist device support are almost non-existent although increasing numbers of patients are supplied with percutaneous circulatory support.

20.2 Historical Development of Surgical Mechanical Circulatory Support

20.2.1 From the First Heart-Lung Machine to the Total Artificial Heart

The first heart-lung machine (HLM) was developed by John H. Gibbon in 1953. In 1966, Michael E. DeBakey implanted a left VAD (LVAD) successfully for the first time, even before the first heart transplantation was performed. The first total artificial heart was implanted by Domingo Liotta and Denton A. Cooley in 1969. Significant advances in the development of VAD systems were seen in the late 1980s: The assist devices of the first generation were pulsatile-flow devices. The systems of the second generation (1990s) were characterized by continuous flow. Similar to the third generation devices, they had a longer half-life and the possibility of intracorporeal implantation.

20.2.2 From Paracorporeal to Intracorporeal Systems

The main representative of the paracorporeal systems is the *Thoratec VAD* system. Both its ventricles and cannulas are placed on the anterior abdominal wall. Still of importance is the *Berlin Heart EXCOR VAD* paracorporeal system. To date, it is the only lifesaving opportunity for children with cardiac decompensation. The first representative of the intracorporeal systems, the *HeartMate I*, is a pulsatile device and only of historical interest today. The modern pumps (e.g., HeartMate II, HVAD) are continuous-flow systems with a higher energy efficiency and a lower wastage. However, a higher rotation speed is needed, which increases the risk of hemolysis. In addition, as complete ventricular unloading by continuous flow devices prevents blood flow via the aortic valve, its loss of function leads to remodeling processes and aortic regurgitation.

20.2.3 Technical Issues of an Intracorporeal VAD Implantation Using the HVAD (HeartWare) Pump

The implantation rates of the HVAD continue to rise because of the small pump size, the technically easy handling and the improved adverse event rates. Surgery can be performed with or without HLM via conventional sternotomy or minimally invasive via two thoracotomies. Apical purse-string sutures are placed at the optimal HVAD inflow site at the apex of the left ventricle. The HVAD sewing ring is attached, the apex is cored and the HVAD pump secured (Fig. 20.1). The outflow graft is anastomosed to the ascending aorta and the patient is weaned from the HLM. Minimally invasive implantation technique is supposed to reduce perioperative right ventricular failure associated with reduced outcomes and may prevent scar and adhesion formation making subsequent heart transplantation easier.

20.3 Contraindications and Adverse Events Under Ventricular Assist Device Support

Contraindications for VAD support are multi-organ failure, sepsis, malignancies with a life expectancy under 2 years, impossibility of therapeutic anticoagulation (e.g., active cerebral or gastrointestinal bleeding), severe vascular disease (e.g., abdominal aortic aneurysm over 5 cm, peripheral artery occlusive disease), patient incompliance and a severe precapillary pulmonary hypertension.

Frequent adverse events after VAD implantation are bleeding, thromboembolic complications, right ventricular failure, infections and arrhythmias. Bleeding complications are often localized in the gastrointestinal tract or nasal mucosa and occur either perioperatively or late in the postoperative course. Right heart failure or acquired von Willebrand disease are often responsible for late bleeding complications. Thromboembolic complications are caused by activation of plasmatic coagulation and thrombocyte aggregation triggered by the contact of the blood with the VAD surface. To minimize the risk of right ventricular failure, preoperative

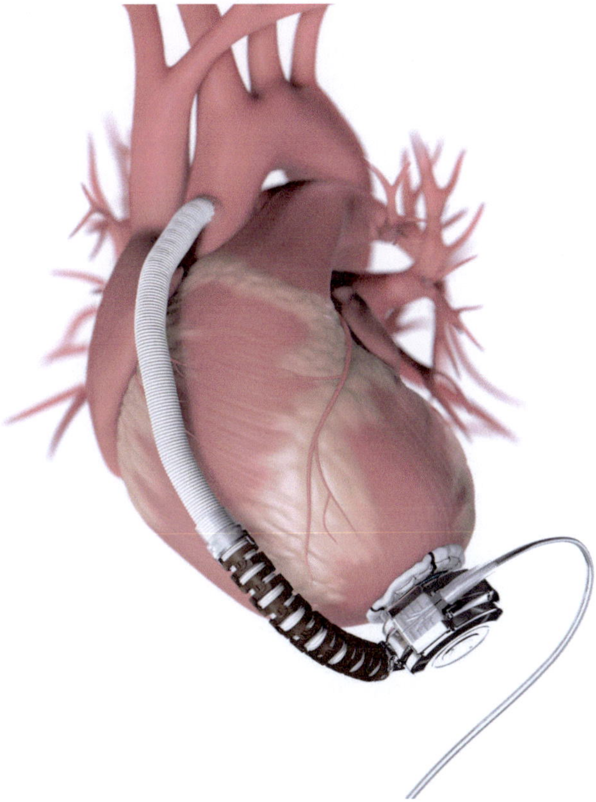

Fig. 20.1 Implanted HVAD pump: The HVAD sewing ring is attached at the apex of the left ventricle and the HVAD pump is secured. The outflow graft is anastomosed to the ascending aorta (Photo courtesy of HeartWare International, Inc. Framingham, MA)

evaluation of the right ventricle is necessary and temporary (about 3–4 weeks) right VAD (RVAD) implantation must be discussed. Beside the perioperative infections as pneumonia and urinary tract infection, device-associated infections (mainly driveline infections) caused by *Staphylococcus* species, rarely *Pseudomonas* species and *Candida* or *Aspergillus* species must be considered. Ventricular arrhythmias are due to the underlying disease, but can also be induced mechanically by the pump. The implantation of an implantable cardioverter defibrillator (ICD), if not already performed, must be discussed.

20.4 Epidemiology of MCS

Most of the current evidence is derived from large registries. The 2011 founded INTERMACS registry is a National Heart, Lung and Blood Institute (NHLBI) sponsored database. The latest 2014 published sixth INTERMACS report [1] summarizes demographical data, survival, adverse event rates and risk factors of over 10,000 patients of about 141 participating centers in the first 8 years (June 2006 to June 2013) of patient enrolment. In patients with continuous-flow assist devices, the current 1-year survival is 80 %, the 2-year survival 70 % [1]. Since 2010, all patients with destination therapy are supported with a continuous-flow system. The destination therapy has increased from 14.7 % in 2006/2007 up to 41.6 % in 2012/2013 and thus represents one of the main indications. Adverse event rates with continuous-flow pumps are significantly lower than for previous pulsatile technology [14]. Multi-organ failure is the main complication in the first four postoperative months, whereas neurological adverse events dominate after 3 months. The risk for multi-organ failure and infections rises after 4–5 years. The overall survival is higher with continuous-flow systems.

20.5 Gender Differences in VAD Support

20.5.1 Imbalance of VAD Implantation to the Disadvantage of Women

Despite the similar prevalence in both sexes, women are hospitalized more frequently and die more often from the consequences of heart failure than men [15]. Nevertheless, VAD placement is far less likely used in women than in men. Women are underrepresented in large multicenter heart failure or mechanical circulatory support studies [16, 17]. In the use of VADs for bridge-to-transplantation (BTT), women comprise only 22 % of individuals in the HeartMate II BTT trial and 28 % in the HVAD ADVANCE trial [18]. This may be explained by anatomical reasons, as women cannot accommodate the huge pumps of the early VAD types because of their smaller intrathoracic volume. Topkara et al. analysed the outcome of heart transplanted patients bridged to transplantation with both HVAD (HeartWare) and HeartMate II (Thoratec) devices [19]. It was shown that HVAD patients had smaller body surface areas and lower body weight and that the HVAD system was implanted significantly more often in women. The preferred use of HVAD pumps in women is also confirmed by European data [20]. The smaller pump size of the HVAD pump and the possibility of intrapericardial implantation enable VAD implantation in individuals with small body surface area. This may also facilitate VAD support in children in the future.

20.5.2 Gender Specific Characteristics in the Perioperative Course

Similar to previous published studies [17, 21], data derived from the European Registry for Patients with Mechanical Circulatory Support (EUROMACS) showed that significantly more male patients received mechanical circulatory support (N=967, 151 women) [20]. As expected, women and men differed in height, weight and body surface area and women were reported to have less ischemic but more dilated and restrictive cardiomyopathy (Fig. 20.2). Female patients bridged to transplantation with continuous-flow systems were shown to present with more advanced states of heart failure [22], having more severe mitral and tricuspid regurgitation and a significantly lower cardiac output [20]. Postoperatively, they needed longer inotropic medication, required longer intensive care therapy and needed more additional right ventricular support. Bogaev et al. showed that fewer women underwent heart transplantation and thus continued longer on assist device support [16].

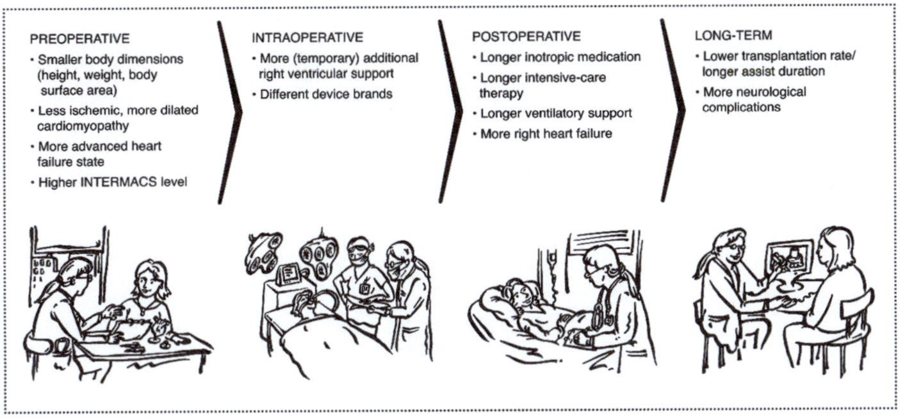

Fig. 20.2 Female specific therapeutic course in VAD support

Gender-specific higher levels of class I panel reactive antibodies were made responsible for the lower transplantation rates, because they are associated with a higher risk for antibody-mediated rejection after heart transplantation.

20.5.3 Gender Differences Concerning Adverse Events and Survival

In several studies, women were described to have more adverse events and a worse outcome after VAD implantation [23, 24]. Adverse events such as bleeding, neurological complications, right heart failure, infections and arrhythmias are different in both genders (Fig. 20.3). In women, more re-operations for bleeding complications were recorded, whereas the prevalence of pump thrombosis or cerebral bleeding was similar [20]. A first gender-specific analysis of the INTERMACS data 2012 revealed no gender differences in time to first infection, bleeding or device dysfunction [21]. Nevertheless, women suffered earlier than men from neurological complications. Female gender alone was described as a significant risk factor for stroke [25]. Bogaev et al. showed a higher rate of hemorrhagic stroke although there were no differences in INR, partial thromboplastin time and thrombocyte count [16]. If the higher rate of neurological complications in women is due to gender differences in pharmacokinetics and pharmacodynamics of the anticoagulation therapy or due to gender-specific differences in thrombotic risk is unknown. Ochiai et al. demonstrated that female gender was a significant risk factor for right heart failure after implantation of a pulsatile-flow system [26]. Data from the EUROMACS registry showed that women more often experienced right heart failure, although the preoperative right heart function was not different in both genders [20]. Additionally, a higher prevalence of arrhythmias and peripheral arterial embolisms and a slightly higher rate of driveline infections were seen in women.

Morgan et al. described a worse survival of women with pulsatile-flow systems [23]. In the EUROMACS database, female patients had a significant shorter survival on LVAD support, which even worsened under BIVAD therapy (Fig. 20.4).

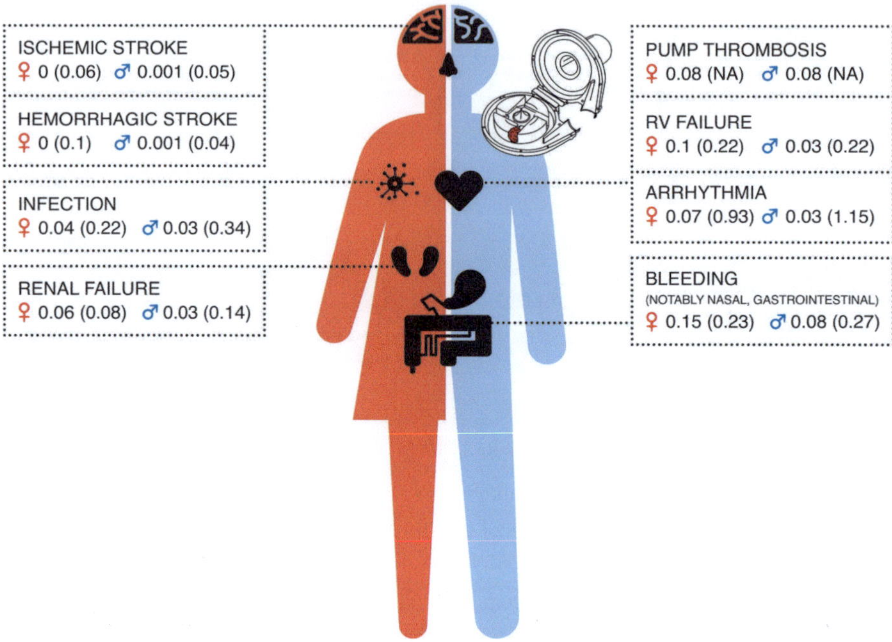

Fig. 20.3 Adverse events and gender-specific prevalence (in events-per-patient-year; *red*: women; *blue*: men); data derived from the EUROMACS registry [20]; in brackets: international data from the HeartMate II clinical trial [16]

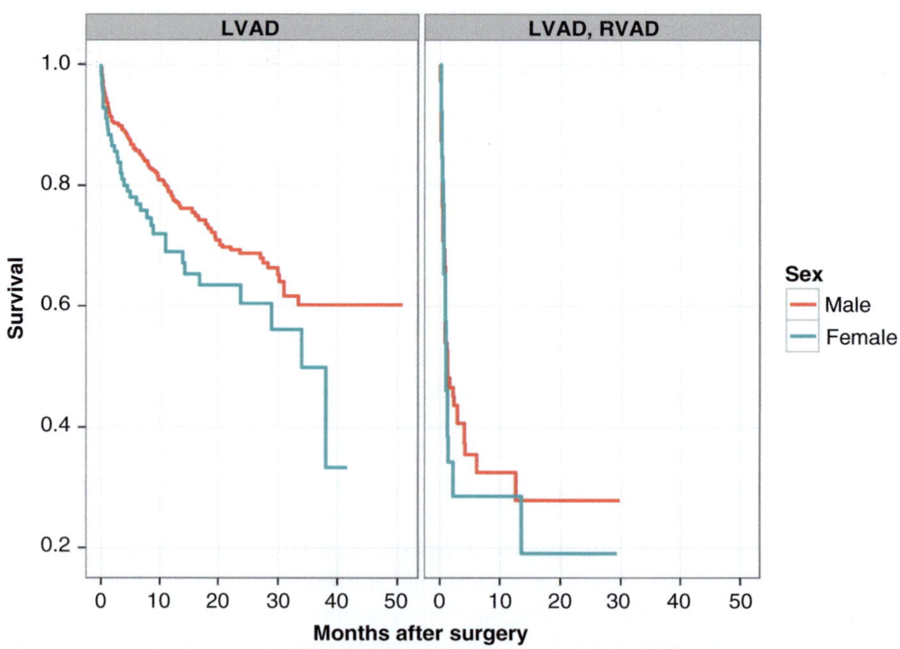

Fig. 20.4 Postoperative gender specific survival on LVAD and BIVAD support (Data derived from the EUROMACS registry [20])

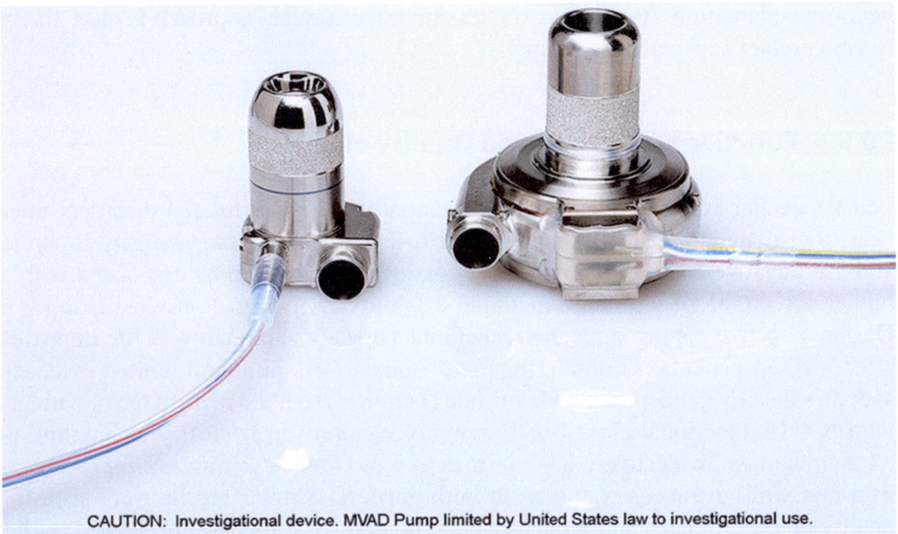

Fig. 20.5 Miniaturization of VAD systems using the example of the MVAD (*left*) and HVAD (*right*) device of HeartWare; the use of the MVAD device is limited to clinical studies (Photo courtesy of HeartWare International, Inc. Framingham, MA)

Further studies examining patients with continuous-flow systems could not show any gender differences in mortality [16, 18, 22]. Also Hsich et al. did not observe differences in mortality [21], although, again, women were more often in cardiogenic shock (INTERMACS level 1) at time of implantation.

20.5.4 Outlook: Will a Ventricular Assist Device Be Developed Specifically for Women?

If the lower VAD implantation rates in women are really due to the female anatomy with smaller body surface area and lower intrathoracic volume, women may benefit from the development of decreasing VAD size. The HeartWare's MVAD pump [27, 28], presently undergoing clinical testing, is about one-third the size of the commonly used HVAD device (Fig. 20.5). The MVAD can be implanted minimally invasive by a transapical access. The MVAD pump is designed to support a wide range of flows to enable both full and partial support. The small pump size and the wide range of flows facilitate right ventricular support and implantation in patients with smaller body surface area. The next generation is the HeartWare Longhorn device, which is presently still in pre-clinical testing [29]. Neither cardiopulmonary bypass nor outflow graft anastomosis will be needed. It is positioned intraventricularly and the outflow cannula is directed to lie in the ascending aorta or in the main pulmonary artery (if the device is used for right ventricular support).

Beside the smaller pump size and the possibility of implantation in smaller persons, the minimally invasive surgical access is supposed to reduce the risk for right ventricular failure and the formation of adhesions facilitating a subsequent heart transplantation. In addition, the less invasive surgical approach is more likely to gain greater acceptance by patients.

20.5.5 Functional Capacity and Quality of Life

Female gender is a risk factor for depression and anxiety-related disorders after heart transplantation [30]. Women appear to experience higher intensity of stress and use negative coping styles. Female gender was shown to be associated with a higher perception of physical functional disability after heart transplantation [31]. Despite negative coping strategies, functional capacity and quality of life improves after VAD implantation in both, men and women [16], although limited evidence specifies data by gender. In the HeartMate II clinical trial, the percentage of patients with NYHA functional class I or II symptoms improved from 0 % at baseline to 83 % in women, respectively 85 % in men at 6 months. A significant improvement in 6-min walk distances was seen in both genders. Similar results were seen for quality-of-life in males and females. As compared with the baseline scores, scores on the Minnesota Living with Heart Failure questionnaire and the Kansas City Cardiomyopathy questionnaires improved by over 30 points in patients with pulsatile- and continuous-flow pumps [16, 32]. Quality-of-life improved irrespective of INTERMACS profile [33].

Conclusions

In summary, women receive less VAD support despite higher rates of heart failure. The reasons are manifold, most evident are anatomical restrictions. In several studies, women had more adverse events and a worse outcome with mechanical circulatory support. Female gender was shown to be associated with longer stay on the intensive care unit and higher prevalence of right heart failure and neurological complications. Decreasing pump size that overcomes often anatomically smaller structures will possibly lead to increasing VAD implantation rates in women. In addition, referral strategies and time of implantation may improve the outcome of mechanical circulatory support in women.

References

1. Kirklin JK, Naftel DC, Pagani FD, Kormos RL, Stevenson LW, Blume ED, Miller MA, Timothy Baldwin J, Young JB. Sixth INTERMACS annual report: a 10,000-patient database. J Heart Lung Transplant Off Publ Int Soc Heart Transplant. 2014;33(6):555–64. doi:10.1016/j.healun.2014.04.010.
2. de By TM, Mohacsi P, Gummert J, Bushnaq H, Krabatsch T, Gustafsson F, Leprince P, Martinelli L, Meyns B, Morshuis M, Netuka I, Potapov E, Zittermann A, Delmo Walter EM, Hetzer R, EUROMACS Members. The European Registry for Patients with Mechanical Circulatory Support (EUROMACS): first annual report. Eur J Cardiothorac Surg Off J Eur Assoc Cardiothorac Surg. 2015;47(5):770–6. doi:10.1093/ejcts/ezv096; discussion 776–7.

3. Rihal CS, Naidu SS, Givertz MM, Szeto WY, Burke JA, Kapur NK, Kern M, Garratt KN, Goldstein JA, Dimas V, Tu T, Society for Cardiovascular Angiography and Interventions; Heart Failure Society of America; Society of Thoracic Surgeons; American Heart Association; American College of Cardiology. 2015 SCAI/ACC/HFSA/STS Clinical Expert Consensus Statement on the Use of Percutaneous Mechanical Circulatory Support Devices in Cardiovascular Care: Endorsed by the American Heart Assocation, the Cardiological Society of India, and Sociedad Latino Americana de Cardiologia Intervencion; Affirmation of Value by the Canadian Association of Interventional Cardiology-Association Canadienne de Cardiologie d'intervention. J Am Coll Cardiol. 2015;65(19):e7–26. doi:10.1016/j.jacc.2015.03.036.
4. O'Gara PT, Kushner FG, Ascheim DD, Casey Jr DE, Chung MK, de Lemos JA, Ettinger SM, Fang JC, Fesmire FM, Franklin BA, Granger CB, Krumholz HM, Linderbaum JA, Morrow DA, Newby LK, Ornato JP, Ou N, Radford MJ, Tamis-Holland JE, Tommaso CL, Tracy CM, Woo YJ, Zhao DX, Anderson JL, Jacobs AK, Halperin JL, Albert NM, Brindis RG, Creager MA, DeMets D, Guyton RA, Hochman JS, Kovacs RJ, Kushner FG, Ohman EM, Stevenson WG, Yancy CW, American College of Cardiology Foundation/American Heart Association Task Force on Practice Guidelines. 2013 ACCF/AHA guideline for the management of ST-elevation myocardial infarction: a report of the American College of Cardiology Foundation/American Heart Association Task Force on Practice Guidelines. Circulation. 2013;127(4):e362–425. doi:10.1161/CIR.0b013e3182742cf6.
5. Thiele H, Zeymer U, Neumann FJ, Ferenc M, Olbrich HG, Hausleiter J, Richardt G, Hennersdorf M, Empen K, Fuernau G, Desch S, Eitel I, Hambrecht R, Fuhrmann J, Bohm M, Ebelt H, Schneider S, Schuler G, Werdan K, I-SIT Investigators. Intraaortic balloon support for myocardial infarction with cardiogenic shock. N Engl J Med. 2012;367(14):1287–96. doi:10.1056/NEJMoa1208410.
6. Smedira NG, Moazami N, Golding CM, McCarthy PM, Apperson-Hansen C, Blackstone EH, Cosgrove 3rd DM. Clinical experience with 202 adults receiving extracorporeal membrane oxygenation for cardiac failure: survival at five years. J Thorac Cardiovasc Surg. 2001;122(1):92–102. doi:10.1067/mtc.2001.114351.
7. Naidu SS. Novel percutaneous cardiac assist devices: the science of and indications for hemodynamic support. Circulation. 2011;123(5):533–43. doi:10.1161/CIRCULATIONAHA.110.945055.
8. Thiele H, Sick P, Boudriot E, Diederich KW, Hambrecht R, Niebauer J, Schuler G. Randomized comparison of intra-aortic balloon support with a percutaneous left ventricular assist device in patients with revascularized acute myocardial infarction complicated by cardiogenic shock. Eur Heart J. 2005;26(13):1276–83. doi:10.1093/eurheartj/ehi161.
9. Lauten A, Engstrom AE, Jung C, Empen K, Erne P, Cook S, Windecker S, Bergmann MW, Klingenberg R, Luscher TF, Haude M, Rulands D, Butter C, Ullman B, Hellgren L, Modena MG, Pedrazzini G, Henriques JP, Figulla HR, Ferrari M. Percutaneous left-ventricular support with the Impella-2.5-assist device in acute cardiogenic shock: results of the Impella-EUROSHOCK-registry. Circ Heart Fail. 2013;6(1):23–30. doi:10.1161/CIRCHEARTFAILURE.112.967224.
10. Perera D, Stables R, Thomas M, Booth J, Pitt M, Blackman D, de Belder A, Redwood S, Investigators B. Elective intra-aortic balloon counterpulsation during high-risk percutaneous coronary intervention: a randomized controlled trial. JAMA. 2010;304(8):867–74. doi:10.1001/jama.2010.1190.
11. Remmelink M, Sjauw KD, Henriques JP, de Winter RJ, Koch KT, van der Schaaf RJ, Vis MM, Tijssen JG, Piek JJ, Baan Jr J. Effects of left ventricular unloading by Impella recover LP2.5 on coronary hemodynamics. Catheter Cardiovasc Interv Off J Soc Cardiac Angiogr Interv. 2007;70(4):532–7. doi:10.1002/ccd.21160.
12. Seyfarth M, Sibbing D, Bauer I, Frohlich G, Bott-Flugel L, Byrne R, Dirschinger J, Kastrati A, Schomig A. A randomized clinical trial to evaluate the safety and efficacy of a percutaneous left ventricular assist device versus intra-aortic balloon pumping for treatment of cardiogenic shock caused by myocardial infarction. J Am Coll Cardiol. 2008;52(19):1584–8. doi:10.1016/j.jacc.2008.05.065.

13. Schwartz BG, Ludeman DJ, Mayeda GS, Kloner RA, Economides C, Burstein S. High-risk percutaneous coronary intervention with the TandemHeart and Impella devices: a single-center experience. J Invasive Cardiol. 2011;23(10):417–24.
14. Kirklin JK, Naftel DC, Kormos RL, Stevenson LW, Pagani FD, Miller MA, Timothy Baldwin J, Young JB. Fifth INTERMACS annual report: risk factor analysis from more than 6,000 mechanical circulatory support patients. J Heart Lung Transplant Off Publ Int Soc Heart Transplant. 2013;32(2):141–56. doi:10.1016/j.healun.2012.12.004.
15. Lloyd-Jones D, Adams R, Carnethon M, De Simone G, Ferguson TB, Flegal K, Ford E, Furie K, Go A, Greenlund K, Haase N, Hailpern S, Ho M, Howard V, Kissela B, Kittner S, Lackland D, Lisabeth L, Marelli A, McDermott M, Meigs J, Mozaffarian D, Nichol G, O'Donnell C, Roger V, Rosamond W, Sacco R, Sorlie P, Stafford R, Steinberger J, Thom T, Wasserthiel-Smoller S, Wong N, Wylie-Rosett J, Hong Y, American Heart Association Statistics C, Stroke Statistics S. Heart disease and stroke statistics – 2009 update: a report from the American Heart Association Statistics Committee and Stroke Statistics Subcommittee. Circulation. 2009;119(3):480–6. doi:10.1161/CIRCULATIONAHA.108.191259.
16. Bogaev RC, Pamboukian SV, Moore SA, Chen L, John R, Boyle AJ, Sundareswaran KS, Farrar DJ, Frazier OH, HeartMate IICI. Comparison of outcomes in women versus men using a continuous-flow left ventricular assist device as a bridge to transplantation. J Heart Lung Transplant Off Publ Int Soc Heart Transplant. 2011;30(5):515–22. doi:10.1016/j.healun.2010.12.009.
17. Hunt SA, Abraham WT, Chin MH, Feldman AM, Francis GS, Ganiats TG, Jessup M, Konstam MA, Mancini DM, Michl K, Oates JA, Rahko PS, Silver MA, Stevenson LW, Yancy CW, Antman EM, Smith Jr SC, Adams CD, Anderson JL, Faxon DP, Fuster V, Halperin JL, Hiratzka LF, Jacobs AK, Nishimura R, Ornato JP, Page RL, Riegel B, American College of Cardiology; American Heart Association Task Force on Practice Guidelines; American College of Chest Physicians; International Society for Heart and Lung Transplantation; Heart Rhythm Society. ACC/AHA 2005 Guideline Update for the Diagnosis and Management of Chronic Heart Failure in the Adult: a report of the American College of Cardiology/American Heart Association Task Force on Practice Guidelines (Writing Committee to Update the 2001 Guidelines for the Evaluation and Management of Heart Failure): developed in collaboration with the American College of Chest Physicians and the International Society for Heart and Lung Transplantation: endorsed by the Heart Rhythm Society. Circulation. 2005;112(12):e154–235. doi:10.1161/CIRCULATIONAHA.105.167586.
18. Birks EJ, McGee Jr EC, Aaronson KD, Boyce S, Cotts WG, Najjar SS, Pagani FD, Hathaway DR, Najarian K, Jacoski MV, Slaughter MS, Investigators AT. An examination of survival by sex and race in the HeartWare Ventricular Assist Device for the Treatment of Advanced Heart Failure (ADVANCE) Bridge to Transplant (BTT) and continued access protocol trials. J Heart Lung Transplant Off Publ Int Soc Heart Transplant. 2015;34(6):815–24. doi:10.1016/j.healun.2014.12.011.
19. Topkara VK, O'Neill JK, Carlisle A, Novak E, Silvestry SC, Ewald GA. HeartWare and HeartMate II left ventricular assist devices as bridge to transplantation: a comparative analysis. Ann Thorac Surg. 2014;97(2):506–12. doi:10.1016/j.athoracsur.2013.08.048.
20. Bernhardt AM, Sill B, Wagner FM, deBy TM, Gummert J, Mohacsi P, Reichenspurner H, Deuse T. (45) – Gender differences in mechanical circulatory support – insights from a European Registry. J Heart Lung Transplant. 2015;34(4, Supplement):S25. doi:http://dx.doi.org/10.1016/j.healun.2015.01.056.
21. Hsich EM, Naftel DC, Myers SL, Gorodeski EZ, Grady KL, Schmuhl D, Ulisney KL, Young JB. Should women receive left ventricular assist device support?: findings from INTERMACS. Circ Heart Fail. 2012;5(2):234–40. doi:10.1161/CIRCHEARTFAILURE.111.963272.
22. Weymann A, Patil NP, Sabashnikov A, Mohite PN, Garcia Saez D, Amrani M, Bahrami T, De Robertis F, Wahlers T, Banner NR, Popov AF, Simon AR. Gender differences in continuous-flow left ventricular assist device therapy as a bridge to transplantation: a risk-adjusted comparison using a propensity score-matching analysis. Artif Organs. 2015; 39(3):212–9. doi:10.1111/aor.12361.

23. Morgan JA, Weinberg AD, Hollingsworth KW, Flannery MR, Oz MC, Naka Y. Effect of gender on bridging to transplantation and posttransplantation survival in patients with left ventricular assist devices. J Thorac Cardiovasc Surg. 2004;127(4):1193–5. doi:10.1016/S0022.
24. Hernandez AF, Grab JD, Gammie JS, O'Brien SM, Hammill BG, Rogers JG, Camacho MT, Dullum MK, Ferguson TB, Peterson ED. A decade of short-term outcomes in post cardiac surgery ventricular assist device implantation: data from the Society of Thoracic Surgeons' National Cardiac Database. Circulation. 2007;116(6):606–12. doi:10.1161/CIRCULATION AHA.106.666289.
25. Boyle AJ, Jorde UP, Sun B, Park SJ, Milano CA, Frazier OH, Sundareswaran KS, Farrar DJ, Russell SD, HeartMate IICI. Pre-operative risk factors of bleeding and stroke during left ventricular assist device support: an analysis of more than 900 HeartMate II outpatients. J Am Coll Cardiol. 2014;63(9):880–8. doi:10.1016/j.jacc.2013.08.1656.
26. Ochiai Y, McCarthy PM, Smedira NG, Banbury MK, Navia JL, Feng J, Hsu AP, Yeager ML, Buda T, Hoercher KJ, Howard MW, Takagaki M, Doi K, Fukamachi K. Predictors of severe right ventricular failure after implantable left ventricular assist device insertion: analysis of 245 patients. Circulation. 2002;106(12 Suppl 1):I198–202.
27. Cheung A, Chorpenning K, Tamez D, Shambaugh Jr C, Dierlam AE, Taskin ME, Ashenuga M, Reyes C, LaRose JA. Design concepts and preclinical results of a miniaturized HeartWare platform: the MVAD system. Innovations. 2015. doi:10.1097/IMI.0000000000000155.
28. McGee Jr E, Chorpenning K, Brown MC, Breznock E, Larose JA, Tamez D. In vivo evaluation of the HeartWare MVAD Pump. J Heart Lung Transplant Off Publ Int Soc Heart Transplant. 2014;33(4):366–71. doi:10.1016/j.healun.2013.10.003.
29. Connellan M, Iyer A, Robson D, Granger E, Dhital K, Spratt P, Jansz P. The HeartWare transvalvular miniature ventricular assist device used for right ventricular support. J Heart Lung Transplant. 2013;32(4):S149. doi:10.1016/j.healun.2013.01.339.
30. Dew MA, Kormos RL, DiMartini AF, Switzer GE, Schulberg HC, Roth LH, Griffith BP. Prevalence and risk of depression and anxiety-related disorders during the first three years after heart transplantation. Psychosomatics. 2001;42(4):300–13.
31. Grady KL, Naftel DC, Young JB, Pelegrin D, Czerr J, Higgins R, Heroux A, Rybarczyk B, McLeod M, Kobashigawa J, Chait J, White-Williams C, Myers S, Kirklin JK. Patterns and predictors of physical functional disability at 5 to 10 years after heart transplantation. J Heart Lung Transplant Off Publ Int Soc Heart Transplant. 2007;26(11):1182–91. doi:10.1016/j.healun.2007.08.001.
32. Slaughter MS, Rogers JG, Milano CA, Russell SD, Conte JV, Feldman D, Sun B, Tatooles AJ, Delgado 3rd RM, Long JW, Wozniak TC, Ghumman W, Farrar DJ, Frazier OH, HeartMate III. Advanced heart failure treated with continuous-flow left ventricular assist device. N Engl J Med. 2009;361(23):2241–51. doi:10.1056/NEJMoa0909938.
33. Grady KL, Naftel D, Stevenson L, Dew MA, Weidner G, Pagani FD, Kirklin JK, Myers S, Baldwin T, Young J. Overall quality of life improves to similar levels after mechanical circulatory support regardless of severity of heart failure before implantation. J Heart Lung Transplant Off Publ Int Soc Heart Transplant. 2014;33(4):412–21. doi:10.1016/j.healun.2013.10.017.

MIX
Papier aus verantwortungsvollen Quellen
Paper from responsible sources
FSC® C105338

If you have any concerns about our products,
you can contact us on
ProductSafety@springernature.com

In case Publisher is established outside the EU,
the EU authorized representative is:
Springer Nature Customer Service Center GmbH
Europaplatz 3, 69115 Heidelberg, Germany

Printed by Libri Plureos GmbH
in Hamburg, Germany